ADDITIONAL VOLUMES IN PREPARATION

Drug Permeation Enhancement

Enhancement

Theory and Applications

edited by
Dean S. Hsieh
Conrex Pharmaceutical Corporation
Malvern, Pennsylvania

Marcel Dekker, Inc.   New York • Basel • Hong Kong

Library of Congress Cataloging-in-Publication Data

Drug permeation enhancement : theory and applications / edited by Dean
S. Hsieh.
    p.   cm.—(Drugs and the pharmaceutical sciences ; 62)
    Includes bibliographical references and index.
    ISBN 0-8247-9015-4 (alk. paper)
    1. Transdermal medication. 2. Skin—Permeability. 3. Nasal
mucosa—Permeability. 4. Cornea—Permeability. I. Hsieh, Dean.
II. Series: Drugs and the pharmaceutical sciences ; v. 62.
  [DNLM: 1. Dosage Forms. 2. Administration, Cutaneous. 3. Skin Ab-
sorption. 4. Administration, Intranasal. W1 DR893B v. 62 1994 / QV 785
D7947 1994]
RM151.D78   1994
615′.7—dc20
DNLM/DLC   93-9043
for Library of Congress   CIP

RM151
.D78
1994

The publisher offers discounts on this book when ordered in bulk quantities.
For more information, write to Special Sales/Professional Marketing at the
address below.

This book is printed on acid-free paper.

Marcel Dekker, Inc.
270 Madison Avenue, New York, New York 10016

Current printing (last digit):
10 9 8 7 6 5 4 3 2 1

PRINTED IN THE UNITED STATES OF AMERICA

Preface

Ever since nitroglycerin-containing transdermal patches were first introduced into the market and achieved commercial success, activities related to the introduction of new transdermal drug delivery systems (TDDSs), including research and development, registration, and regulation, have been greatly intensified in academic institutions, industrial sectors, and governmental agencies. Currently, more than twenty versions of TDDSs containing nitroglycerin, isosorbide dinitrate, scopolamine, clonidine, estradiol, fantanyl, and nicotine have been commercialized. It is well known that, because of the skin barrier, many drugs are unsuitable for TDDSs if no permeation enhancers or other physical means are incorporated in the formulation or devices. Most researchers agree that if the percutaneous absorption of drugs through the skin can be enhanced by either chemical or physical means (or both), the spectrum of drug candidates for transdermal delivery can be increased greatly. Furthermore, peptide drugs definitely require some sort of permeation enhancement for noninvasive administration, because the size and charge of the molecules themselves hinder absorption. The need for developing permeation enhancement technology is urgent, and the potential applications are enormous. However, our understanding of how to overcome the biological barriers (skin, mucosa, and cornea) is still at the rudimentary stage. The objective of this book is to cover the fundamental aspects of both

iii

physical and chemical enhancement for the transport of drugs, both peptides and nonpeptides, across skin, mucosa, and cornea.

This book is divided into five parts: "General Introduction to Drug Permeation Enhancement" (Chapters 1–3), "Drug Permeation Enhancement via the Skin: Chemical Means" (Chapters 4–10), "Drug Permeation Enhancement via the Skin: Physical Means" (Chapters 11–15), "Drug Permeation Enhancement via the Nasal Route" (Chapters 16 and 17), and "Drug Permeation Enhancement via the Ocular Route" (Chapters 18 and 19). Some chapters deal with fundamental principles of drug permeation enhancement (Chapters 1–5 and 11), some with toxicology (2, 3, 4, and 17), and some with examples of applications (8, 9, 13–16, 18, and 19).

This book provides a definitive overview of drug permeation enhancement from the perspectives of both theory and application. It will be useful not only for those who are unfamiliar with this field but also for those who are interested in further exploring this emerging technology.

Dean S. Hsieh

Contents

Contributors

BRUCE J. AUNGST, Ph.D.   The DuPont Merck Pharmaceutical Company, Wilmington, Delaware

CHARAN R. BEHL, Ph.D.   Pharmaceutical Research and Development, Hoffmann–La Roche, Inc., Nutley, New Jersey

H. E. BODDÉ, Ph.D.   Center for Bio-Pharmaceutical Sciences, Leiden University, Leiden, The Netherlands

HING CHAR, Ph.D.   Pharmaceutical Research and Development, Hoffmann–La Roche, Inc., Nutley, New Jersey

GEORGE C. Y. CHIOU, Ph.D.   Institute of Ocular Pharmacology, Department of Medical Pharmacology and Toxicology, Texas A&M University College of Medicine, College Station, Texas

GIUSEPPE CICCONE, M.S.   Pharmaceutical Research and Development, Hoffmann–La Roche, Inc., Nutley, New Jersey

JOHN DEVANE, Ph.D.   Elan Pharmaceutical Research Corporation, Gainesville, Georgia

MICHAEL A. DORATO, Ph.D.   Lilly Research Laboratories, Division of Eli Lilly and Company, Greenfield, Indiana

WILLIAM R. GOOD, Ph.D.   CIBA-GEIGY Corporation, Summit, New Jersey

F. H. N. DE HAAN, Ph.D.   Center for Bio-Pharmaceutical Sciences, Leiden University, Leiden, The Netherlands

MARGO B. HABERKAMP, Ph.D.   Grosse Point, Michigan

NANCY J. HARPER, Ph.D.   Pharmaceutical Research and Development, Pfizer Central Research, Groton, Connecticut

DEAN S. HSIEH, Ph.D.   Conrex Pharmaceutical Corporation, Malvern, Pennsylvania

H. E. JUNGINGER, Ph.D.   Center for Bio-Pharmaceutical Sciences, Leiden University, Leiden, The Netherlands

SARAN KUMAR, Ph.D.   Pharmaceutical Research and Development, Hoffmann–La Roche, Inc., Nutley, New Jersey

TAMIE KURIHARA-BERGSTROM, Ph.D.   CIBA-GEIGY Corporation, Summit, New Jersey

E. LEE, Ph.D.   ALZA Corporation, Palo Alto, California

YI-JING LIN, M.S.   School of Pharmacy, University of Southern California, Los Angeles, California

JUE-CHEN LIU, Ph.D.   Topical Formulation and Drug Delivery Research Center, Johnson and Johnson, Skillman, New Jersey

WASEEM MALICK, Ph.D.   Pharmaceutical Research and Development, Hoffmann–La Roche, Inc., Nutley, New Jersey

MARY MARTIN, Ph.D.   Elan Corporation, Monskland, Athlone, County Westmeath, Ireland

DEEPAK MEHTA, Ph.D.   Pharmaceutical Research and Development, Hoffmann–La Roche, Inc., Nutley, New Jersey

B. ROBERT MEYER, M.D.   Department of Medicine, Albert Einstein College of Medicine, Bronx, New York

MICHAEL MEZEI, Ph.D.   College of Pharmacy, Dalhousie University, Halifax, Nova Scotia, Canada

SHIRLEY M. NG, Ph.D.   The R. W. Johnson Pharmaceutical Research Institute, Raritan, New Jersey

SUNIL B. PATEL, Ph.D.   Pharmaceutical Research and Development, Hoffmann–La Roche, Inc., Nutley, New Jersey

JOYCE Y. PEI, M.B.A.   Bristol–Myers Squibb, Princeton, New Jersey

DAVID PIEMONTESE Pharmaceutical Research and Developn. `nt, Hoffmann–La Roche, Inc., Nutley, New Jersey

YONGYUT ROJANASAKUL, Ph.D.   School of Pharmacy, West Virginia University, Morgantown, West Virginia

VINOD P. SHAH, Ph.D.   Center for Drug Evaluation and Research, Food and Drug Administration, Rockville, Maryland

WEI-CHIANG SHEN, Ph.D.   School of Pharmacy, University of Southern California, Los Angeles, California

YING SUN, Ph.D.   Topical Formulation and Drug Delivery Research Center, Johnson and Johnson, Skillman, New Jersey

L. TASKOVICH, M.S.   ALZA Corporation, Palo Alto, California

F. THEEUWES, D.Sc.   ALZA Corporation, Palo Alto, California

OOI WONG, Ph.D.   Cygnus Therapeutic Systems, Redwood City, California

S. YUM, Ph.D.   ALZA Corporation, Palo Alto, California

YU-QUN ZHENG   Institute of Ocular Pharmacology, Department of Medical Pharmacology and Toxicology, Texas A&M University College of Medicine, College Station, Texas

Drug Permeation Enhancement

I

GENERAL INTRODUCTION TO DRUG PERMEATION ENHANCEMENT

1

Understanding Permeation Enhancement Technologies

Dean S. Hsieh
Conrex Pharmaceutical Corporation, Malvern, Pennsylvania

I. INTRODUCTION

From the onset of drug delivery research, scientists have investigated the enhancement of drug absorption to improve efficacy of treatment and to reduce the toxicities associated with systemic therapy. One of the first studies was with DMSO, and it was followed closely by a study with Azone. However, none of the permeation enhancers have yet been commercialized [1]. Actually, there is a tremendous need for compounds to enhance drug absorption across the biological barriers of the skin, mucosa, and cornea and the blood–brain barrier, the failure of these compounds to reach commercialization is due primarily to concerns about their related toxicities. Our understanding of permeation enhancement of drugs is still very uneven and limited, although efforts have been made to elucidate the mode of action of penetration enhancers in human skin [2]. Nonetheless, the time will soon come when we can design a drug delivery system in combination with a permeation enhancement technology to achieve better therapeutic efficacy along with the reduction of systemic toxicities.

This volume, comprising 19 chapters written by scientists from the pharmaceutical industry and from academic and governmental institutions, was written to provide a framework for this new technology for immediate and future applications. As an introduction, I would like to point out 12 important questions for readers to ponder. The answers to these questions may or may not be found within this volume, but the questions themselves are crucial when we consider practical applications of permeation enhancement.

1. What is permeation enhancement?
2. What kinds of permeation enhancement technologies exist?
3. Because of the differences in biological membranes (skin, mucosa, cornea, nail, blood–brain barrier, etc.), should the permeation enhancement technologies be tailored to the needs of each application?
4. What factors must we consider when developing a dosage form in combination with a permeation enhancement technology?
5. Is a permeation enhancer an excipient (an inert vehicle), a device, or a new drug?
6. What constitutes a "good" enhancer or a "bad" enhancer?
7. What is the mechanism of action of each permeation enhancement technology?
8. Is the mode of action of a particular enhancer general or specific?
9. Is there any synergistic effect between enhancers, solvents, and vehicles?
10. What would be considered a permeation "inhibitor" as compared with a permeation "enhancer"?
11. Is the enhancer under consideration compatible with other excipients, device components, and the drug itself?
12. Finally, can enhancers be used to achieve formulation objectives?

Chapter 2 of this volume, by Vinod P. Shah of the Center for Drug Evaluation and Research, Food and Drug Administration (FDA), is a very good starting point for those who are interested in skin permeation enhancement technologies. I hope this volume provides a sound basis for scientists, formulators, engineers, and medical practitioners to explore the dimensions of this new technology and that it also sheds new light for those innovators designing permeation enhancement technologies for practical applications.

II. BASIC MECHANISMS IN PARACELLULAR AND TRANSCELLULAR TRANSPORT

Mammalian cell membranes separate cells from their environment and from one another. Cell membranes are barriers to macromolecules and to most polar molecules, but they are relatively permeable to water and small hydrophobic molecules. Many pharmacologically important molecules and drugs cannot readily move across cell membranes. Under physiological conditions, there are several mechanisms governing the transport of molecules across cell membranes (please refer to Chapter 3 for details). Under pathological conditions, will it be possible to use the same mechanism to deliver the drug into the cell to correct the abnormality of the cell function(s)?

Table 1 Basic Mechanisms of
Transepithelial Transport of
Drugs

Passive diffusion
Active diffusion
Endocytosis
Transcytosis

Methods of facilitating the transport of molecules, either small or large, across the epithelial cells can be categorized into two major groups: paracellular and transcellular transport [3].

A. Paracellular Transport

Paracellular transport is the transport of molecules around or between the cells. Tight junctions or similar situations exist between cells. At the tight junctions, the cell membranes are brought into extremely close apposition, but are not fused, so as to occlude the extracellular space. Consequently, ions or molecules may not be able to pass through the membranes. Because of the perception that proteolytic activity is deficient in the paracellular space, it was once commonly assumed that peptides and proteins could not be absorbed via the paracellular pathway [3]. Therefore in recent times the investigation of paracellular transport of peptides and proteins has gained great interest. Without the employment of physical or chemical permeation enhancement techniques, the absorption of the majority of peptides or proteins is negligible or minimal (Chapter 16). Both Chapters 3 and 16 describe the intranasal administration of peptides and proteins. The uses of chemical enhancers and metabolism inhibitors are discussed. Chapters 18 and 19 discuss further the ocular absorption of peptides in combination of chemical enhancers for systemic application, while Chapters 12–15 discuss physical means (i.e., iontophoresis and phonophoresis) to enhance the transdermal absorption of peptides and proteins. The increases in peptide/protein absorption across the epithelium are attributed to paracellular transport. How the physical or chemical agents affect paracellular transport is still unknown. Further investigation of the mechanism is undoubtedly needed.

B. Transcellular Transport

Table 1 lists the mechanisms of transport of drugs and macromolecules across epithelial cellular membrane. These include passive transport of small molecules, active transport of ionic and polar compounds, and endocytosis and transcytosis of macromolecules. Passive transport is the movement of a solute along its concentration gradient. Active transport differs from passive transport in that the transport process is mediated by membrane transport proteins coupled to an energy source. In active transport, the solutes can be transported against a concentration gradient. The transport of macromolecules is different from the transport of small molecules across epithelial cells. Most of the transport of macromolecules is mediated by endocytosis and transcytosis. In these processes, macromolecules are progressively enclosed by the cell membranes. They then migrate within membrane-bound vehicles to the perinuclear region of the cell, where the vehicles coalesce with lysosomes in which intracellular digestion occurs. In transcytosis, macromolecules bind to receptors on the surface of epithelial cells, then the receptor–macromolecule complex is incorporated into vehicles and carried into the cell. The complex remains intact in endosomes and is retrieved in transport vehicles that fuse with the membranes of the opposite side of the cell monolayer. Therefore, intact macromolecules can be transported across the epithelial barrier.

III. BIOLOGICAL BARRIERS TO DRUG PERMEABILITY

Common sites of drug administration include the eye, skin, nasal cavity, mouth, intestines, and rectum, and there are also the parenteral routes of administration: intravenous, intramuscular, intraperitoneal, and subcutaneous. Each site or route of application presents biological barriers to the delivery of drugs to target organs and tissues. These barriers may function in a physical, chemical, or biological fashion, and any combination of barriers may be present, depending on the specific mode and site of application of a given drug delivery system. In general, biological barriers are site-specific and are related to the histological organization of the specific site [4]. Biological barriers are an important issue in drug delivery, especially for peptide or protein drugs [2,5,6; see also Chapter 16].

A. The Skin

The skin forms the continuous external surface of the body and, among the different regions of the body, varies in thickness, color, and the presence of hairs, glands, and nails. Despite these variations, which reflect different functional demands, all types of skin have the same basic structure. The external surface of the skin consists of a keratinized squamous epithelium called the epidermis. The epidermis is supported and nourished by a thick underlying layer of dense, fibroelastic connective tissue called the dermis. The dermis is highly vascular and contains many sensory receptors. It is attached to underlying tissues by a layer of loose connective tissue called the hypodermis or subcutaneous layer, which contains variable amounts of adipose tissue. Hair follicles, sweat glands, subaceous glands, and nails are epithelial structures, which are termed epidermal appendages because they originate during embryological development from downgrowth of the epidermal epithelium into the dermis and hypodermis.

It is generally agreed that the stratum corneum, the outermost layer of the skin, is the barrier to the passage of drugs across the epidermis [4,7,8]. The stratum corneum consists of 15–20 layers of densely packed, flattened, metabolically inactive cells, followed by several histologically distinguishable layers of closely packed cells forming a tight cellular continuum 50–100 μm in thickness. Epidermal cell membranes are tightly joined, and there is little to no intercellular space for ions and polar nonelectrolyte molecules through which to diffuse.

In the case of toenails or fingernails, the keratinized tissue is a very thick and dense barrier to drug penetration for the treatment of infections occurring at the nail bed. The delivery of antifungal agents underneath the nail to reach the nail bed is a very challenging problem for pharmaceutical scientists to explore. An alternative approach is to abrade the infected region of the nail before applying the antifungal formulation. In this approach, the biological barrier to drug permeability would be similar to that of the stratum corneum.

B. The Mucosae

The terms mucous membrane and mucosa are generally used to describe the moist linings of the gastrointestinal and respiratory tracts. These terms always refer to both the epithelium and its supporting lamina propria. Another connective tissue layer called the submucosa usually connects the mucosa to the underlying structure. On the surface of the mucosal epithelium, there exists a layer of mucus composed of mucopolysaccharides secreted from goblet cells in the mucosa. The types of epithelium among different mucosae are discussed below.

1. *Mucosa of the nasal cavity* [4,9]. The mucosal membranes of the nasal cavity include several types of epithelia. A small portion extending into the nasal cavity from the nares is a stratified squamous epithelium. The remainder of the nasal membrane is made up of the respiratory epithelium, which is composed of ciliated cuboidal and columnar cells; goblet cells; and the olfactory epithelium, a pseudostratified neuroepithelium.
2. *Mucosa of the lower respiratory tract* [4,10]. The respiratory epithelium undergoes progressive transition from a tall, pseudostratified, columnar, ciliated form in the larynx and trachaea to a simple, cuboidal, nonciliated form in the smallest airways. Goblet cells are numerous in the trachea but decrease in number in the lungs and are absent from the terminal bronchioli.
3. *Mucosa of the oral cavity* [5]. The epithelium of the oral mucosa is of the stratified squamous type, which tends to be keratinized in areas subject to great friction.

Table 2 Mucosal Barriers to Paracellular Peptide/Protein Permeation

	Nasal	Buccal	Intestinal	Rectal
Type of epithelium	Ciliated, cuboidal, and columnar	Stratified squamous	Simple columnar	Simple columnar
Barrier factor	Intercellular matrix derived from the membrane coating granules	Keratinized epithelium	Tight junctions	Tight junctions
Effect of calcium chelator	NO	NO	YES	YES
Effect of glycocholate	YES	YES	YES	YES
Effect of peptidase inhibitors	YES	YES	YES	YES

4. *Mucosa of the small intestine.* The intestinal villi are lined with a simple, columnar epithelium that is continuous with that of the crypts. The cells of this epithelium are of two main types: enterocytes and goblet cells. The enterocytes, which are involved in membrane digestion and absorption, are tall columnar cells with basally located nuclei; goblet cells are scattered among the enterocytes. The lamina propria extends between the crypts and into the core of each villus and contains a rich vascular and lymphatic network into which digestive products are absorbed.

5. *Mucosa of the large intestine (cecum, colon, and rectum).* The mucosa of the entire large intestine consists of closely packed, straight, tubular glands containing cells of two main types: absorptive cells and goblet cells. The simple tubular glands extend from the luminal surface to the muscularis mucosa and are separated from each other by their plats of lamina propria. The lamina propria is rich in capillaries and diffusely infiltrated by leukocytes.

Table 2 compares the differences in type of epithelium, predominant barrier factor, and the responses to treatment among different mucosae.

C. The Cornea

The cornea is the thick, transparent portion of the corneoscleral layer enclosing the anterior one-sixth of the eye. The outer surface is lined by a stratified squamous epithelium about five cells thick. The epithelium is supported by a specialized basement membrane known as Bowman's membrane. The bulk of the cornea, the substantia propria, consists of a highly regular form of dense collagenous connective tissues. Fibroblasts and occasional leukocytes are scattered in the corneal ground substance. The inner surface of the cornea is lined by a layer of flattened endothelial cells that are supported by a very thick elastic basement membrane known as Descemet's membrane.

D. The Blood–Brain Barrier (BBB)

The brain is protected by an endothelial capillary commonly known as the blood–brain barrier [11]. This barrier consists of the brain capillary endothelial cells, which are bound by tight junctions, and their supporting basement membrane. This barrier is effective in protecting the brain from potentially harmful chemicals but renders the administration of potentially beneficial drugs to the afflicted brain difficult, if not impossible, when the brain suffers from infection, tumor, or dysfunction. The perivascular feet of astrocytes in the BBB probably play a less important role in drug transport.

IV. PERMEABILITY ENHANCEMENT: OVERCOMING TRANSPORT THRESHOLDS ACROSS BIOLOGICAL BARRIERS

Regardless of the means of enhancement used, the common goal of permeability enhancement is to reduce the "threshold" of the biological barriers. The input of electric energy in iontophoresis provides the driving force (or energy) for facilitating the transport of ionic molecules across the skin (Chapter 11). The incorporation of chemical enhancers in a formulation is intended to lower the "activation energy" of drug transport across the skin by modifying either the diffusibility parameters or the solubility parameters of drugs in the skin (Chapters 4–8).

No matter which methods we use to enhance permeability across the biological membranes, we have to bear in mind that the primary concern is safety. Chapter 17 illustrates a toxicological evaluation program for transnasal delivery of peptide and protein drugs when permeation enhancers are incorporated into the nasal spray formulation. It provides a complete outline for toxicological evaluation and can be used as a model for similar technologies that enhance peptide and protein drug across biological membranes.

These issues include at least three aspects: permeability, enzyme (e.g., peptidase) degradation, and incompatibility. Chapter 16 addresses permeability and metabolism as barriers to transmucosal delivery of peptides and proteins. Because of the low bioavailability of transmucosally administered peptides and proteins, commercialization of mucosal delivery of peptide and protein drugs is not yet advanced.

Table 3 Examples of
Permeation Enhancement
Technologies

Physical means
  Iontophoresis
  Phonophoresis
  Thermal modulation
  Magnetic modulation
  Mechanical modulation
Chemical means
  Permeation enhancers
  Prodrug design
Biological means
  Receptors
Combinations

V. MEANS OF ENHANCING PERMEABILITY

The methods of enhancing drug transport across the biological barriers described
in this volume can be divided into two major categories: physical and chemical
means. Biological means of permeation enhancement have recently been discussed elsewhere [12] and thus are not included here. Future studies could possibly investigate the combination of methods of physical, chemical, or biological
means for the facilitation of drug transport across biological barriers. Chapters
13 and 14 describe the clinical investigation of iontophoretic transdermal
patches, which enhance the transport of drugs across the skin by electric forces.
Chapter 8 describes the use of ethanol as permeation enhancer for enhancing
the percutaneous absorption of estradiol, and Chapter 9 deals with the use of
liposomes as penetration enhancers for localized dermal treatment, a method
that has already been commercialized.

An increase in bioavailability in the transmucosal delivery of peptides and
proteins will make the delivery systems meaningful from a commercial per-
spective. Chapter 16 discusses the use of permeation enhancers and metabolism
inhibitors to increase this bioavailability. Uses of iontophoresis and phonophoresis are the subject of discussion in Chapters 12–15.

Table 3 lists the means that can be employed to facilitate the transport of
drugs across the biological barriers.

VI. CHEMICAL PERMEATION ENHANCERS

In 1988 I reviewed the chemical permeation enhancers reported in the literature
in Chapter 8 of Ref. 1. Later on, I further classified these chemical permeation

enhancers according to their chemical classes [13], their mode of action, and their solubility parameters [14,15].

It is generally agreed that the percutaneous absorption of most drugs is a passive diffusion process that can be described by Fick's first law of diffusion. This principle is illustrated in equation (1), in which the amount of drug transported through a unit area of skin per unit time, the flux (J), is the product of the diffusion coefficient of the drug in the skin (D), the skin–vehicle partition coefficient of the drug (K), and the drug concentration in the vehicle or delivery system (C) divided by the thickness of the skin (h).

$$J = DKC/h \qquad (1)$$

In principle, enhancers act on skin so that drug diffusibility or drug solubility or both in the skin is modified, leading to an increase in transport. Equation (2) illustrates this relationship: Drug transport through the skin (J) is the product of skin permeability (P) and drug concentration at saturation in the skin (C), provided there is an excess supply of drug in the delivery system.

$$J = PC \qquad (2)$$

As equations (1) and (2) indicate, permeability can be enhanced by altering the structure of the skin (modifying the diffusion coefficient) or by increasing the solubility of the drug in the skin. In other words, enhancers such as DMSO and Azone can increase diffusibility in the stratum corneum by acting as solvents to dissolve the skin lipids or to denature skin proteins. Azone, a seven-member ring lactim (discussed in Chapter 7), is a typical example of enhancers that modify the diffusion coefficient of the drug in the process of skin permeation. Their action somewhat damages the integrity of the skin. It can take 2 weeks for the skin to recover to its original state after Azone has been in contact with it for as short a time as 1 min. In other cases, enhancers can modify drug solubility parameters (i.e., the partition coefficient from the vehicle to the skin, K_m, and the permeability coefficient in the skin, K_p), which may not damage the integrity of the skin structure. Two examples of enhancers of this type are ethanol (Chapter 9) and macrocyclic ketones and lactones [Hsieh, unpublished data; 14]. Their action on the skin, if any, is transient and reversible (Chapters 4 and 8).

VII. DIFFERENCES BETWEEN TRANSDERMAL AND TOPICAL DRUG DELIVERY (16,17)

For transdermal products, the goal of dosage design is to maximize the flux through the skin into the systemic circulation and simultaneously minimize the retention and metabolism of the drug in the skin. In contrast, topical products are developed to minimize the flux of the drug through the skin while maximizing its retention in the skin. However, for both transdermal and topical products, drugs must penetrate across the stratum corneum, the outermost layer of the skin. With this in mind, we should consider the increase of drug penetration across the stratum corneum as well as the increase of drug retention in the stratum corneum and/or epidermis when we develop topical drug delivery systems. The drug metabolism in the skin should also be minimized. There is a clear distinction between transdermals and topicals. Thus, the selection of permeation enhancement technology should be evaluated according to the objective of delivery.

A. Transdermals (14,15)

The selection of enhancers for use in transdermal products should be based on well-established efficacy for enhancing the release of the drug from the dosage form; promotion of its percutaneous absorption; demonstrated compatibility with the pressure-sensitive adhesives and system components to ensure a suitable balance among tack, adhesion, and cohesive strength; and ease of system activation upon removal of the release liner. Newer transdermal systems requiring enhancers will provide the formulation scientists with new challenges in formulation optimization and design, in which the important triad of formulation components—drugs, enhancers, and adhesives—must be compatible. The success of early formulation development may depend upon the proper selection of the system components and the configuration of the enhancer in the system to facilitate percutaneous absorption of the drug.

B. Topicals

There is growing interest in the optimization of drug delivery targeting the drug to the pathological site in the skin. Two consecutive AAPS/FDA/industry cosponsored workshops on dermatological therapeutic products were held in Arlington, Virginia, in March 1990 and December 1991 to address these issues [16,17]. The major objectives of these workshops were to develop the principles and criteria involved in the establishment of bioavailability and bioequivalence of dermatological therapeutic products. The primary goal of dermatological therapeutic products is to increase the retention of therapeutic drugs in the skin rather than the penetration of drug through the skin.

VIII. DEVELOPING PERMEATION ENHANCEMENT TECHNOLOGIES

A. For Topical Use

Many drugs useful for dermal conditions are still administered orally or via other systemic applications. Some examples are methotrexate for psoriasis, 13-cis-retinoic acid for acne, griseofulvin for fungal infection, and steroids for dermatitis. There are many side effects associated with these systemic drugs. Several attempts have been made to develop topical formulations containing drugs such as methotrexate for psoriasis treatment [18]. Unfortunately, the physicochemical characteristics of these drugs do not allow them to permeate well across the skin.

There are three major barriers to the topical delivery of drugs:

1. Most of the drugs permeate poorly across the stratum corneum.
2. If the drugs permeate across the stratum corneum, they are not easily retained in the skin for localized therapy.
3. Many drugs are too irritating to the skin to deliver topically.

Therefore, the strategy to develop permeation enhancement technologies for the treatment of dermal conditions should be to use the stratum corneum and/or the epidermis as a drug reservoir for the slow release of drugs to the targeted pathological site(s). In this way, permeation enhancement technologies are used not only to facilitate the permeation of drugs across the stratum corneum, but also to increase the retention time of the drugs in the stratum corneum and/or epidermis. This targeted drug delivery system will become important for skin care product development in the area of dermatologicals and cosmeceuticals.

To date, no general guidelines have been developed for pharmaceutical scientists to follow on how to develop topical formulations that can increase drug retention in the skin. Most formulations are still produced through trial and error. It is imperative that we investigate the analysis of drug retention and penetration in a systematic way.

B. For Transdermal Use

As discussed in Section VI, drugs delivered transdermally are intended for systemic treatment. The permeation enhancement technologies should be able to facilitate the transport of a drug across the skin so that the drug enters into the blood circulation. There is a large body of literature related to the development of permeation enhancers for percutaneous absorption through the skin [12,15,19]. The criteria for selecting ideal chemical permeation enhancers are discussed elsewhere [14,15]. The permeation enhancers should also be compatible with the components of transdermal patches, and the triad relationship among drug, enhancer, and system component should be optimized.

C. For Mucosal Use

Potential sites of mucosal drug administration are the mucosa of the nasal cavity, lower respiratory tract, oral cavity, small intestine, and large intestine. This section will be limited, however, to the mucosa in the nasal cavity and the choice of peptide/protein drugs for systemic treatment [20]. In contrast to invasive methods such as subcutaneous, intravenous, or intramuscular injection, a non-

Table 4 Peptide Products for Intranasal Administration Across the Nasal Mucosa

Brand name	Peptide	Therapeutic indications	Manufacturer
Synarel (Nafarelin)	LHRH analogue	Endometriosis	Syntex
Buserelin	Gonadotropin-releasing hormone and LHRH antagonist	Endometritis, prostate carcinoma, testis retention	Hoescht AG
Minirin	Desmopressin (DDAVP)	Primary nocturnal enuresis, release Factor VIII, diabetes insipidus	Rorer
Diapid	Vasopressin lypressin (lysine-8-vasopressin)	Diabetes insipidus	Sandoz
Partocon	Oxytocin	Induction of labor	Ferring AB
Syntocinon	Oxytocin	Initial milk let-down	Sandoz

invasive method of mucosal delivery boasts the following features: (1) self-medication, (2) noninvasiveness, (3) patient acceptance, and (4) pharmaceutical compatibility. Recently, five peptide drugs with intranasal delivery systems were introduced into the market for various medical indications (Table 4). Four of these peptides are oxytocin, vasopressin lypressin, desmopressin (DDAVP), and LHRH analogue. It is worthwhile to note that all four are small, containing fewer than 10 amino acid residues. It is conceivable that the majority of peptide drugs cannot permeate across the mucosal membranes (see Chapter 16), owing to the existence of tight junctions between epithelial cells.

The major advantage of nasal delivery of a peptide/protein drug is its noninvasiveness, resulting in improved patient compliance, ease of use, and convenience of administration. The requirements for toxicity evaluation are discussed in detail in Chapter 17. Both systemic and local toxicity of permeation enhancement technologies should be investigated. Those who have an interest in the nasal toxicity of permeation enhancement technologies should refer to Chapter 17.

In addition to toxicity, the efficacy of the drugs should also be considered. The low bioavailability of peptides in nasal delivery will limit economic feasibility as compared with injectable systems. In the case of a nasal spray of insulin, a system with bioavailability below 20% as compared with injectable insulin will not be able to compete with injectables in the marketplace. Without the use of permeation enhancers in the nasal insulin formulation, bioavailability is below

1% in the tested animal models. Obviously, permeation enhancers are needed in nasal insulin delivery systems.

Consequently, developers of a nasal peptide and protein drug delivery system containing permeation enhancers should address the:

Biological issues: including permeability, enzymatic degradation, and compatibility

Physiological issues: including rapid plasma clearance, immunogenicity, and rhythmical release kinetics

Peptide stabilization issues: including covalent and noncovalent modifications of peptides

D. For Blood-Brain Barrier Use

Two principal features distinguish brain endothelial cells from other endothelial cells. These features define the BBB:

1. *Tight junctions.* The endothelial cells of the brain's capillaries are tightly joined to create a virtually impenetrable barrier. Endothelial cells in the rest of the body are joined together by permeable junctions that allow diffusion of small and large molecules between the bloodstream and peripheral organs.

2. *Regulated transport.* Despite the existence of tight junctions that prevent the free passage of blood constituents to brain tissues, the brain requires many molecules found in the bloodstream. Brain capillary endothelial cells are further distinguished from those in the rest of the body by their ability to regulate the traffic of specific molecules into and out of the brain, which is accomplished by receptors located on the endothelial cell surface. Glucose, for example, is transported by a selective transporter from the bloodstream, where it is in high concentration, across the endothelial cell into the brain, where it is present at a lower concentration.

Tight junctions and regulated transport enable the BBB to protect the CNS from the transient changes in the composition of the bloodstream, to selectively transport molecules into and out of the brain for maintenance of brain metabolism, and to exclude many compounds such as anticancer chemotherapeutics, anti-infectives, peptides, and proteins creates a significant problem in treating disorders of the CNS.

From the viewpoint of enhancing drugs across the BBB, at least two approaches should be considered:

1. The increase in permeability of the BBB should be transient and reversible. Selection of suitable permeation enhancers is being investigated.

2. Preferably, the transport of neuropharmaceutical compounds should be selective and targeted. The use of specific carriers such as receptor-mediated carriers has been proposed [12].

IX. CONCLUSION

Drug permeation enhancement technology is a new and emerging field. The potential applications are enormous. However, the optimization of each application requires substantial effort to understand the histological barrier, to design the drug delivery system with enhancing ability to overcome the barrier, and preferably, to target the drug to the pathological sites. Physical, chemical, and biological means of enhancing permeability have been investigated. Further refinement of these techniques will be crucial for commercial success.

REFERENCES

1. D. S. T. Hsieh, *Controlled Release Systems: Fabrication Technology*, Vol. 1, CRC Press, Boca Raton, FL, 1988, pp. 167–188.
2. J. M. Anderson and S. W. Kim, Eds., *Advances in Drug Delivery Systems*, Vol. 3, Elsevier, New York, 1987, pp. 85–97.
3. V. H. L. Lee, *Peptide and Protein Drug Delivery*, Marcel Dekker, New York, 1991, pp. 13–16.
4. P. R. Wheater, H. G. Burkitt, and V. G. Daniels, *Functional Histology: A Text and Color Atlas*, Churchill Livingstone, New York, 1979.
5. J. M. Anderson and S. W. Kim, Eds., *Advances in Drug Delivery Systems*, Vol. 3, Elsevier, New York, 1987, pp. 123–131.
6. P. F. Bai, P. Subramanian, H. I. Mosberg, and G. L. Amidon, Structural requirements for the intestinal mucosal-cell peptide transporter: the need for N-terminal alpha-amino group, *Pharm. Res. 8* (5), 593–599 (1991).
7. A. F. Kydonieus and B. Berner, Eds., *Transdermal Delivery of Drugs*, Vol. 1, CRC Press, Boca Raton, FL, 1987, pp. 29–42.
8. Y. W. Chien, *Novel Drug Delivery Systems: Fundamentals, Developmental Concepts and Biomedical Assessments*, Marcel Dekker, New York, 1982, pp. 149–218.
9. Y. W. Chien, Ed., *Transnasal Systemic Medications: Fundamentals, Developmental Concepts and Biomedical Assessments*, Elsevier, New York, 1985, pp. 100–106.
10. P. R. Byron, Ed., *Respiratory Drug Delivery*, CRC Press, Boca Raton, FL, 1990, pp. 1–38.
11. S. I. Rapoport, *Blood Brain Barrier in Physiology and Medicine*, Raven, New York, 1976.
12. W. C. Shen, J. S. Wan, and H. Ekrami, Enhancement of polypeptide and protein absorption by macromolecular carriers via endocytosis and transcytosis, *Adv. Drug Delivery Rev. 8*, 93–113 (1992).
13. D. S. L. Chow and D. S. T. Hsieh, Structure–activity relationship of permeation enhancers and their possible mechanisms, *Pharm. Tech. Conference 1989 Fall Proceedings*, Aster Publishing, Eugene, OR, 1989, pp. 233–247.

14. W. R. Pfister and D. S. T. Hsieh, Permeation enhancers compatible with transdermal drug delivery systems, part I: selection and formulation considerations, *Pharm. Technol.*, September 1990.

15. W. R. Pfister and D. S. T. Hsieh, Permeation enhancers compatible with transdermal drug delivery systems, part II: system design considerations, *Pharm. Technol.*, October 1990.

16. AAPS Workshop cosponsored by U.S. Food and Drug Administration, Principles and Criteria for the Development and Optimization of Topical Therapeutic Products, Mar. 26–28, 1990, Hyatt Regency Crystal City, Arlington, VA.

17. AAPS Workshop cosponsored by U.S. Food and Drug Administration, The Establishment of Bioavailability and Bioequivalence of Dermatological Products, Dec. 3–5, 1991, Hyatt Regency Crystal City, Arlington, VA.

18. G. D. Weinstein, J. L. McCullough, and E. Olsen, Topical methotrexate therapy for psoriasis, *Arch. Dermatol. (U.S.)*, *125*, 227–230 (1989).

19. K. Walters and J. Hadgraft, Eds., *Skin Penetration Enhancement*, Marcel Dekker, New York, 1990.

20. D. S. T. Hsieh and Z. H. Cai, Permeation enhancers and intranasal delivery of peptides, Pharm. Tech. Conference 1990 Proceedings, pp. 91–101.

21. D. S. T. Hsieh, U.S. Patent 5,023,252, Transdermal and trans-membrane delivery of drugs.

2

Skin Penetration Enhancers: Scientific Perspectives

Vinod P. Shah
Center for Drug Evaluation and Research, Food and Drug Administration, Rockville, Maryland

I. INTRODUCTION

Since the recognition of skin as a portal of drug entry into the body, a major challenge in developing dermatological products has been to increase drug delivery (and drug absorption) through the skin in a reproducible and reliable manner. The stratum corneum (SC), the outermost layer of the skin, forms the rate-limiting lipophilic barrier. Much research has been focused on discovering methods for enhancing drug penetration through the skin. Two types of principles have been employed to increase drug penetration (and absorption) through skin: chemical and physical. When employing these methods of enhancement, certain scientific issues must be considered and should be addressed at the time of product development and evaluation.

Dermatological drug products can be grouped into two major categories: (1) dermal or topical drug products intended for a localized pharmacological effect and (2) transdermal drug products intended for the treatment or prevention of a systemic disease. Considerable research effort is being invested in dermatological products, especially in transdermals, to enhance drug penetration through the SC to achieve the desired pharmacological effects [1–9].

II. SKIN STRUCTURE AS IT RELATES TO DRUG PENETRATION

The skin is a multilayered organ, complex in structure and function. It is composed of the outer epidermis and the inner dermis. The outermost layer of epidermis is the stratum corneum, which is formed by continuous differentiation of the adjacent viable epidermis. Anatomically, the stratum corneum is a coherent multilaminated membrane consisting of lipids and proteins arranged in a complex interlocking structure similar to bricks and mortar that is highly impermeable. It is breached by hair follicles and sweat ducts, which provide parallel diffusion pathways through the SC. The viable epidermis, on the other hand, has been characterized as an aqueous gel and is thought not to present a significant barrier to penetration in most circumstances [10].

III. ENHANCERS

Three pathways are suggested for drug penetration through the skin: polar, nonpolar, and polar/nonpolar. The enhancers act by altering one of these pathways. The key to altering the polar pathway is to cause protein conformational change or solvent swelling. The key to altering the nonpolar pathway is to alter the rigidity of the lipid structure and fluidize the crystalline pathway (this substantially increases diffusion). The fatty acid enhancers increase the fluidity of the lipid portion of the SC [11,12]. Some enhancers (binary vehicles) act on both polar and nonpolar pathways by altering the multilaminate pathway for penetrants. Enhancers can increase the drug diffusivity in the SC by dissolving the skin lipids or by denaturing skin proteins. The type of enhancer employed has a significant impact on the design and development of the product.

The success of dermatological drug products that are intended for systemic drug delivery, such as the transdermals, depends on the ability of the drug to penetrate through skin in sufficient quantities to achieve its desired therapeutic effect. The methods employed for modifying the barrier properties of the SC to enhance drug penetration (and absorption) through the skin can be categorized as (1) chemical and (2) physical methods of enhancement [8].

A. Chemical Enhancers

Chemicals that promote the penetration of topically applied drugs are commonly referred to as accelerants, absorption promoters, or penetration enhancers. A prime research objective is to identify chemicals that significantly enhance drug penetration through the epidermis but do not severely irritate or damage the skin. Some of the properties of such chemical permeation enhancers and the desirable attributes have been described by Barry [1]. These chemicals ideally should be safe and nontoxic, pharmacologically inert, nonirritating, and nonallergic [13]. In addition, the skin tissue should revert to its normal integrity and barrier properties upon removal of the chemical.

What do enhancers do? They

- Increase drug permeability through the skin by causing reversible damage to the SC.

- Increase (and optimize) thermodynamic activity of the drug when functioning as cosolvent.
- Increase the partition coefficient of the drug to promote its release from the vehicle into the skin.
- Operate by conditioning the SC to promote drug diffusion.
- Promote penetration and establish drug reservoir in the SC.

Many of the vehicles, in spite of being great enhancers, are limited in their functions as vehicles because of their deleterious effect on the skin; an example is dimethyl sulfoxide (DMSO). DMSO is a powerful solvent, and it increases drug penetration, but at the same time, it alters the biochemical and structural integrity of the skin and operates by direct insult to the SC [1]. Ethanol is often used as an enhancer/cosolvent, for example in estrogen patches, to increase drug penetration [7].

What is the fate of enhancers in the body? Are these enhancers irritant? What is the effect of repeat application of enhancers at the same site? Does it alter the integrity of the SC and drug penetration properties? Use of strong enhancers may leach other components from the patch, which may penetrate the SC, in case one should be concerned about the fate of such chemicals in the body.

The ability of the enhancer to increase drug penetration is important, but it is critical that this task be accomplished without skin irritation or sensitization. The goal is to find an enhancer that will disrupt the impermeable SC barrier membrane without altering the fragile living tissue underneath [6].

B. Physical Enhancers

The iontophoresis and ultrasound (also known as phonophoresis or sonophoresis) techniques are examples of physical means of enhancement that have been used for enhancing percutaneous penetration (and absorption) of various therapeutic agents.

One of the major concerns in the usage of iontophoresis is that the device may cause painful destruction of the skin with high current settings. It is essential to use high quality electrodes with adequate skin adhesion, uniform current distribution, and well-controlled ionic properties. The mechanism of transdermal penetration by this technology is still not clear.

IV. POINTS TO CONSIDER WHEN USING ENHANCERS IN THE PRODUCT

Penetration enhancers usually increase the permeation of not only the drug, but also other formulation excipients. In addition, their own intrinsic skin diffusivity can be increased. These effects must be carefully evaluated to avoid toxicological implications, especially in terms of irritation potential. Irritation from transdermal drug products appears to be a function of occlusion. It is linked to SC hydration and decreased diffusional resistance to formulation components such as enhancers. Enhancers should be evaluated for irritancy potential under conditions of long-term occlusion. Development of models with the use of solubility parameters to predict drug–vehicle–skin interactions and flux rate may aid in optimal selection of an enhancer [14].

In light of the above discussion, when chemical enhancers are used, the following points should be considered and evaluated:

What is the mechanism of action?
Does it cause irritation and damage to the skin?
Is the action reversible?
What is the effect on multiple application under occlusion?
What is the fate of the enhancer in the body? Is it metabolized? What is the influence of the degraded moieties from the enhancer, if any?
Is the enhancer powerful enough to increase penetration of other excipients?
Is the effect of the enhancer constant over the full duration of dosage form application?
What are the interaction potentials?
Does the enhancer maintain the structural integrity of the SC?
Does the enhancer selectively enhance permeation?
Is the enhancer inert, or does it cause contact irritation or promote bacterial growth?
What is the basic understanding of the interactions of chemical agents with proteins and lipids?
How safe is the enhancer? Does it cause any toxicity?

Attempts should be made to address these scientific questions during the development and evaluation of dermatological drug products, especially those that are intended for systemic drug delivery such as transdermals containing enhancers. The physical methods for enhancing drug penetration raises different types of concerns, which need to be addressed during the development and evaluation of iontophoretic and ultrasound enhancement techniques.

REFERENCES

1. B. W. Barry, Properties that influence percutaneous absorption, in *Dermatological Formulations, Percutaneous Absorption*, B. W. Barry, Ed., Marcel Dekker, New York, 1983, pp. 127–233.
2. E. R. Cooper, Vehicle effects on skin penetration, in *Percutaneous Absorption*, R. L. Bronaugh and H. I. Maibach, Eds., Marcel Dekker, New York, 1985, pp. 525–530.

3. C. L. Gummer, Vehicles as penetration enhancers, in *Percutaneous Absorption*, R. L. Bronaugh and H. I. Maibach, Eds., Marcel Dekker, New York, 1985, pp. 561–570.

4. Y. W. Chien, Development concepts and practice in TTS, in *Transdermal Controlled Systemic Medications*, Y. W. Chien, Ed., Marcel Dekker, New York, 1987, pp. 25–82.

5. E. R. Cooper, Alterations in skin permeability, in *Transdermal Controlled Systemic Medications*, Y. W. Chien, Ed., Marcel Dekker, New York, 1987, pp. 83–91.

6. E. R. Cooper and B. Berner, Penetration enhancers, in *Transdermal Delivery of Drugs*, Vol. 2, A. F. Kydonieus and B. Berner, Eds., CRC Press, Boca Raton, FL, 1987, pp. 57–62.

7. K. A. Walters, Penetration enhancers and their use in transdermal therapeutic systems, in *Transdermal Drug Delivery*, J. Hadgraft and R. H. Guy, Eds., Marcel Dekker, New York, 1989, pp. 197–246.

8. D. Rolf, Chemical and physical methods of enhancing transdermal drug delivery, *Pharm. Technol. 12*(Sept.), 131–140 (1988).

9. W. R. Pfister and D. S. T. Hsieh, Permeation enhancers compatible with transdermal drug delivery systems, *Pharm. Technol. 14*(Sept.), 132–138 (1990).

10. R. J. Scheuplein, Mechanisms of percutaneous absorption. II. Transient diffusion and the relative importance of various rates of skin penetration, *J. Invest. Dermatol. 48*, 79–88 (1967).

11. K. Knutson, R. O. Potts, D. B. Guzek, G. M. Golden, J. E. McKie, W. J. Lambert, and W. I. Higuchi, Macro- and molecular physical-chemical considerations in understanding drug transport in the stratum corneum, *J. Controlled Release 2*(10), 67–87 (1985).

12. R. O. Potts, Physical characterization of the stratum corneum: the relationship of mechanical and barrier properties to lipid and protein structure, in *Transdermal Drug Delivery*, J. Hadgraft and R. H. Guy, Eds., Marcel Dekker, New York, 1989, pp. 23–58.

13. M. Kat and B. J. Poulsen, in *Handbook of Experimental Pharmacology*, Vol. 28, B. B. Brodie and J. Gillette, Eds., Springer-Verlag, New York, 1971, Part 1, p. 103.

14. K. B. Sloan, S. A. M. Koch, K. G. Silvers, and F. L. Fowlers, Use of solubility parameters of drug and vehicle to predict flux through skin, *J. Invest. Dermatol. 87*, 244–252 (1986).

3

Basic Mechanisms in Transepithelium Transport Enhancement

Wei-Chiang Shen and Yi-Jing Lin
School of Pharmacy, University of Southern California, Los Angeles, California

I. POLARITY AND JUNCTIONS IN EPITHELIAL CELLS

The structural and functional characteristics of epithelial cells are their polarity and the differential composition of the apical, lateral, and basal membranes [1].

The apical membrane is the membrane facing the luminal surface. This membrane is usually associated with enzymes such as disaccharidase, alkaline phosphatase, and leucine aminopeptidase. The microvilli on the apical plasma membranes are special organelles that greatly increase the surface area of membrane exposed to the lumen. Many of the epithelial apical surfaces are covered by a viscous glycoprotein coat that can protect against mechanical and chemical damage to the cell. Most of the glycoproteins have terminal sialic acid residues that confer a negative charge to the apical surface. Therefore, the negative charge of the apical surface prevents the binding of the negatively charged drugs from attaching to the membrane.

The basolateral membrane is opposed to adjacent epithelial cells and to the basement membrane and interior of the organism. The basal membrane is usually the location of Na^+-K^+ ATPase [2], receptors for hormones and growth factors, and nutrient transport systems [3]. The basal membrane is also active in endocytosis for the transepithelial transport of macromolecules such as immunoglobulins [4]. The most unusual feature of the lateral surface of epithelial cells is the presence of various functionally and morphologically distinct intercellular junctions. These junctions can be divided into three major types: (1) tight junctions that occlude the intercellular spaces and thus play a major role in determining transepithelial permeability; (2) adhering junctions that link membranes and the cytoskeletal elements between cells to allow mechanical force to be distributed; and (3) gap junctions that permit ions and other molecules to pass between cells.

The development of junctions and the degree of tightness can be expressed by the electrical resistance of the cell monolayers. Madara measured fluxes of inulin, mannitol, and sodium and the magnitude of the increments of transepithelial resistance. It was found that restriction of transjunctional permeability accounted for the observed resistance rise, and T_{84} junctional strands have finite permeability to molecules with radii less than 3.6 Å but are essentially impermeable to molecules with radii greater than 15 Å [5,6]. Therefore, resistance determination can be used as a good index of the tightness of intercellular junctions on confluent monolayers in cell cultures [7].

II. EPITHELIAL TRANSPORT OF DRUGS AND MACROMOLECULES

There are several ways that drugs and macromolecules can cross the epithelial cells: passive transport of small molecules, active transport of ionic and polar compounds, and endocytosis and transcytosis of macromolecules.

A. Passive Transport

Passive transport is the movement of a solute along its concentration and electrical gradients. Small and nonionic molecules usually cross cell monolayers by passive transport. The rate at which a molecule diffuses across the lipid bilayer of cell membranes depends largely on the size of the molecule and its relative lipid solubility. In general, the smaller and more hydrophobic the molecule, the more rapidly it will diffuse across the bilayer. Cell membranes, however, are also permeable to some small water-soluble molecules, such as ions, sugars, and amino acids. They can be passively transported across the cell monolayers either by specialized transport protein or by the water-filled channels at the tight junctions [8,9].

B. Active Transport

Active transport differs from passive transport in that the transport process is mediated by membrane transport proteins coupled to an energy source. In active transport, the solutes can be transported against a concentration gradient. Many active transport systems are driven by the energy stored in ion gradients. Na^+ is the usual cotransported ion whose electrochemical gradient provides the driving force for the active transport of a second molecule, such as glucose, amino acid, and dipeptide. Hydrolysis of ATP or other high-energy compounds on the surface of the protein also provides the energy for active transport, as is the case for the Na^+-K^+ ATPase [10], which pumps Na^+ out and K^+ into a cell against their electrochemical gradients. The cross-epithelial transports of many drugs, for example, L-Dopa [11], 5-fluorouracil [12], and cephalexin [13], are mediated by active transport.

C. Endocytosis and Transcytosis

The transport of macromolecules is different from the transport of small molecules across epithelial cells. Most of the transport of macromolecules is mediated by endocytotic and transcytotic processes [14]. In endocytosis drugs or macromolecules are progressively enclosed by the cell membranes. After invagination, macromolecules migrate within membrane-bound vesicles to the perinuclear region of the cell, where the vesicles coalesce with lysosomes in which intracellular digestion occurs. The absorption of ferritin, ricin [15], and horseradish peroxidase [16] by epithelial cells occurs by this process.

Macromolecules and drugs can also be transported across epithelial cells by transcytosis. The process of transcytosis combines elements of the pathways for endocytosis and exocytosis. Macromolecules bind to receptors on the surface of epithelial cells, and then the receptor–macromolecule complex is incorporated into vesicles and carried into the cell. The complex remains intact in endosomes and is retrieved in transport vesicles that fuse with the membranes of the opposite side of the cell monolayer. Therefore, intact macromolecules can be transported across the epithelial barrier [17,18].

III. MECHANISMS OF ACTION OF PENETRATION ENHANCERS

Penetration enhancers are compounds that can increase the absorption of coadministered drugs by increasing the mucosal membrane permeability and hence the absorption of poorly permeable drugs. For example, therapeutic amounts of insulin can be absorbed across the human nasal mucosa when administered as a nasal spray using bile salts as a penetration enhancer [19]. Sodium salicylate can enhance the absorption of water-soluble compounds and polypeptides from the rectum and small intestine [20,21]. Other compounds such as surfactants [22], chelating agents, nonsteroidal anti-inflammatory drugs [23], hyperosmolar stimuli [5], and fatty acids [24] have also been shown to alter the permeability of epithelial membranes.

Several possible mechanisms of action of transepithelial penetration enhancers have been proposed. The promotional effects of bile salts and fatty acids may be due to their surface activity as well as their chelating activity [25,26]. Salicylates enhance membrane permeability in vitro in everted colonic experiments due to the interaction of salicylate with membrane components [27]. Generally, there are two mechanisms of action of transepithelial penetration enhancers; they change the permeability of the membrane or the physicochemical properties of the drug.

A. Change in the Permeability of Membranes

A penetration enhancer can influence the mucosa in five ways: (1) by acting on the mucus layers (e.g., bile salts), (2) by action on the tight junction (e.g., chelating agents), (3) by acting on the membrane components (e.g., the fatty acids or salicylic acid type of penetration enhancers), (4) by acting on the vesicular transport (e.g., hyperosmotic solutions), and (5) by acting on the activity of proteases (e.g., surfactants).

1. Action on the Mucus Layer

Penetration enhancers may enhance intranasal absorption of proteins by dispersing the mucous barrier [28]. The mucous layer covering the cell surface of the mucosa can be seen as an unstirred layer, acting as a barrier to the diffusion of drug molecules. Ionic surfactants are able to reduce the mucus viscosity and elasticity. Consequently, the barrier function of the layer is reduced, and an increase in the permeability of the mucosa can be achieved [29].

2. Action on Tight Junction

The intercellular tight junction is one of the major barriers to paracellular transport of macromolecules and polar compounds. It has been found that tight junction structure and permeability can be regulated by many potential physiological factors including concentration of cyclic AMP [30], intercellular calcium concentrations [31,32], and transient mucosal osmotic loads [5,33]. Several studies have shown that one of the possible mechanisms of penetration enhancers is due to their effect on tight junctions of epithelial membranes [34,35]. The effects of penetration enhancers on the tight junctions results in a loosening of the tight junctions and an increase in paracellular transport of poorly absorbed drugs.

The promotion of absorption by many chelators, such as EDTA, depends on their chelating activities. Calcium ions play an important role as cross-linking agents in mucous structure and in the cellular junctions between epithelial cells [7]. Removal of endogenous calcium from the intestinal epithelial cells by the formation of a calcium–EDTA complex loosens the cellular barrier, especially the intercellular tight junctions. Murakami et al. [34] proposed that ethyl acetoacetate enamine derivatives of phenylglycine and ampicillin, which are membrane-permeable and have calcium-binding abilities, enhance the rectal absorption of water-soluble β-lactam antibiotics. However, the promoting ability of the enamine derivatives for rectal absorption of ampicillin decreases when calcium chloride is coadministered [34]. Therefore, the mechanism by which chelating-type penetration enhancers increase absorption is probably due to the interaction between the enhancers and the calcium ions in the epithelial surface. This interaction can cause a temporary change in the integrity of the membrane and increase paracellular transport.

3. Action on the Membrane Components

The membranes of epithelial cells contain proteins and phospholipids. The hydrophobic interactions between the acyl chains of lipid molecules result in the formation of a well-organized phospholipid bilayer. These ordered bilayers are poorly permeable for both macromolecules and highly polar compounds. Therefore, many highly polar drugs and macromolecules cannot cross the bilayers because of insufficient lipophilicity and large molecular size. Numerous studies have shown that penetration enhancers can increase the permeability of membranes by affecting the biological membrane components, such as proteins and lipids. Fatty acids [36], monoglycerides [37], fatty acid–bile salt micelles [38], surfactants [39], and nonsteroidal anti-inflammatory drugs such as indomethacin, aspirin, and phenylbutazone [21,23] have been shown to increase epithelial membrane permeability by affecting the membrane proteins or lipids [23]. The most likely mechanism by which detergents enhance absorption of poorly absorbable drugs is the solubilization of phospholipids and membrane proteins by detergents [39]. The extraction of membrane components by detergents causes an increase in membrane permeability, so drug absorption can be markedly increased [39]. The action of nonsteroidal anti-inflammatory drugs on the absorption of marker drugs and the accumulation of the enhancer were particularly decreased by pretreatment of the rectal membrane with mercuric chloride or papain [23]. In liposomes prepared from lipids extracted from rectal tissues, the permeability of the lipid layers was markedly increased in the presence of nonsteroidal anti-inflammatory drugs [23]. These results indicate that the interaction of anti-inflammatory drugs with membrane components (proteins and lipids) plays an important role in the mechanism of action.

The effect of fatty acids and monoglycerides on barrier properties of liposome membranes prepared from egg phosphatidylcholine was investigated by Muranishi et al. [37]. It was reported that the incorporation of fatty acids and monoglycerides with the membranes enhanced the permeability of liposomal membranes and that such a change in permeability was induced by the disordering effect on the interior and the interaction of the polar region of the membranes. The interaction of fatty acids with the membrane may trigger a transient, ''corn''-shaped lipid complex in which the polar head-group region is smaller than the one subtended toward the end of the acyl chain; the bilayer configuration is destabilized as a result. Thus, an increase in membrane permeability associated with membrane perturbation by fatty acids is thought to be the essential mechanism.

Recently the contribution of membrane-bound proteins to enhancement of intestinal permeability was investigated [40]. The promoted absorption effect by oleic acid was reduced by pretreating the mucosa with several sulfhydryl (SH) reagents. The results suggest that the intact SH group of membrane-associated protein is necessary for the enhanced permeation by fatty acids.

These studies suggest that the interaction of penetration enhancers with epithelial components results in the perturbation of cell membranes and the promoted absorption of poorly absorbed drugs. The perturbation of epithelial membranes results in increased transcellular permeability.

4. Action on the Vesicular Transport

A minimal transport of macromolecules across epithelial cells can be accomplished by the vesicular transport process. In this process, pinocytotic vesicles derived from the apical surface of the epithelial cells are transported to the lateral cell surface, where they deposit their contents into the intercellular space. Therefore, an increase in the rate of pinocytosis may lead to an enhanced transport of drug across epithelial cells. A hyperosmotic solution load may alter the sensitivity of the microvillar plasma membranes to adsorbed compounds and thereby produce an enhanced rate of pinocytosis [41]. The possible effects of luminal hyperosmolality on the integrity of the intestinal macromolecular barrier of the rat jejunum was investigated. It was found that the passage of macromolecules across the jejunal epithelium of the rat is enhanced under conditions of luminal hyperosmotic stress. This may be due to alteration in the functional integrity of the tight junctional macromolecular barrier and to an enhanced rate of pinocytosis.

5. Action on the Enzymatic Activity

It is well known that polypeptides such as enkephalins are subject to degradation by proteolytic enzymes during passage through the mucosal membrane [42]. This degradation has limited the development of nonparenteral administration of protein and peptide drugs. Thus, a significant inhibition of the degradation may result in an increase in the absorption of protein and peptide drugs [43,44].

The promoting effect of surfactants on the nasal absorption of insulin was attributed not only to their direct effect on the nasal mucosa, but also to their inhibitory effect on proteolytic enzymes. The addition of surfactants, especially bile salts, results in an 80% inhibition of the enzymatic degradation of insulin and of the enzymatic activity of leucine aminopeptidase, which rapidly breaks down the B-chain of insulin from the hydrophobic N-terminal end [43].

B. Change in the Physicochemical Properties of Drugs

A penetration enhancer can also promote absorption by action on the drug solubility and dissolution rate, dispersion protein aggregation, and formation of micelles.

1. Action on Drug Solubility and Dissolution Rate

In water-insoluble drugs, such as glutethimide, griseofulvin, and hexestrol, the extent of absorption is usually controlled by the drug solubility and dissolution rate. Therefore, a penetration enhancer may exert its effects by increasing solubility and dissolution of the drug. Penetration enhancers, such as sodium salicylate and bile salts, are thought to increase absorption by this effect [45–47]. In the presence of 1.5 M sodium salicylate, an approximate 8,000-fold increase in the solubility of insulin has been reported. Thus, it may substantially contribute to the improved drug bioavailability mediated by salicylate [46].

2. Dispersion of Protein Aggregation

A high proportion of aqueous insulin molecules are present as either microcrystals or polymers in commercial preparations [48]. Bile salts are thought to disperse these microcrystals and aggregates and to completely solubilize insulin as monomers, thereby increasing the insulin monomer concentrations at the absorptive surface [49].

3. Formation of Micelles

A significant change in the ability of a drug to permeate a biological membrane may result from an interaction with a penetration enhancer. A molecular complex consists of constituents held together by weak forces such as hydrogen bonds. The properties of drug–enhancer complexes, including solubility, molecular size, diffusiveness, and lipid–water partition coefficient, can differ significantly from the properties of the respective free drugs. Mixed micelle formation is thought to provide a high juxtamembrane concentration of soluble insulin that facilitates the flow of insulin monomers. Reverse micelles act as transmembrane channels or mobile carriers for insulin to move down an aqueous concentration gradient through mucosal cells [49].

The enhanced intestinal absorption of a drug by bile salt–fatty acid micelles is mostly due to the increase in the permeability of the mucosal membrane caused by the incorporation of the lipid component of mixed micelles [50]. Westergaard and Dietschy suggested a mechanism whereby bile salt micelles facilitate solute uptake into the intestinal mucosal cell [51]. The principal role of bile salt micelles is to overcome the resistance of the aqueous diffusion layer and maintain a maximum concentration of free solute at the membrane–solute interface.

IV. FACTORS INFLUENCING THE EFFICACY OF PENETRATION ENHANCERS

Numerous studies have shown that increased absorption by penetration enhancers can be influenced by many factors [52], such as route of administration [53,54], lipophilicity of enhancers [22,49,55], physicochemical properties of the compounds absorbed [52], and the ability of penetration enhancers to increase membrane permeability [35,38].

Penetration enhancers can be used in a variety of administration routes including oral, rectal, and vaginal administration. However, the efficacy of a penetration enhancer may be different in each administration route. For instance, ceftriaxone absorption was enhanced 8-fold following oral administration and 30-fold following rectal administration using a suspension formulation of a vehicle containing mono- and diglycerides of caprylic acid as enhancers [54]. Muranishi [36] further demonstrated that the mucosal sensitivity of the enhancers along the gastrointestinal tract is in the following order: rectum > colon > small intestine > stomach.

Numerous studies show that the lipophilicity of penetration enhancers can affect the enhancement activity. Gordon et al. [49] reported structure–function studies on a series of natural bile salts by testing their ability to enhance insulin absorption across the human nasal mucosa. Dramatic differences in insulin absorption were observed between closely related bile salt species. Similarly, Kim et al. [55] used various enamine derivatives as penetration enhancers to study the rectal absorption of insulin in dogs and rabbits. They found that the absorption-enhancing ability of the phenylalanyl derivative of ethyl acetoacetate was 4 times as high as that of its less lipophilic glycyl counterpart.

The efficacy of penetration enhancers also depends on the nature of the solute. The coadministration of various peptides, leuprolide [53], insulin [19], and metkephamide [56], with 1% sodium glycocholate brings about the greatest increase in the absorption of a poorly absorbed peptide, leuprolide, while having no effect on the absorption of a relatively well absorbed peptide, metkephamide. Furthermore, even in the presence of the penetration enhancer, the bioavailability of insulin is far from complete [19].

V. EPITHELIAL CELL CULTURES FOR THE STUDY OF PENETRATION ENHANCERS

A. Models for the Study of Penetration Enhancers

The permeability of epithelial cells and the efficacy of penetration enhancers have been investigated in numerous in vivo and in vitro models. In vivo and in situ models are still the most popular systems in the investigation of penetration enhancers. In vivo study of the effects of penetration enhancers is usually performed by administering the drugs noninvasively with or without a penetration enhancer to experimental animals. Blood samples from the animals are subsequently collected, and the amount of absorbed drugs is analyzed. In situ absorption experiments can be performed by recirculation [57] or single-pass perfusion [40] techniques. The experimental animals are anesthetized, and the experimental organ is exposed and cannulated. A solution containing a penetration enhancer and a poorly absorbed drug is perfused into the organ. To determine the efficacy of the penetration enhancer, blood samples are collected from the animals after drug administration. Currently, animals are the major models for the study of the effects of penetration enhancers. However, using the whole animal as an experimental model presents many complicating factors that preclude interpretation and characterization of the cellular and molecular phenomena in the epithelia. Furthermore, it is very difficult to investigate the mechanisms of action of penetration enhancers in an animal model system.

Brush border membrane vesicles from gastrointestinal tract membrane labeled with fluorescent probes have been used to elucidate the mechanism of enhancers. Using brush border membrane vesicles prepared from the small intestine, with their protein and lipid components labeled by fluorescent probes, the perturbing actions of salicylic acid on the membrane were studied [21,58]. The use of a brush border membrane vesicle containing fluorescence makes it possible to study the membrane permeability effectively and easily. However, the preparation of brush border membrane vesicles is laborious.

Ussing chambers have been used to study the transport of low-permeability solutes across the nasal mucosa and small intestine with and without penetration enhancers [59]. Experimental mucosa mounted in an Ussing chamber exhibits normal electrophysiology and histology. The alteration of paracellular and transcellular permeabilities can be measured by the electrophysiological techniques developed by Gordon et al. [49] to study the mechanisms of nasal drug absorption with and without an enhancer. The method provides a useful technique to investigate the nasal transport of drugs and allows evaluation of the effects of penetration enhancers on both absorption and tissue integrity. However, the process is laborious, and the potential utility of this method is limited.

Isolated intestinal epithelial cells have been used in the pursuit of a better understanding of the intestinal mucosa at the cellular level [60]. However, the potential utility of this method is substantially reduced by the limited viability of isolated intestinal epithelial cells. Furthermore, cell isolation procedures result in loss of cell polarity and of the different epithelial components in determining membrane permeability [61].

Cultured epithelial cell lines have been developed as an in vitro model for the study of drug transport and metabolism at biological barriers [61–63]. Several recent studies have used cultured epithelial cells to elucidate the possible mechanisms of action of penetration enhancers.

Several general factors should be considered in developing a cell-cultured model system for drug transport and metabolism studies, which include not only the nature of the cells but also the type of microporous membrane and the supporting matrix, the culturing and experimental conditions, and the diffusion apparatus [61]. Several types of culture apparatus are now available commercially; examples are Transwells (Costar, Cambridge, MA) and Millicells (Millipore, Bedford, MA). An in vitro cell culture model has many advantages over conventional methods for the study of transepithelial penetration enhancers; including the following:

1. A rapid assessment of the permeability of a drug can be achieved.
2. Mechanisms of the various pathways in transepithelial transport can be elucidated.
3. Strategies for enhancing drug transport can be rapidly evaluated.
4. Dose–response curves can be easily constructed.
5. A high degree of reproducibility can be obtained.
6. Time-consuming and expensive animal studies can be minimized.

B. Epithelial Cell Lines in Drug Transport Studies

Several cultured epithelial cell lines have been used for drug transport studies. The most common cell lines for penetration enhancer studies are the Caco-2 and MDCK cell lines [62,63].

1. Caco-2 Cell Line

The Caco-2 cell line is one of the human colon carcinoma cell lines that can be routinely grown as confluent monolayers on microporous membranes. The cell monolayers display a number of characteristics of intestinal cells, including signs of structural and functional differentiation [64,65], polarization [66,67], expression of many brush border enzymes [67,68], and nutrient and macromolecular transport systems, for example, transcellular transport of cobalamin [64]. Therefore, Caco-2 cells seem to be a better model for the study of drug absorption by the intestinal epithelium. However, Caco-2 cells develop leaky intercellular junctions and exhibit low transepithelial electrical resistance (TEER) [68]. Under standard conditions Caco-2 cells grown on microporous membranes can express these properties in approximately 15–20 days. The integrity of the cell monolayers can be monitored by measuring the transepithelial electrical resistance. A confluent cell monolayer normally displays electrical resistance of between 150 and 400 ohm·cm^2. Therefore, the Caco-2 cell line is not very sensitive for the study of paracellular transport. However, Caco-2 cells are useful for metabolism studies as they have many of the brush border enzymes of small intestinal mucosa in quantities similar to those found in vivo. Caco-2 cells are also very useful as a model to study the intestinal absorption of drugs.

2. MDCK Cell Line

The Madin-Darby canine kidney (MDCK) cell line is one of the best characterized epithelial cell lines. It was originally derived from the kidney of a normal male cocker spaniel. MDCK cells retain several physiological properties of mammalian epithelial cells [69]. They form cell monolayers with a characteristic morphology of polarized epithelial cells (brush border, apical cell–cell junctions, and lateral spaces) [70,71]. Biochemical polarity of the cellular plasma membranes is evident from the demonstration of the asymmetric composition of the apical and basolateral membranes [72]. MDCK cells also retain the specific binding protein for mineralocorticoids and renal hormones. Strain I MDCK cells form good tight junctions with a high electrical resistance (>1500 ohm·cm^2) that are barriers for paracellular transport [62]. Under normal conditions, macromolecules and highly hydrophilic compounds do not cross MDCK cell monolayers easily [62]. These characteristics have led several groups to use MDCK cells grown on permeable supports as models for transepithelial transport studies [62]. Because of the tightness of cell junctions, this in vitro model of MDCK cells can be used to study the effects, mechanisms, and toxicities of penetration enhancers. However, strain I MDCK cells do not possess measurable activities of many enzymes associated with membranes of other types of epithelial cells [73].

C. Studies of Penetration Enhancers in Cell Cultures

1. DMSO

Dimethyl sulfoxide (DMSO) has been considered a classic penetration enhancer. It can significantly increase transdermal absorption of many drugs [74,75]. The possible mechanisms of enhancing ability and cytotoxicity of DMSO as a penetration enhancer have been studied in cultured MDCK cell monolayers [76]. The enhancing ability of DMSO can be determined by measuring the transport rate of compounds with poor permeability such as HRP and [^{14}C]sucrose. The integrity and cytotoxicity can be determined by TEER measurement and by a vital dye (e.g., trypan blue) staining method, respectively. It has been found that at nontoxic doses (e.g., <15%) DMSO can reversibly decrease transepithelial electrical resistance of the cell monolayers and increase transport of the fluid phase markers HRP and [^{14}C]sucrose. The enhanced transport of HRP and [^{14}C]sucrose is most likely due to an increase of the paracellular process; no increase of cell-associated HRP or [^{14}C]sucrose was found [76].

2. Surfactants

Surfactants have been the most frequently employed penetration enhancers for the nasal route of drug administration. Several mechanisms have been proposed for their action; they may inhibit protease activity [19,43], decrease the resistance of the mucous layer [25], increase paracellular transport [29], and/or increase transcellular transport [49].

The possible mechanisms of enhancement of bile salts have been studied in cultured MDCK cell monolayers. A reversible decrease of TEER has been found in MDCK cell monolayers treated with 0.05% deoxycholate. Under similar conditions, no effect was observed with cholate and an intermediate effect was observed with chenodeoxycholate [77,78]. The changes in TEER are consistent with the reported efficacies of these three bile salts for the enhancement in the nasal absorption of insulin in humans: deoxycholate > chenodeoxycholate > cholate [49].

From the investigation in cultured MDCK cell monolayers, it is suggested that deoxycholate may exert its effect on epithelia by at least two different mechanisms. The exact action of deoxycholate as a penetration enhancer is dependent on the concentrations of the bile salt and on the nature of the drug. At low concentrations, the enhancement of HRP transport is largely due to an increase in the cellular uptake of this protein [77,78]. At higher concentrations, deoxycholate can loosen the tight junction and increase the paracellular leakage of fluid in epithelial monolayers. Furthermore, the cytotoxicity of deoxycholate on the epithelial cells depends on the concentration of deoxycholate as well as the duration of exposure to the cell monolayers [77,78].

The enhancing effects of other surfactants—sodium taurodihydrofusidate, sodium dodecyl sulfate, and lopysorbate 80—have been investigated in Caco-2 cells [79]. In this in vitro model, the integrity of the cell monolayers was determined by measurements of the TEER and by scanning electron microscopy. Furthermore, the cytotoxicity was measured by the MTT method based on intracellular dehydrogenase enzyme activities, and the enhancing ability of the surfactants was determined by measuring the transport rate of mannitol and polyethylene glycol. At a concentration close to critical micelle concentration, relatively sharp decreases were observed in intracellular dehydrogenase activities and TEER of the cell monolayers. A significant increase in absorption of marker drugs was also found. The minimal concentration that caused absorption enhancement was similar to the concentrations that caused a decrease in intracellular enzyme activities and TEER of the cell monolayers. Thus, the results indicate that the absorption enhancement induced by surfactants probably is due to the action of surfactants on the cell membranes and intercellular junctions.

3. Chelators

Citric acid has been shown to promote the mucosal absorption of heparin and growth hormone [53,80]. Confluent MDCK cells have been used to study the possible mechanism of enhancing the activity of citric acid [81]. In the presence of a Ca^{2+} chelating agent, for example, citrate or EGTA, a decrease in TEER of cell monolayers and an increase in transport of [^{14}C]sucrose were observed. Ca^{2+} plays a very important role in the maintenance of the integrity and function of intercellular tight junctions [82]. As a Ca^{2+} chelator, citrate may loosen the tight junction of the epithelium and enhancing the paracellular transport of drugs.

VI. CONCLUSION

Penetration enhancers have been shown to promote the absorption of various types of drugs, particularly proteins and peptides, across epithelial barriers. In general, an enhancer can promote drug absorption by way of either the transcellular route or the paracellular route. However, owing to the lack of an in vitro model of the epithelium, the exact mechanisms of action of penetration enhancers at the molecular and cellular levels are still largely undetermined. Recent developments in cell cultures of epithelial cell lines grown on microporous filters are potentially applicable to the investigation of drug transport across epithelial barriers. Cultured epithelial cell monolayers can be used to measure the alteration of tight junctions, cellular uptake of drugs, and cell viability in the presence of enhancers. Because of the simplicity and reproducibility of the cell culture systems, this in vitro model may provide important information regarding the basic mechanisms in the enhancement of transport across epithelial barriers. Such information can be useful for the design of effective and safe penetration enhancers in the future.

Acknowledgment We are grateful to Robert B. Blakeslee for critically reading the manuscript.

REFERENCES

1. J. S. Handler, *Annu. Rev. Physiol. 51*, 729 (1989).
2. M. J. Caplan and J. D. Anderson, *Cell 46*, 632 (1986).
3. A. L. Hubbard and B. Stieger, *Annu. Rev. Physiol. 51*, 755 (1989).
4. H. J. Geuze, H. W. Slot, G. J. A. M. Strous, J. Peppard, and K. von Figura, *Cell 37*, 195 (1984).
5. J. L. Madara, *J. Cell Biol. 97*, 125 (1983).
6. J. L. Madara and K. Dharmsathaphorn, *J. Cell Biol. 101*, 2124 (1985).
7. A. Martinez-Palomo, I. Meza, G. Beaty, and M. Cereijido, *J. Cell Biol. 87*, 736 (1980).
8. M. Kasahara and P. C. Hinkle, *Proc. Natl. Acad. Sci. U.S.A. 73*, 396 (1976).
9. H. Ginsburg, *Biochim. Biophys. Acta 506*, 119 (1978).
10. K. J. Sweadner and S. M. Goldin, *N. Engl. J. Med. 302*, 777 (1980).
11. H. Shindo, T. Komai, and K. Kawai, *Chem. Pharm. Bull. 21*, 2030 (1973).
12. L. S. Schanker and J. J. Jeffrey, *Nature 190*, 727 (1961).
13. E. Nakashima, A. Tsuji, H. Mizuo, and T. Yamana, *Biochem. Pharmacol. 33*, 3345 (1984).
14. J. S. Rodman, R. W. Mercer, and P. D. Stahl, *Current Opinion Cell Biol. 2*, 664 (1990).

15. M. R. Neutra, N. G. Guerina, T. L. Hall, and G. L. Nicolson, *Gastroenterology 82*, 1137 (1982).
16. W. A. Walker, R. Cornell, L. M. Davenport, and K. J. Isselbacher, *J. Cell Biol. 54*, 195 (1972).
17. A. L. Warshaw, W. A. Walker, and K. J. Isselbacher, *Gastroenterology 66*, 987 (1974).
18. K. E. Mostov and N. E. Simister, *Cell 43*, 389 (1985).
19. S. Hirai, T. Yashiki, and H. Mima, *Int. J. Pharm. 9*, 165 (1981).
20. T. Nishihata, J. H. Rytting, and T. Higuchi, *J. Pharm. Sci. 71*, 865 (1982).
21. H. Kajii, T. Horie, M. Hayashi, and S. Awazu, *J. Pharm. Sci. 75*, 475 (1986).
22. G. S. M. J. E. Duchateau, J. Zuidema, and F. W. H. M. Merkus, *Int. J. Pharm. 31*, 193 (1986).
23. K. Nakanishi, H. Saitoh, M. Masada, A. Tatematsu, and T. Nadai, *Chem. Pharm. Bull. 32*, 3187 (1984).
24. E. J. van Hoogdalem, M. A. Hardens, A. G. de Boer, and D. D. Breimer, *Pharm. Res. 5*, 453 (1988).
25. R. W. Freel, M. Hatch, D. L. Earnest, and A. M. Goldner, *Am. J. Physiol. 245*, G816 (1983).
26. T. Ishizawa, M. Hayashi, and S. Awazu, *J. Pharm. Pharmacol. 39*, 892 (1987).
27. T. Nishihata and T. Higuchi, *Biochim. Biophys. Acta 775*, 269 (1984).
28. C. Marriott, D. T. Brown, and M. F. Beeson, *Biorheology 20*, 71 (1983).
29. G. P. Martin, C. Marriott, and I. W. Kellaway, *Gut 19*, 103 (1978).
30. M. E. Duffey, B. Hainau, S. Ho, and C. J. Bentzel, *Nature (Lond.) 204*, 451 (1981).
31. D. R. Pitelka, B. N. Taggart, and S. T. Hamamoto, *J. Cell Biol. 96*, 613 (1983).
32. C. E. Palant, M. D. Duffey, B. K. Mookerjee, S. Ho, and C. J. Bentzel, *Am. J. Physiol. 245*, C203 (1983).
33. M. W. Brightman, M. Hori, S. I. Rapoport, T. S. Reese, and E. Westergaard, *J. Comp. Neurol. 152*, 317 (1973).
34. T. Murakami, N. Yata, H. Tamauchi, and A. Kamada, *Chem. Pharm. Bull. 30*, 659 (1982).
35. T. Murakami, Y. Sasaki, R. Yamajo, and N. Yata, *Chem. Pharm. Bull. 32*, 1948 (1984).
36. S. Muranishi, *Pharm. Res. 2*, 108 (1985).
37. N. Muranushi, N. Takagi, S. Muranishi, and H. Sezaki, *Chem. Phys. Lipids 28*, 269 (1981).
38. P. Tengamnuay and A. K. Mitra, *Pharm. Res. 7*, 127 (1990).
39. D. Lichtenberg, R. J. Robson, and E. A. Dennis, *Biochim. Biophys. Acta 737*, 285 (1983).
40. M. Murakami, K. Takada, T. Fuji, and S. Muranishi, *Biochim. Biophys. Acta 939*, 238 (1988).
41. M. Cooper, S. Teichberg, and F. Lifshitz, *Lab. Invest. 38*, 447 (1978).
42. S. Dodda-Kashi and V. H. L. Lee, *Life Sci. 38*, 2019 (1986).
43. S. Hirai, T. Yashiki, and H. Mima, *Int. J. Pharm. 9*, 173 (1981).
44. V. H. L. Lee, D. Gallardo, and J. P. Longenecker, *Proc. Intn. Symp. Controlled Release Bioact. Mater. 14*, 55 (1987).

45. E. Touitou and P. Fisher, *J. Pharm. Sci. 75*, 384 (1986).
46. E. Touitou, F. Alhaique, P. Fisher, A. Memoli, F. M. Riccieri, and E. Santucci, *J. Pharm. Sci. 76*, 791 (1987).
47. T. R. Bates, M. Gibaldi, and J. L. Kanig, *J. Pharm. Sci. 55*, 191 (1966).
48. T. L. Blundell, J. F. Cutfield, S. M. Cutfield, E. J. Dodson, G. G. Dodson, D. C. Hodgkin, and D. A. Mercola, *Diabetes 21*, 492 (1972).
49. G. S. Gordon, A. C. Moses, R. D. Silver, J. S. Flier, and M. C. Carey, *Proc. Natl. Acad. Sci. U.S.A. 82*, 7419 (1985).
50. N. Muranushi, M. Kinugawa, Y. Nakajima, S. Muranishi, and H. Sezaki, *Int. J. Pharm. 4*, 271 (1980).
51. H. Westergaard and J. M. Dietschy, *J. Clin. Invest. 58*, 97 (1976).
52. V. H. L. Lee and Y. Yamamoto, *Adv. Drug Delivery Rev. 4*, 171 (1990).
53. H. Okada, I. Yamazaki, Y. Ogawa, S. Hirai, T. Yashiki, and H. Mima, *J. Pharm. Sci. 71*, 1367 (1982).
54. G. Beskid, J. Unowsky, C. R. Behl, J. Siebelist, J. L. Tossounian, C. M. McGarry, N. H. Shah, and R. Cleeland, *Chemotherapy 34*, 77 (1988).
55. S. Kim, A. Kamada, T. Higuchi, and T. Nishihata, *J. Pharm. Pharmacol. 35*, 100 (1983).
56. K. S. E. Su, K. M. Campanale, L. G. Mendelsohn, G. A. Kerchner, and C. L. Gries, *J. Pharm. Sci. 74*, 394 (1985).
57. K. Higaki, I. Kishimoto, H. Komatsu, M. Hashida, and H. Sezaki, *Int. J. Pharm. 36*, 131 (1987).
58. H. Kajii, T. Horie, M. Hayashi, and S. Awazu, *Life Sci. 37*, 523 (1985).
59. M. A. Wheatley, J. Dent, E. B. Wheeldon, and P. L. Smith, *J. Controlled Release 8*, 167 (1988).
60. F. Hartmann, R. Owen, and D. M. Dissell, *Am. J. Physiol. 242*, G147 (1982).
61. K. L. Audus, R. L. Bartel, I. J. Hidalgo, and R. T. Borchardt, *Pharm. Res. 7*, 435 (1990).
62. M. J. Cho., D. P. Thompson, C. T. Cramer, T. J. Vidmar, and J. F. Scieszka, *Pharm. Res. 6*, 71 (1989).
63. P. Artursson, *J. Pharm. Sci. 79*, 476 (1990).
64. G. Wilson, I. F. Hassan, C. J. Dix, I. Willianson, R. Shah, and M. Mackay, *J. Controlled Release 11*, 25 (1990).
65. I. J. Hidalgo, T. J. Raub, and R. T. Borchardt, *Gastroenterology 96*, 736 (1989).
66. E. M. Grasset, M. Pinto, E. Dussaulx, A. Zweibaum, and J.-F. Desjeux, *Am. J. Physiol. 247*, C260 (1984).
67. M. Pinto, S. Robine-leon, M. D. Appay, M. Kedinger, N. Triadou, E. Dussaulx, B. Lacroix, P. Simon-Assmann, K. Haffen, J. Fogh, and A. Zweibaum, *Biol. Cell 47*, 323 (1983).
68. M. Rousset, *Biochimie 68*, 1035 (1986).
69. J. Leighton, Z. Brada, L. W. Estes, and G. Justh, *Science 163*, 472 (1969).
70. D. S. Misfeldt, S. T. Hamamoto, and D. R. Pitelka, *Proc. Natl. Acad. Sci. U.S.A. 73*, 1212 (1976).
71. M. Cereijido, E. S. Robbins, W. J. Dolan, C. A. Rotunno, and D. D. Sabatini, *J. Cell. Biol. 77*, 853 (1978).

72. J. C. W. Richardson and W. L. Simmons, *FEBS Lett. 105*, 201 (1978).
73. J. C. W. Richardson, V. Scalera, and N. L. Simmons, *Biochim. Biophys. Acta 673*, 26 (1981).
74. S. L. Spruance, M. B. McKeough, and J. R. Cardinal, *Ann. N.Y. Acad. Sci. 411*, 28 (1983).
75. D. J. Freeman and S. L. Spruance, *J. Infect. Dis. 153*, 64 (1986).
76. Y. J. Lin, J. Wan, and W.-C. Shen, *Pharm. Res. 6*, S-115 (1989).
77. Y. J. Lin and W.-C. Shen, *Proc. Int. Symp. Controlled Release Bioact. Mater. 17*, 343 (1990).
78. Y. J. Lin and W.-C. Shen, *Pharm. Res. 8*, 498 (1991).
79. E. K. Anderberg, C. Nystrom, and P. Artursson, *Proc. Intn. Symp. Controlled Release Bioact. Mater. 17*, 345 (1990).
80. T. K. Sue, L. B. Jaquew, and E. Yuen, *Can. J. Physiol. Pharmacol. 54*, 613 (1976).
81. M. J. Cho, J. F. Scieszka, and P. S. Burton, *Int. J. Pharm. 52*, 79 (1989).
82. B. Gumbiner, *Am. J. Physiol. 253*, c749 (1987).

II

DRUG PERMEATION ENHANCEMENT VIA THE SKIN: CHEMICAL MEANS

4

Skin Permeation Enhancement Reversibility

Margo B. Haberkamp

Grosse Pointe, Michigan

I. INTRODUCTION

The acceptance of skin penetration enhancers as adjuvants will depend on the degree to which their effects are transient. Data on the reversibility of their effects, including information on the speed and mechanisms of repair, are of considerable interest. Much of what is known, or assumed, about enhancement reversibility is based on a knowledge of skin structure, kinetics, and damage repair mechanisms and the mechanism of action of the various enhancers.

There are two extremes to be considered when determining whether skin permeation enhancement is "reversible" or not. Owing to the dynamics of the skin repair mechanisms, almost any damage to the stratum corneum can be eventually repaired or reversed by replacement of the damaged tissues. The epidermis is a unique tissue with its programmed replacement and constant renewal of its barrier. Enhancers that permanently damage the basic structure of the skin may have to await replacement of the damaged tissue to be "reversible." At the other end of the spectrum are enhancers that investigators hope will only temporarily alter the barrier function of the skin. It is hoped that the increased permeability is simply due to the presence of the enhancer molecules within the stratum corneum and subsequent "fluidizing," "randomizing," or "opening" effects on the skin barrier. These "enhancers" are more correctly referred to as vehicle additives that optimize presentation to and partitioning into the surface of the skin. It is thought that penetration enhancement due to this type of effect should be completely reversible upon removal of the enhancer molecule.

Skin permeation enhancers can be divided into many categories according to their structure, mechanism of action, the type of drugs whose permeation they enhance, etc. As far as reversibility of enhancement is concerned, the most important characteristic of an enhancer is its mechanism of action.

Penetration enhancers have been credited with various mechanisms of action including alteration of the cell content or intercellular lipid composition, a direct effect on the cell membrane such as increased membrane fluidity, effects on the cohesiveness between cells, dissolution of stratum corneum lipids, disruption of the water structure of the stratum corneum, and alteration of the conformation or denaturation of stratum corneum proteins (keratin). Enhancers have also been credited with formulation-related mechanisms of enhancing drug permeation. Such enhancers basically facilitate drug penetration by increasing the penetrant's thermodynamic activity in the vehicle. They act simply as solvents and are therefore formulation optimizers, not true penetration enhancers. This distinction is important, for with these additives reversibility has no meaning as there is no damage to the skin barrier. Because penetration enhancers and these vehicle additives all lead to greater drug bioavailability, many researchers lump them together. For the purposes of this discussion, however, it is very helpful when the mechanism of permeation enhancement is known, for it is often directly linked to the reversibility of the enhancement.

The structure and biochemistry of the skin is integral to its barrier function. If the skin's ability to maintain its barrier and thus permit easier penetration of pharmaceuticals is truly altered, it is likely due to impairment of the skin's structural or biochemical integrity. Therefore, modification of the barrier function of the epidermis is reversible only upon reversal of the structural/biochemical changes caused by the enhancer. To understand how the barrier can be damaged and repaired it is necessary to understand the skin's structure, kinetics, and repair mechanisms. This discussion focuses on the stratum corneum, the outermost layer of the epidermis, wherein lies the major barrier to skin permeation and consequently the site of action of most permeation enhancers.

II. SKIN STRUCTURE AND BIOCHEMISTRY

The major cellular components of the epidermis are keratinocytes organized into differentially distinct layers, with the terminal, outermost cells fully keratinized, dead, and embedded in a lipid matrix consisting of products produced during differentiation. It is this terminal layer, the stratum corneum, that presents the major barrier to penetration by the various drug products. The two routes thought to be of importance for the penetration of most drugs are the intracellular polar route and the intercellular lipid route. Consequently, the biochemical makeup and/or physical characteristics of these two pathways are thought to be modified by penetration enhancers.

The structure and function of the stratum corneum is best understood in its context as the end product of epidermal differentiation. The cells begin their life in the stratum germinativium, the basal layer of the epidermis, where mitotically active keratinocytes attached to the basement membrane give rise to the more superficial layers of the epidermis. These basal stem cells produce committed proliferative cells that will divide into postmitotic, migratory basal cells that differentiate as they move toward the skin's surface. These basal cells contain a large nucleus and all the usual cell organelles. They also contain keratin (mol wt 46,000–58,000) filaments in fine bundles located around the nucleus and desmosomes, the junctions between keratinocytes [1]. When stimulated by epidermal injury or insult, more of the basal stem cells enter the mitotic cycle to produce the necessary committed basal cells that will eventually replace the injured tissue from below.

After leaving the basal cell portion of the epidermis the keratinocytes adopt the typical spine-like appearance of the stratum spinosum. This spine-like appearance is due to the joining of adjacent keratinocytes by the now more prominent desmosomes and accompanying shrinking back of the cell membranes. The spinous keratinocytes also contain more prominent keratin (mol wt 55,000–65,000) filament bundles, still located near the desmosomes and nucleus [1]. Spinous keratinocytes begin to synthesize involucin, an insoluble protein that eventually forms an integral part of the cell wall of the fully differentiated keratinocyte. These cells contain the usual cell organelles and are capable of remarkable endocytic and phagocytic activity, especially after epidermal injury. Indigestible material is incorporated into these cells and shed with the cell. In the upper cell layers of the stratum spinosum the cells are slightly larger and more flattened and lamellar granules begin to appear in the cytoplasm. The granules contain several classes of lipids, neutral sugars conjugated to proteins and lipids, and acid hydralases such as acid phosphatase [2,3]. Elias [2] has suggested that the lamellar granule, or "membrane coating granule," has multiple functions including augmentation of the barrier function of the stratum corneum, synthesis and storage of cholesterol, provision of epidermal lipids, and desquamation of the fully differentiated keratinocyte.

Cells, progressing through the stratum spinosum stage next enter the stratum granulosum, where the keratin filaments now contain high molecular weight (63,000–67,000) fractions [1]. The granular keratinocytes still contain the typical cytoplasmic organelles, and they begin to concentrate and cross-link the involucrin that was formed in the spinous layer. An obvious feature of the stratum granulosum is the basophilic keratohyaline granules. Characteristic of this epidermal strata, these granules contain an early, high molecular weight form of filaggrin, a matrix protein that is responsible for embedding and promoting the aggregation of the keratin filaments in the fully cornified keratinocyte [4,5]. The transition from a granular to cornified keratinocyte involves severe dehydration of the cell and an abrupt loss of the nucleus and cellular components. The keratin filaments remain in the cell as it forms a large flattened surface ideal for protecting the underlying cells.

As the granular keratinocytes approach the stratum corneum, the lamellar bodies aggregate, fuse, and release their contents into the intercellular space. As they journey further toward the skin surface, the lipid contents of this exudate are organized into lipid-rich sheets of neutral, polar lipids, possibly with the aid of a few enzymes that remain [2]. The cells slightly overlap and are joined by modified desmosomes. Keratins, interlocked by disulfide bonds, along with filaggrin, form most of what remains of the cell. The final end product of epidermal differentiation has a unique architecture that helps maintain the permeability barrier and allows for orderly desquamation of the surface cells. The cells are stacked in columns with lipid-rich intercellular domains, resulting in three distinct physicochemical domains: cell interior, cell walls, and the intercellular space. This structure is not present after wounding or in some disease states. A stratum corneum that lacks this structure permits greater transepidermal water loss [6].

Triglycerides are the single most abundant lipids found in the skin, but the composition of the surface triglycerides is very different from the composition of those found within the epidermis. Triglycerides are cleaved via lipase activity of normal cutaneous bacterial flora to form the free fatty acids of the surface film. The composition of the lipid myelin is critical to the skin's proper function. Deficiency of essential fatty acids is associated with increased mitosis and disturbed keratinization. Topical application of linoleic acid may correct these problems [7,8]. Although phospholipids constitute a major fraction of the epidermal lipids commonly found within the viable epidermis, they are essentially absent from the stratum corneum. Here one finds another type of polar lipid, ceramides, which also form bilayer configurations. Cholesterol and cholesterol sulfate are also found in the stratum corneum. The lipid content of the epidermis may vary between sites on the animal, and apparently this may play a role in explaining the variation in permeability from site to site. It has been shown that quantitative differences in lipid content correlate better with regional variations in skin permeability than does stratum corneum thickness or cell number [6].

III. EPIDERMAL KINETICS

The overall unidirectional movement of the epidermal keratinocytes helps the skin maintain its barrier integrity. The time required for an average cell to travel from the basal cell layer to the surface of the skin is known as the turnover time or renewal time and, for normal human skin, has been estimated with radiotracer techniques to be between 26 and 28 days. By the same measure, the journey from the basal layer to the stratum corneum takes approximately 14 days. The cell takes another 14 days to traverse the stratum corneum and desquamate. This time may be considerably shortened in hyperplasic disease states such as psoriasis or when the skin is injured or irritated. One might guess that this would lead to an altered form of horny tissue, and there is evidence that hyperproliferating skin possesses a defective barrier as shown by increased absorption of chemicals [9]. It is noteworthy that these are local effects, and repair is limited to the damaged surface. The epidermal turnover time is known to vary from species to species. For instance, hairless mouse skin epidermal turnover time, approximately 4–5 days in normal, uninjured skin, is much shorter than the equivalent human time of 15 days [10]. The epidermal turnover time may also vary from site to site on an animal [11].

The integrity of the upper epidermal layers is dependent upon the replication taking place in the basal cell layer. Mitosis of the basal cells is thought be under a type of negative feedback inhibition. Chalones, "local hormones" present in the epidermis, act as chemical inhibitors of mitosis [12]. This inhibition, normally at least minimally present, is apparently removed when the skin is injured. It is not yet understood exactly where and how chalones are produced by the epidermis.

IV. INJURED SKIN

There are many types of injuries that the skin must endure because of its external location and protective role. The skin responds to all injuries, including chemical insult, through complex immunological processes involving the vascular system and the mast cells and fibroblasts present in the tissue, and by the invasion of circulatory proteins and cells. This inflammatory response, involving both vascular and cellular components, results in swelling, reddening, heat, and pain at the site. During the vascular phase of the response there is an increase in capillary permeability, whereas the cellular response includes the formation of chemical mediators and chemotaxis. The skin's response to epidermal injuries is more constrained because these are injuries to dead tissue, which is programmed to desquamate, and therefore the response is dependent on how these injuries affect the underlying tissue and the barrier function of the skin. The effects of, and repair response to, physical tape stripping injury and chemical irritation injuries are described below.

A. Tape Stripping Injury

Stripping injuries are interesting because they allow study of the skin's recovery from a relatively large, well-circumscribed, homogeneous injury. They allow the researcher to examine the response of the skin to the removal of its protective barrier layer, the stratum corneum, in the absence of *direct* harm to underlying tissues. Stripping is performed by pressing an adhesive tape to the skin and removing it. This process is repeated until the skin surface is pink and glistening. This process removes the stratum corneum but apparently leaves the deeper layers physically intact. Nevertheless, an electron microscopic examination of human epidermis after tape stripping revealed major changes in the keratinocytes [13]. Within 4–12 hr following stripping there is widespread withdrawal and separation between the cells. The desmosome–tonofilament complexes that anchor the keratinocytes together disintegrate and clump around the nuclei. Superficial keratinocytes undergo parakeratosis (loss of the nucleus), and basal cells begin to rapidly proliferate. Within 72 hr there is regeneration of a keratin layer. However, it appears that the cells are driven through the differentiation too rapidly, thus resulting in incomplete keratinization [14]. It is obvious that although the layers beneath the stratum corneum may be intact after tape stripping, they are nevertheless adversely affected. Desiccation of the tissue resulting from excessive water evaporation from the site may set the repair processes in motion. It is of great importance to replace the removed stratum corneum, and this is done at the expense of proper keratinization.

Several studies have been conducted to determine the precise effect of skin stripping on the turnover of the epidermis. There is an initial depression in DNA synthesis after severe stripping and an initial accumulation of cells in the G_2 phase of mitosis [15–17]. This is followed by a "regenerative" increase is mitosis with mean basal cell cycle time of about 12 hr as compared to the normal time of about 80 hr [17]. It has been noted that the "regenerative activity is proportional to the deficit of cells produced by the stripping" [16]. The peak response time varies from 20–24 hr to 30–36 hr, dependent upon the severity of the stripping [15,16].

Evidence of the damage done to the barrier function of the epidermis by tape stripping is readily available. Studies have shown increased permeability of compounds [18,19]. Also, when the integrity of the skin is breached by an insult such as the removal of the stratum corneum, the transepidermal water loss (TEWL) increases. Tape stripping studies in which the entire stratum corneum was removed have shown that the stratum corneum is the major barrier to water loss. The restoration of this barrier as the stratum corneum regenerates itself is well documented. There appear to be two phases to its renewal. Shortly after stripping, a temporary barrier to TEWL is formed, with granular layer cells converted into parakeratotic cells. As this layer thickens, the TEWL decreases. When the regenerating epidermis is capable of forming normally keratinized cells, the true barrier is re-formed [20]. TEWL measurements obtained after a stripping injury confirm this biphasic renewal of the barrier to water loss. After complete removal of the stratum corneum, the temporary barrier will form and reduce the increased water loss to 50% of its original value within 14 days. This is followed by a much slower decline in the observed TEWL values [21]. It has been estimated that after a less severe stripping, one that does not remove the entire horny layer, it takes about 3.6 days for the increased TEWL to drop to half of its original value [22]. It has also been demonstrated that the return to normal barrier property on fully stripped mice follows first-order kinetics with a half-life of about 55 hr [23]. Figure 1 illustrates the recovery of the barrier function in hairless mouse skin that has been stripped 15 times [23].

It is logical to expect that an action, such as application of a penetration enhancer, that compromises the epidermal barrier to water loss will cause a repair response similar to this one. This is, of course, dependent on the extent of damage and whether the penetration enhancer does any direct damage to the layers beneath the stratum corneum, thereby impairing their ability to respond. If the enhancer has a toxic effect on the basal stem cells, it can be expected to cause severe, long-term, if not irreversible, damage to the barrier. An enhancer that exerts an influence on the cell layers between the stem cells and the stratum corneum will have a more readily reversible, but possibly still very severe, effect. This type of injury may be caused by ultraviolet B (UV-B; 280–320 nm) irradiation of the skin. Light of this wavelength effectively passes through the stratum corneum and is absorbed by the underlying epidermis. Immediately after burning, the TEWL (skin permeability) is normal because the stratum corneum is unharmed. However, if the TEWL is measured 2–5 days after the burn, it may be greatly elevated, depending on the severity of the burn. Figure 2 presents the average increase in TEWL seen after exposure of hairless mouse skin to UV-B burns of varying intensity [24]. This effect is accompanied by increased cell turnover as the skin attempts to repair the damage. The increase in permeability is a direct result of the damage wrought by the UV-B radiation, reflecting the impaired ability of the damaged and hyperproliferating cells to form a competent barrier once they reach the surface [23–25].

B. Chemical Irritation

Evidence of the effect of chemical irritants on the skin abounds. There are thousands of case reports of dermatitis and other cutaneous reactions to chemical exposure. Cutaneous irritation can be produced by a large number of substances. The type of irritation may vary; some compounds cause acute reactions whereas others demonstrate an irritating effect only after repeated exposure, that is, they are cumulative irritants. Known irritants include metal ions, gases, surfactants, acidic and basic inorganic and organic substances, and petroleum products and solvents. Any chemical that is permeable enough to measurably alter the biochemical environment of the living epidermis is likely to be irritating. Thus one observes that normally innocuous, poor penetrants are irritating when placed on barrier-deficient skin.

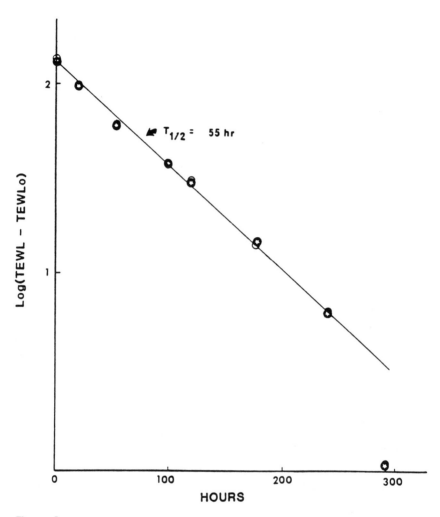

Figure 1

Anionic surfactants, known penetration enhancers, provide a good illustration of the skin's response to chemical irritation. They are among the best known and most ubiquitous irritants. The topical irritant potential of such surfactants has been assessed by several investigators. Early studies on the effect of surfactants on skin pointed to the ability of these compounds to denature skin proteins as a possible mechanism of their irritant effect [26,27]. Later studies

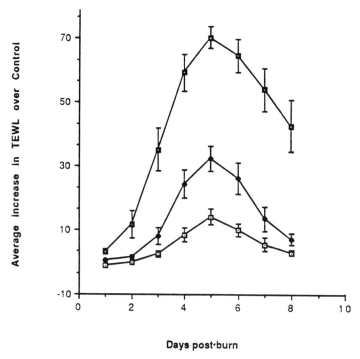

Figure 2

focused on the increased permeability of surfactant-irritated skin. They pointed out that surfactants change the composition of the lipid matrix of the stratum corneum. The quantity of lipids present in the stratum corneum does not change, but rather the relative composition of the various lipids is altered [28,29]. These investigators suggest that the surfactant-caused increase in skin permeability is due to this change in lipid composition. The total percent of lipid is the same before and after surfactant treatment; therefore this is not a simple extraction of the stratum corneum. Several studies have indicated that there is an increase in the rate of transepidermal water loss in surfactant-irritated skin [29–31]. Surfactants appear to increase the amount of free cholesterol present in the stratum corneum and to change the ceramide and free fatty acid profile [32].

Work by Imokawa and Mishima [33–35] suggests that the irritant potential of surfactants is related to their ability to influence intercellular adhesion and cause membrane rupture. Electron microscopic studies of surfactant-irritated skin have shown that it is thicker than normal skin [36]. It is possible that the ability of surfactants to influence intercellular adhesion, possibly due to surfactant-induced changes in the interstitial lipids, leads to a change in desquamation of the irritated skin. It is also possible that the increase in epidermal thickness may simply be due to an increase in cell production. Presumably the proliferating basal cells, though undamaged themselves by the surfactant, sense the increase in permeability of the skin and are triggered to proliferate in an effort to normalize the permeability and maintain homeostasis. This hypothesis is supported by the fact that the whole epidermis, not just the stratum corneum, thickens following irritation by surfactants [2].

The influences of certain topically applied chemicals on the mitotic index and incorporation of tritiated thymidine have also been investigated. After prolonged treatment with vitamin A acid and hexadecane, investigators found increases in epidermal thickness and an acceleration of turnover comparable to that seen in psoriasis [16]. However, they did not see the parakeratosis prominent in psoriasis [37] and in the early barrier formed after tape stripping [12,16]. Hairless mouse skin treated with a single application of DMSO gives a response similar to that seen with skin massage [38], an increase in cell proliferation for 3 days following treatment but no discernible subsequent hyperplasia. The augmented cell production is apparently balanced by an increased cell loss. In comparison, treatment of hairless mouse skin with the known hyperplasia-producing substances benzene and cantharidin and the carcinogen 20-methylcholanthrene results in an increase in mitotic rate followed by observable hyperplasia [39]. The effect on the epidermis resembles that seen with "regenerative" skin reactions compensating for sudden cell loss, like that elucidated with tape stripping. In some cases an initial irritation of the skin with a chemical will lead to a poorly formed stratum corneum, which allows greater penetration of subsequently applied irritant and thus increased irritation. The end result is a vicious cycle of increasing irritation and permeability.

The fact that many of the suspected mechanisms of action of penetration enhancers are also suspected mechanisms of skin irritation should not be overlooked. The skin will view a mechanism that increases permeability as a compromise of its barrier function, will usually be irritated by it, and will act to correct it. In this way the mechanism of action, skin irritability, and reversibility of the penetration enhancement are linked. Enhancers that increase penetration of agents via true structural modification of the stratum corneum are likely skin irritants (at least at high concentrations or with prolonged contact times) and are unlikely to produce a readily or wholly reversible penetration enhancement. Those enhancers that do produce a quickly reversible change in the skin barrier are likely to have achieved it through maximizing the thermodynamic activity of the formulation. It is not, of course, impossible that true penetration enhancement may be reversible. Permeability changes may be partly or wholly reversed upon removal of the enhancer from the tissue, due to possible renaturation of solvent-denatured keratin, recrystallization of fluidized lipids, removal of "defect" sites in the interfacial bilayer [40], etc. Reversibility may then be dependent on the type of binding, if any, between the altered stratum corneum constituents and the enhancer. It will also depend on possible removal of the enhancer by degradation, enzymatic activity, or applied solvent flux.

V. ENHANCER REVERSIBILITY

A. Dimethyl Sulfoxide

Dimethyl sulfoxide (DMSO) is one of the more extensively studied penetration enhancers. Early studies by Kligman [41,42] indicated that DMSO increases permeability but does not produce irreversible damage to the stratum corneum. Twice-daily unoccluded exposure produced only a mild dermatitis in some patients. Further, Kligman found that the skin became tolerant to this irritant effect upon continuous exposure to DMSO. Later, other authors disagreed with these results. Sweeney et al. [43] found that the increased water loss caused by application of concentrated (60–100%) aqueous solutions of DMSO was permanent in vitro. After in vivo application of pure DMSO for 30 min, Baker [44] observed an 8–17-fold increase in water loss 90 min postexposure. This effect was reduced to a three- to fourfold increase 6.5 hr post-treatment, but the barrier did not return to normal within the 24-hr experimentation period. Baker observed a milder effect and more complete reversal with both dimethylformamide (DMF) and dimethylacetamide (DMA) application.

Another group of researchers monitored the penetration enhancement due to 80% DMSO treatment in vitro on guinea pig skin [45]. Subsequent washout of the DMSO-modified tissue with buffer led them to conclude that the DMSO caused an irreversible modification within the stratum corneum. A later study, also with DMSO but on human skin, found the increased permeability partially reversible following complete extraction with water [46]. As illustrated in Figure 3, Kurihara [47] reported a similar result, with partial (one-third) reversal of DMSO-induced permeability enhancement following 48 hr of resolvation of the tissue with saline solution. Further resolvation did not have any greater effect. These studies strongly support the conclusion that DMSO causes a certain degree of irreversible biological damage to the stratum corneum as well as a more reversible physicochemical damage to the barrier that may be rescinded by removing the enhancer. A histopathologic study of nude mouse skin treated with 100% DMSO under occlusion found evidence of severe irritation including hyperkeratosis, marked acanthosis, disorganization of the prickle cell layer, intraepidermal vasiculation, and severe cell infiltration throughout the dermis and

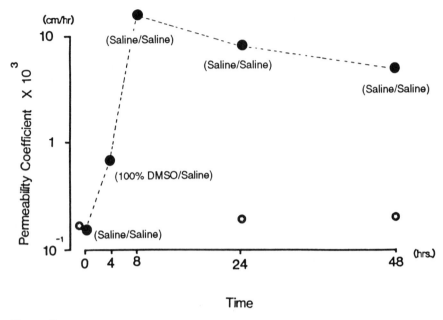

Figure 3

into the epidermis [48]. Therefore, DMSO's effects may be somewhat modified by removal of DMSO from the stratum corneum, but complete reversal must wait for actual regeneration of the barrier by the underlying epidermis.

B. Azone

Azone is another relatively well studied penetration enhancer. Studies have shown dose-dependent enhancing (mechanistic) effects and that Azone's penetration-enhancing effect is dependent on the amount of it present in the skin [49,50]. Treatment of skin with Azone followed by repeated doses of drug clearly showed that the increased permeability remained for several days [51]. However, this in vitro effect may not be seen in vivo. It has been demonstrated that Azone-induced skin penetration enhancement is not readily reversible and that pretreatment (vs. concurrent treatment) of the skin with Azone promotes skin penetration of drug but eliminates the lag time [51–54]. It is unclear whether this is due to simple retention of Azone (and therefore its effects) within the skin or to permanent damage to the skin lipids and keratins. A histopathologic study of nude mouse skin treated for 24 hr with 10% Azone under occlusion rated the Azone-treated skin as unacceptably irritated, with crusting of the stratum corneum and extensive cell infiltration in the upper dermis [48]. An enhancer such as Azone that produces alteration of the keratin structure and is a known irritant to mouse skin is an unlikely candidate as a readily reversible penetration enhancer in humans. The increased skin penetrability seen in several studies over an extended period of time indicates that it is likely that Azone causes biological changes in the stratum corneum that are reversible only upon replacement of the damaged stratum corneum from below.

C. Surfactants

Many different surfactants have been suggested as skin penetration enhancers; however, only a few have been studied for the reversibility of their effects. Decylmethyl sulfoxide (DCMS) has been shown to produce an initial high flux of 5-Fu that is reversible as the DCMS is washed out of the skin [55]. Another study also found a great initial enhancement effect that was rapidly reversible [53]. A pretreatment study of hexamethylene lauramide and its homologues found that the longer the period since application of these enhancers, the smaller the flux of subsequently applied hydrocortisone [56]. These effects were seen in vivo but not in vitro. The authors concluded that it takes the enhancers longer to penetrate dead skin and therefore they remain active longer in dead skin than in living skin. This is one possible explanation, but it might also be true that actively metabolizing skin repairs itself within the given time period or is capable of removing the enhancer through some enzymatic or other neutralizing pathway. Whatever the explanation, it is likely that this agent also effects a quite readily reversible enhancement of skin penetration.

There have been a couple of very interesting studies on the effects of surfactants and bile salts as nasal membrane penetration enhancers. These studies are especially interesting because they have been performed on living animals, and it is quite likely that the response and recovery of living tissue is different from what one would expect to see from excised tissue. Hirai et al. [57] studied the effects of several surfactants and bile salts on the nasal absorption of insulin and monitored the recovery from the ''hyperabsorptive'' state. In spite of nearly the same absorption-promoting effects, the recovery was significantly faster (4 hr) for membrane treated with the bile salt sodium glycocholate than for the surfactant polyoxylethylene 9-lauryl ether (8 hr). A microscopic study of the tissue showed complete recovery of the bile-salt-treated tissue by 24 hr whereas the observed damage was much greater and recovery not complete by 24 hr in the surfactant-treated tissue. A subchronic study in which doses were administered three times a day for one month showed no change in the morphology of the bile-salt-treated tissue, whereas the surfactant-treated tissue showed slight morphological changes. Tengamnuay and Mitra [58] studied the effect of bile salt–fatty acid mixed micelles on the nasal absorption of peptides. They observed increased membrane permeability with the micelles. After removal of the micelles and flushing of the nasal cavity with normal saline solution for 20 min followed by reperfusion with the peptide, the membrane returned to its original impermeable state within 20–40 min.

There has been very little direct investigation of the reversibility of skin penetration enhancers. Much of what is assumed is simply inferred from a knowledge of the mechanism of action of the enhancer or its other effects on the skin. For instance, it is often assumed that a compound's ability to enhance the skin penetration of a drug may be related to its ability to irritate the skin, which may also be related to its reversibility or the ability of the skin to recover from the effects of the enhancer. However, a 1989 study [59] showed that there was a poor correlation between the effectiveness of fatty acid isomers at enhancing naloxone flux and their irritation indices. The mechanism by which a given enhancer might irritate the skin may be different from the mechanism by which it aids penetration of a drug, or it may be the same. Some other general assumptions (and possible traps) that may mislead an investigator in determining the reversibility of a given enhancer include the effects of the enhancer on the histology of the skin, whether the enhancer is washable/rinsable from the skin, and whether it is a specific or nonspecific enhancer. It is sometimes assumed that an enhancer that is specific for a particular drug or class of drugs works by a vehicular or solvent effect and should therefore be readily reversible. With some enhancers it is also possible that reversibility may be concentration-dependent. This has been suggested as a possibility with Azone; it is thought that the mechanism of action of Azone is compounded by a protein-denaturing effect at high concentrations.

It is extremely important to note that most of the work done with enhancers is performed on excised or ''dead'' skin. Although the stratum corneum presents the major barrier to drug penetration and the stratum corneum is also ''dead,'' it is possible that the reversibility of some enhancers may very well be dependent on the animal being intact. The enzymes present in the epidermis or stratum corneum may be washed out, diluted, or inactivated by the diffusion cell apparatus. Some studies have proposed ''biodegradable'' enhancers and are therefore dependent upon intact enzymes [60,61]. ''Reversibility'' based on washout of the enhancer with large buffer or saline fluxes through fully hydrated tissue may not turn out to be real or obtainable in situ. All of the above are possible complicating factors and should be kept in mind when evaluating the reversibility of skin penetration enhancement. In the final analysis, all penetration enhancers, as long as they are not directly toxic to the basal stem cells, should be reversible within the turnover time of the tissue due to the dynamics of stratum corneum replacement and the ability of the skin to repair itself.

REFERENCES

1. S. C. G. Tseng, M. J. Jarvinen, W. G. Nelson, J. W. Huang, J. Woodcock-Mitchel, and T. T. Sun, *Cell 30*, 361 (1982).
2. P. M. Elias, *J. Invest. Dermatol. 80*, 44 (1983).
3. R. K. Freinkel and T. N. Traczyk, *J. Invest. Dermatol. 80*, 441 (1983).
4. J. D. Lonsdale-Eccles, J. A. Haugen, and B. A. Dale, *J. Biol. Chem. 255*, 2235 (1980).
5. B. A. Dale, K. A. Holbrook, and P. M. Steinert, *Nature 276*, 729 (1978).
6. P. M. Elias, E. R. Cooper, A. Korc, and B. E. Brown, *J. Invest. Dermatol. 76*, 297 (1981).
7. N. J. Lowe and R. B. Stoughton, *Brit. J. Dermatol. 96*, 155 (1977).
8. N. J. Lowe, *Brit. J. Dermatol. 97*, 39 (1977).
9. A. E. Solomon and N. J. Lowe, *J. Arch. Dermatol. 114*, 1029 (1978).
10. S. T. R. Han, M. Haberkamp, and G. L. Flynn, *J. Toxicol.-Cut. Ocular Toxicol. 8*, 539 (1990).
11. C. S. Potten, *J. Invest. Dermatol. 65*, 488 (1975).
12. S. Bertsch, K. Csotas, J. Schweizer, and F. Marks, *Cell Tissue Kinet. 9*, 445 (1976).
13. Y. Mishima and H. Pinkus, *J. Invest. Dermatol. 50*, 89 (1968).
14. C. S. Potten, *J. Cell. Sci. 17*, 413 (1975).
15. H. Hennings and K. Elgio, *Cell Tissue Kinet. 3*, 243 (1970).
16. E. Christophers and O. Braun-Falco, *Br. J. Dermatol. 82*, 268 (1970).
17. O. P. F. Clausen and T. Lindmo, *Cell Tissue Kinet. 9*, 573 (1976).
18. R. L. Bronaugh and R. F. Stewart, *J. Pharm Sci. 74*, 1062 (1985).
19. G. L. Flynn, H. Durrheim, and W. I. Higughi, *J. Pharm. Sci. 70*, 52 (1980).
20. A. G. Matoltsy, A. Schragger, and M. N. Matoltsy, *J. Invest. Dermatol. 38*, 251 (1962).
21. T. Frodin and M. Skogh, *Acta Derm. Venereol. (Stockh.) 64*, 537 (1984).
22. D. Spruit and K. E. Malten, *J. Invest. Dermatol. 45*, 6 (1965).
23. S. K. Govil, Selected studies on the barrier properties of skin, Doctoral Dissertation, Univ. Michigan, 1984.
24. S. T. R. Han, Relationship of epidermal turnover kinetics to qualities of the skin barrier: novel approach to assessment of cutaneous injury, Doctoral Dissertation, Univ. Michigan, 1988.
25. M. B. Haberkamp, The effect of physical and chemical injuries on transepidermal water loss and turnover time of hairless mouse skin, Doctoral Dissertation, Univ. Michigan, 1989.
26. S. P. Harrold, *J. Invest. Dermatol. 32*, 581 (1959).
27. E. J. Van Scott and J. B. Lyon, *J. Invest. Dermatol. 21*, 199 (1963).
28. P. M. Elias, *Arch. Dermatol. Res. 270*, 95 (1981).
29. J. H. Hassing, J. P. Nater, and E. Bleumink, *Dermatologica 164*, 314 (1982).
30. P. G. M. Van Der Valk, J. P. Nater and E. Bleumink, *J. Invest. Dermatol. 82*, 291 (1984).
31. C. Prottey, P. J. Hartop, J. G. Black, and J. I. McCormack, *J. Invest. Dermatol. 94*, 13 (1976).
32. A. W. Fulmer and G. J. Kramer, *J. Invest. Dermatol. 86*, 598 (1986).

33. G. Imokawa and Y. Mishima, *ContactDerm. 5*, 357 (1979).
34. G. Imokawa, *J. Soc. Cosmet. Chem. 31*, 45 (1980).
35. G. Imokawa and Y. Mishima, *ContactDerm. 7*, 65 (1981).
36. P. W. A. Tovell, A. C. Weaver, J. Hope, and W. E. Sprott, *B. J. Dermatol. 90*, 501 (1974).
37. G. D. Weinstein and E. J. Van Scott, *J. Invest. Dermatol. 45*, 257 (1965).
38. K. Elgjo and O. P. F. Clausen, *Cell Tissue Kinet. 16*, 343 (1983).
39. K. Elgjo, *Eu. J. Cancer 3*, 519 (1968).
40. M. L. Francoeur, G. M. Golden and R. O. Potts, *Pharm. Res. 7*, 621 (1990).
41. A. M. Kligman, *J. Am. Med. Assoc. 193*, 796 (1965).
42. A. M. Kligman, *J. Am. Med. Assoc. 193*, 923 (1965).
43. T. M. Sweeney, A. M. Downes and A. G. Matoltsy, *J. Invest. Dermatol. 46*, 300 (1966).
44. H. Baker, *J. Invest. Dermatol. 50*, 283 (1968).
45. S. G. Elfbaum and K. Laden, *J. Soc. Cosmet. Chem. 19*, 841 (1968).
46. S. K. Chandrasekaran, P. S. Campbell, and A. S. Michaels, *Am. Inst. Chem. Eng. 23*, 810 (1977).
47. T. Kurihara, Physicochemical study of the accelerant effects of DMSO on percutaneous absorption of an antiviral drug and other chemical prototypes, Doctoral Dissertation, Univ. Michigan, 1983.
48. U. T. Lashmar, J. Hadgraft, and N. Thomas, *J. Pharm. Pharmacol. 41*, 118 (1989).
49. W. J. Lambert, W. I. Higuchi, K. Knutson, and S. L. Krill, *Pharm. Res. 6*, 798 (1989).
50. Y. Morimoto, K. Sugibayashi, K. Hosoya, and W. I. Higuchi, *Int. J. Pharm. 32*, 31 (1986).
51. P. K. Wotton, B. Mollgaard, J. Hadgraft, and A. Hoelgaard, *Int. J. Pharm. 24*, 19 (1985).
52. B. W. Barry and S. L. Bennett, *J. Pharm. Pharmacol. 39*, 535 (1987).
53. M. Goodman and B. W. Barry, *J. Invest. Dermatol. 91*, 323 (1988).
54. H. Okamoto, M. Ohyabu, M. Hashid, and H. Sezaki, *J. Pharm. Pharmacol. 39*, 531 (1987).
55. E. R. Cooper, in *Solution Behavior of Surfactants: Theoretical and Applied Aspects,* Vol. 12, K. L. Mittel and E. J. Fendler, Eds., Plenum, New York, 1982, p. 1505.
56. D. Mirejovsky and H. Takruri, *J. Pharm. Sci. 75*, 1089 (1986).
57. S. Hirai, T. Yashiki, and H. Mima, *Int. J. Pharm. 9*, 173 (1981).
58. P. Tengamnuay and A. K. Mitra, *Pharm. Res. 7*, 127 (1990).
59. B. J. Aungst, *Pharm. Res. 6*, 244 (1989).
60. O. Wong, J. Huntington, R. Konishi, J. H. Rytting, and T. Higuchi, *J. Pharm. Sci. 77*, 967 (1988).
61. O. Wong, J. Huntington, T. Nishihata, and J. H. Rytting, *Pharm. Res. 6*, 286 (1989).

5

Visualization of Drug Transport Across Human Skin and the Influence of Penetration Enhancers

H. E. Junginger, H. E. Boddé, and F. H. N. de Haan
Center for Bio-Pharmaceutical Sciences,
Leiden University, Leiden,
The Netherlands

I. INTRODUCTION

In the design and development of novel drug delivery systems, increasing attention has to be paid to their interactions with the membranes they will be applied to. This holds especially for drug delivery systems for the dermal and transdermal routes of application. The exact knowledge of skin structure is an important prerequisite to the development of strategies to induce changes in the skin barrier (horny layer) and to exploit these possibilities for improved drug permeation by means of (trans)dermal drug delivery systems to optimize drug therapy.

Figure 1 shows a cross section of the skin, the four layers of which are the stratum corneum (horny layer), the viable epidermis, the dermis, and the subcutaneous fat. In principle, five routes of drug penetration can be differentiated:

1. The transeccrine route
2. The transsebaceous route
3. The transfollicular route
4. The intercellular route
5. The transcellular route

The fractional areas of these routes are quite different [1,2], being about 99% for the transepidermal route (intercellular and transcellular routes combined), about 1% for the transfollicular and transsebaceous routes, and less than 0.1%

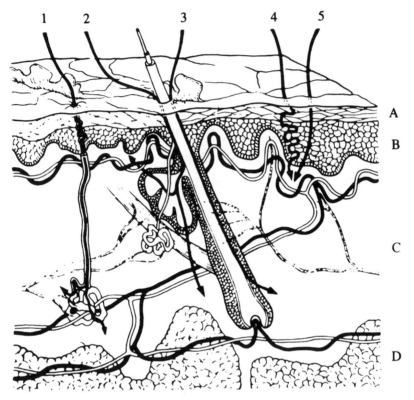

Figure 1 Cross section through skin. A, stratum corneum; B, viable epidermis; C, dermis; D, subcutaneous fat. *1*, transeccrine route; *2*, transsebaceous route; *3*, transfollicular route; *4*, intercellular route; and *5*, transcellular route. (According to [16].)

for the transeccrine route. The fractional area of the last route is sufficiently small to discount transeccrine diffusion contributions in the general treatment. Also, the routes along the skin appendages (shunt routes: transsebaceous and transfollicular routes) may contribute only slightly to the long-term overall drug penetration but may contribute significantly to the short-term penetration of a suitable drug into the skin. It is assumed that transepidermal diffusion pathways are the most prominent penetration routes of transdermally applied drugs.

Many investigators have contributed to a better understanding of the structure and function of the skin [1–16]. Today the stratum corneum is recognized to be the predominant diffusional barrier for transdermal drug delivery. It is built up of stacked layers of horny cells (corneocytes), which are composed mainly of various types of keratins. The corneocytes are embedded in an intercellular

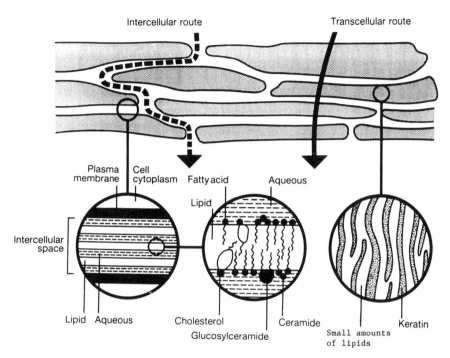

Figure 2 Diagram of possible permeation routes through the stratum corneum, together with idealized representation of intracellular keratin and intercellular bilayer lipids; not to scale. Note that the presence of significant amounts of intracellular lipid is now questionable and that the intercellular domain is probably of greater value than was once thought. (According to Elias [3] and Barry [10].)

matrix (Fig. 2). The intercellular matrix is built up of lipid bilayers that consist above all of free fatty acids, cholesterol, and ceramides. Due to this lipid bilayer structure, lipophilic and hydrophilic domains can be differentiated within the intercellular matrix as possible pathways for drug diffusion.

Skin penetration enhancers, being compounds that increase drug transport across the skin, usually interact with components of the stratum corneum [5, 10–16]. They are thought to disturb the structure of the lipid bilayers by increasing their fluidity and/or by hydration of their polar head groups. In addition, hydration of the corneocytes may occur. Although many speculations have been made [17–24], the pathways of drug diffusion across the stratum corneum (intercellular, transcellular) and the modes of action of the different types of skin penetration enhancers still have to be elucidated and clarified for many cases. For that purpose, visualization of drug transport across the stratum corneum seems to be a logical and straightforward approach to gaining answers to the following questions:

1. Which transport routes (e.g., inter- or intracellular) across the stratum corneum are followed by hydrophilic, amphiphilic, and lipophilic compounds?
2. Where are the penetration barriers located in the stratum corneum?

Having answered these questions, we can try to alter the barriers by hydrating the stratum corneum (e.g., by occlusion) and/or by using penetration enhancers or drug solvents and determining their effects on the transport routes.

Combining these results with results obtained with other sophisticated techniques will lead to a rational design of effective skin penetration enhancers, which can be incorporated in novel drug carrier systems such as microemulsions, liposomes, and niosomes either to achieve high flux rates across the stratum corneum or to create drug depots inside the stratum corneum.

In the following sections, sample preparation and visualization methods on an ultrastructural level developed at the Department of Pharmaceutical Technology of the Center for Bio-Pharmaceutical Sciences are described, and future perspectives about improvement and alternative methods are presented.

II. VISUALIZATION OF NORMAL AND ENHANCED HgCl₂ TRANSPORT THROUGH HUMAN SKIN IN VITRO*

One of the most direct ways to study the route of skin penetration is the microscopic technique with which skin structures can be visualized and, given the proper marker, the diffusible compound (the drug) can be visualized and localized inside that structure. Various attempts have been made to accomplish this, using light microscopy in combination with autoradiography [26], metachromatic staining [27,28], and fluorimetry [29]. Furthermore, electron microprobe analysis has been used to visualize transepithelial sodium transport [30] at the ultrastructural level. The skin penetration of nickel and chromate ions has been studied by Malmqvist et al. [31] using proton-induced X-ray emission (PIXE). They determined transepidermal gradients of Ni^{2+} and Cr^{2+} with about 30-μm intervals between measurements. A simple technique used by some authors to visualize transport of diffusible compounds through skin is the so-called in situ precipitation [32–35].

This study was aimed at visualizing routes of penetration through human skin, using mercuric chloride as a marker and applying transmission electron microscopy. A further aim was the elucidation of the modes of action of some

*From Ref. 25.

penetration enhancers, including Azone and some newly synthesized derivatives thereof.

A. Materials and Methods

1. Skin

Fresh human mamma skin, obtained from mamma operations, was kept overnight on a moist gauze at 4°C. On the second day, the skin was dermatomed to 110 ± 20 μm using an electrodermatome (Padgett). The dermatomed skin samples were cut in circular pieces (18 mm in diameter) and used for diffusion experiments on the same day.

2. Pretreatments

In some cases, before starting a diffusion experiment, the skin was pretreated with one of the following compounds: dimethyl sulfoxide (DMSO), propylene glycol (PG), 1-hexyl-aza-cycloheptane-2-one (hexyl Azone), 1-dodecyl-aza-cycloheptane-2-one (dodecyl Azone), 1-hexadecyl-aza-cycloheptane-2-one (hexadecyl Azone). DMSO and PG were used neat, the azones were applied in a 10% (v/v) solution in PG. Twenty-four hours before starting a diffusion experiment, the skin samples were placed on petri dishes (stratum corneum side up, dermis side down), and the enhancer solution was cast on top of the skin (about 200 μL/cm^2) and left without occlusion; the treated skin samples were then allowed to stand for 24 hr at 4°C (except in the case of DMSO, where the samples were kept at room temperature to prevent crystal formation).

PBS-treated samples were used as controls.

3. Diffusion Experiments

The pretreated skin samples were clamped inside a two-compartment diffusion cell (made of polycarbonate), using dialysis membranes (cutoff at 5000 D) on both sides of the skin for support. The donor chamber (facing the stratum corneum) was filled with 1.5 mL of a 5% (w/v) solution of mercuric chloride (HgCl$_2$) in PBS, pH 7.4. The acceptor chamber contained PBS, pH 7.4. Both chambers were closed. The diffusion experiments were carried out at 33°C. After 1/4, 3/4, 1, 2, 10, and 48 hr the skin samples were rinsed with PBS for 15 sec, wiped dry with a tissue, and divided into 3-mm-diameter samples for electron microscopy. In some cases skin samples were completely immersed in a donor solution (containing 5% HgCl$_2$ in PBS at pH 7.4) and analyzed after 1/2 and 1 hr. Furthermore, a number of 10-hr diffusion experiments were done with the dermis facing the donor chamber, in order to study the influence of the direction of transport.

4. Electron Microscopy

All samples were exposed to the vapor of a 25% ammonium sulfide solution to provoke the precipitation of mercuric sulfide (HgS) and thus obtain fixation and visualization of the mercury, rinsed twice for 5 min in a 0.1 M cacodylate buffer (pH 7.4) at 4°C, and fixed for 7 hr in a 1.5% glutaraldehyde solution in 0.1 M cacodylate buffer (pH 7.4) at 4°C. After two 5-min rinses with cacodylate buffer, the tissue was fixed for about 10 hr in a 1.0% osmium tetroxide/2.1% potassium hexacyanoferrate(II) solution in 0.1 M cacodylate buffer at 4°C. After two more 5-min rinses with 0.1 M cacodylate buffer, dehydration was carried out using an alcohol gradient of 30–50–70–80–90–100% (two times 5 min for each step up to 90%; two times 15 min for the 100%). Subsequently the tissue was impregnated for 30 min with propylene oxide at room temperature, then impregnated with a 50/50 propylene oxide/Epon 812 (DDSA:MNA ratio of 3:7.5) using DMP-30 as a hardener for 30 min, and finally impregnated with pure Epon 812 (DDSA:MNA ratio of 1:2.5) for 3.5 hr. Care was taken to orient the skin samples flat and horizontally in the embedding material. After 4 days of hardening at 60°C, the samples were cut on an LKB microtome using a diamond knife (Diatome); 70-nm (yellow-gray) sections were collected on collodion-coated copper grids (100 mesh) and examined in a Philips EM 201 electron microscope operated at 80 kV. Additional staining agents were not used.

5. Validation of the In Situ Precipitation Method

To verify the quality of fixation with the in situ precipitation method, a number of control experiments were carried out. First, PBS-treated specimens were subjected to a diffusion experiment (40 hr), then washed for 20 hr with PBS, then treated with ammonium sulfide, etc. (''washed *before* precipitation''). A second series of PBS-treated specimens received a PBS wash *after* completion of the ammonium sulfide treatment (''washed *after* precipitation''). To verify the accuracy of localization obtained with the method, some specimens were deliberately overexposed to the electron beam in the electron microscope, so as to allow sublimation of the mercuric sulfide to determine whether the precipitates were on top of or inside the section. Furthermore, the presence of mercury in the precipitates was verified by the use of x-ray microanalytical spot analysis. Measurements were performed with a Tracor TN 1310 energy-dispersive x-ray microanalyzer attached to a Philips EM 400 electron microscope. The specimens were placed in a low-background beryllium holder at an angle of 18° relative to the electron beam. Measurements were done during 200 sec lifetime with a spot size of 100 nm and an accelerating voltage of 80 kV.

B. Results

The x-ray emission spectrum was taken at the site of a precipitate in a randomly chosen section and shows intense emission lines at 2241, 9968, and 11,847 eV, corresponding to the M_α, L_α, and L_β lines of mercury. The osmium M_α emission line at 1890 eV, however, is rather small relative to the mercury line. This result goes to prove that the precipitates consist predominantly of a mercuric compound, with potentially only traces of osmium in it.

Washing experiments show that washing *before* in situ precipitation removed most of the mercury with the exception of some intracellular material. However, washing *after* the precipitation did not have any significant effect on the distribution of mercury in the stratum corneum and epidermis as compared to an unwashed control. When the specimens were overexposed to the electron beam and the mercuric sulfide was sublimated, all previously opaque sites (precipitates) became completely transparent, while the immediately surrounding tissue retained its electron density. This result shows that the precipitates were all *embedded inside* the section, which virtually excludes any delocalization of precipitates due to the cutting procedure.

1. PBS-Treated Controls

The 1/4-hr micrograph (Fig. 3) clearly shows that initially the intercellular route predominates. The compound first enters the skin along interdigitations between apical corneocytes, and it seems to be impeded in its diffusion in regions further away from these interdigitations.

After 1 hr (Fig. 4a), apical corneocytes have taken up mercury; however, lower down, the marker is more abundant in intercellular space and/or bound to corneocyte membranes. After 10 hr (Fig. 4b), the bimodal distribution of mercury in the stratum corneum becomes more pronounced. There is appreciable accumulation of homogeneously distributed mercury in apical corneocytes; directly underneath there is a zone where the mercury is present only patchwise in some cells, and further down in the stratum corneum the mercury is abundant *between* the cells and along the cell membranes. After 10 hr of diffusion in the reverse direction (Fig. 4c), there is an almost "reverse" image: predominant uptake of mercury by granulocytes and proximal corneocytes, further "upwards" an intermediate zone showing intercellular abundance, and finally an apical zone with some intracellular uptake.

Immersion for 1 hr, interestingly, shows a similar distribution of mercury: intracellular uptake in apical corneocytes, proximal corneocytes, and granulocytes and intercellular presence in between. Further downward in the spinous layer, mercury has accumulated chiefly along cell membranes and (to a lesser extent) in nuclear envelopes. In fact, the characteristic undulations of the spinous cell membranes are beautifully visualized due to the mercury "staining."

2. Effect of DMSO

After a DMSO treatment there is (after 1 hr diffusion, Fig. 5) a significant increase in the progression of the diffusion front with respect to the PBS-treated control. In fact, the mercury has already reached the stratum spinosum, and there seems to be an increase in both the intracellular mercury content in apical cor-

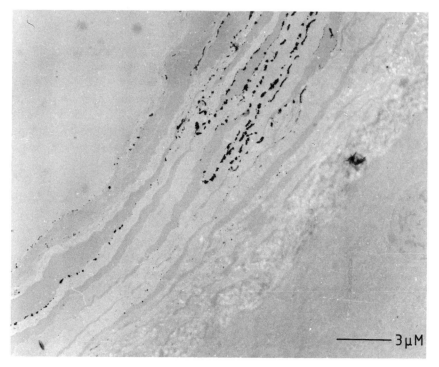

Figure 3 Distribution of mercury in the stratum corneum after 1/4 hr of diffusion of mercuric chloride, showing the intercellular route of penetration (right-hand side). Where interdigitations are absent, there is poor penetration through the stratum corneum (left-hand side).

neocytes and the intercellular mercury concentration between medial and proximal corneocytes. The overall pattern very much resembles the controls obtained after 10 hr of diffusion (compare with Fig. 4b).

3. Effect of Propylene Glycol

The propylene glycol case does not differ significantly from the control, either qualitatively or quantitatively (Fig. 6).

4. Effect of Propylene Glycol–Azone Mixtures

The effect of hexyl Azone (not shown) is similar to that of DMSO in the stratum corneum, in that both the intracellular accumulation of mercury in apical corneocytes and its intercellular presence between medial and proximal corneocytes are enhanced with respect to the control. However, mercury has substantially penetrated into the viable epidermis (unlike the control) and has also penetrated

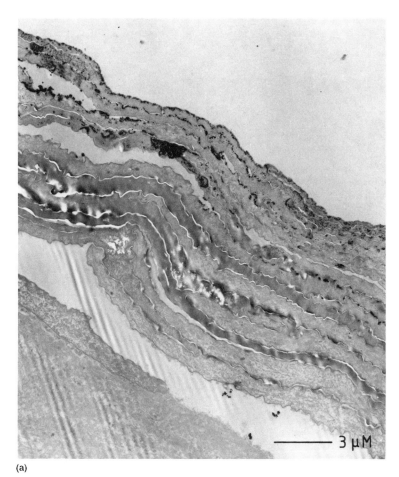

(a)

Figure 4 (a) Diffusion for 1 hr results in mercury uptake in apical corneocytes. (b) Bimodal distribution of mercury after 10 hr of diffusion. Apically, most of the mercury is present in the corneocytes; medially and proximally, the mercury predominates between the cells. (c) Reverse diffusion for 10 hr yields intracellular uptake in proximal and apical corneocytes and intercellular predominance of mercury between medial cells.

heavily into the viable cells and is present inside the cytoplasm (unlike the control or PG- and DMSO-treated specimens).

Hexadecyl Azone qualitatively shows a pattern similar to that of the control: accumulation inside apical corneocytes and predominance of mercury between medial and proximal corneocytes. Dodecyl Azone acts differently from the others (Fig. 7). Whereas in all other cases there was always incorporation of

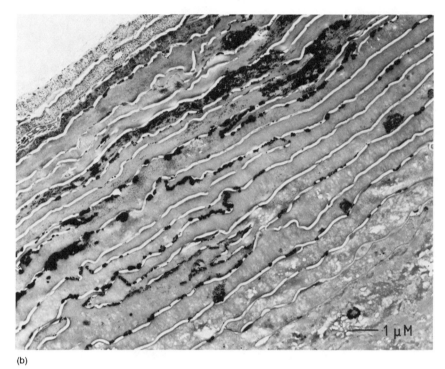

(b)

Figure 4 Continued

mercury into apical corneocytes, here we have an enhanced intercellular presence of mercury throughout the stratum corneum. Massive intercellular precipitates are visible both apically and proximally in the stratum corneum.

C. Discussion

A striking observation in most cases is the bimodal distribution of mercury within the stratum corneum: intracellular accumulation in apical corneocytes and intercellular presence lower down. With longer diffusion or immersion times there is also uptake into proximal corneocytes. Since this phenomenon occurs in various different cases, we suggest that it is related to a difference in the properties of the cells and/or their membranes. Apical and (especially after long diffusion times) proximal corneocytes apparently take up the model compound more easily than medial ones, either because they provide more free binding sites for the mercuric ion (possibly sulfhydryl groups) or because their cell membranes are more permeable to Hg^{2+}. This bimodality may well be associated with the distinction Bowser and White [7] made between the stratum disjunction

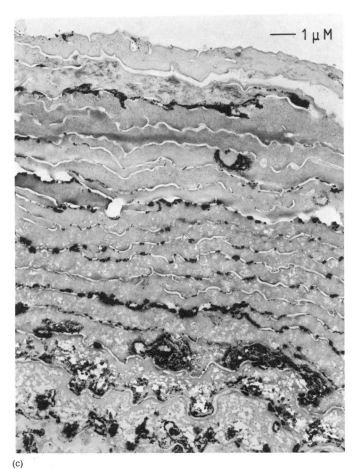

(c)

Figure 4 Continued

and the stratum compactum; in fact, on account of their lipid analyses and water vapor transport measurements, they suggested that the stratum disjunctum (the apical stratum corneum) would have a reservoir function associated with material uptake in cells, and the stratum compactum (the inner stratum corneum) would have a barrier function associated with transport of material between the cells.

From our results we can almost ''reconstruct'' the diffusion pathway the model compound has chosen: first, intrusion through apical interdigitations, then slow uptake into apical corneocytes; subsequently, further diffusion through intercellular spaces down the stratum corneum, into the viable layers; given more

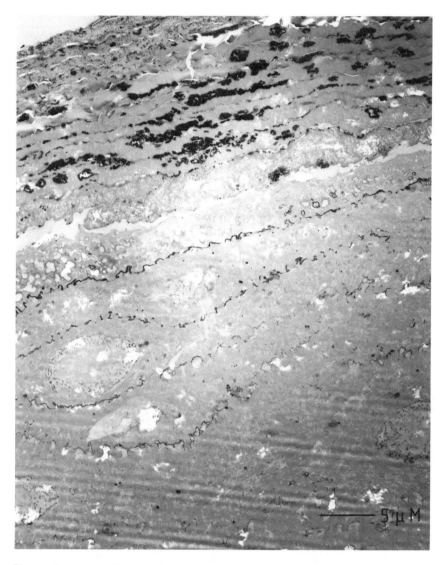

Figure 5 Result after DMSO pretreatment, showing increased mercury penetration, without affecting the bimodal distribution observed in unpretreated skin.

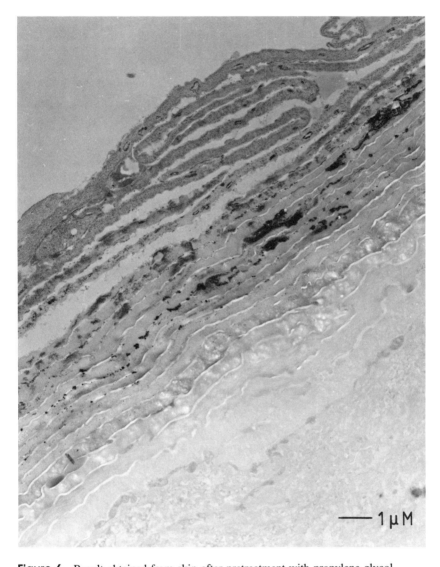

Figure 6 Result obtained from skin after pretreatment with propylene glycol.

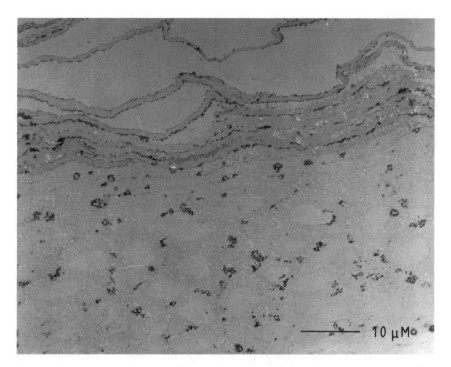

Figure 7 Result obtained from skin pretreated with dodecyl Azone showing enhanced intercellular transport across the entire section.

time, some uptake in the proximal corneocytes and eventually in the medial corneocytes. The effect of time is especially noticeable in the "washing" experiments: After long-term washing, which extends the diffusion time, most of the intercellular material has gone, showing once again the predominance of intercellular channels as transport routes. The relatively small amounts of mercury already present in the cells is retained and possibly increased by additional uptake during 20 hr of washing, confirming the presence of strong binding sites inside the cells.

The fact that a hydrophilic compound permeates through lipid-rich spaces seems peculiar at first. However, it should be borne in mind that the intercellular lipids have a lamellar structure in which lipophilic bilayers and hydrophilic layers alternate [4]. It may well be that $HgCl_2$, and probably any other small hydrophilic compound, chooses the interlamellar hydrophilic channels (see Fig. 2). This would imply that the intercellular pathway is *bicontinuous*, consisting of both lipophilic and hydrophilic routes, the choice depending on the lipophilicity of the drug. The existence of two continuous diffusion pathways between the corneocytes (one polar and one nonpolar) has also been assumed by Barry [5,10,13,36] in addressing the possible effects of penetration enhancers in the intercellular space.

Insofar as mercuric chloride has penetrated into the viable epidermis, it shows a strong tendency to accumulate at the cell membranes. This tendency is possibly due to complexation of the mercuric ion with the phosphate groups of the phospholipids. A remarkable result from these studies is that DMSO, although enhancing the overall penetration, does not change the distribution pattern qualitatively.

Another interesting observation is the enhanced intercellular presence of mercury after treatment with dodecyl Azone. This may be explained as follows: given the fact that both azones have a strong influence on the intercellular lipid fluidity and structure [10,15,36,37], it is assumed that Azone has a strong affinity for the lipid bilayers and enters these bilayers with its hydrocarbon tail, while allowing (part of) its hydrophilic head group to stick into the hydrophilic layer. After a PG/Azone pretreatment, this interlamellar hydrophilic layer most likely consists of a propylene glycol–water mixture. The increased fluidity of the lipid bilayer may also enhance the mobility of the hydrated lipid head groups and thereby increase the diffusivity of the hydrophilic interlamellar layers.

To explain the synergistic effect of PG and dodecyl Azone, Cooper [38] and Barry [10,36] proposed that (1) PG may solubilize dodecyl Azone in the aqueous intercellular regions; and (2) Azone may enhance the PG flux. The present data are in line with that view.

At first sight, it may seem remarkable that a hydrophilic compound such as mercuric chloride can be enhanced in its permeation through the stratum corneum by a lipid fluidizer such as dodecyl Azone. However, it should be kept in mind that the intercellular lipids serve as a *barrier*, first and foremost to prevent water loss and also to keep toxic agents out. Hence it follows that the hydrophilic pathways, which according to the literature and the data presented here may well be the intercellular interlamellar water channels, are not entirely continuous but occasionally may form "blind alleys," possibly near interdigitations where the lipid lamellae are most likely folded around the corneocyte edges [4]. In fact, careful examination of Figure 3 shows that the initial diffusion behavior of the $HgCl_2$ at interdigitations is such that the marker tends to bend around the edges of *one* of the adjacent cells rather than spread out in all directions available at that site. This observation supports the likelihood of the aforementioned blind alleys near corneocyte edges. These may well be the sites where lipid bilayer perturbation would strongly enhance the flux of a polar compound by allowing it to "jump" from one hydrophilic channel to another across the lipid bilayer.

III. CRYOTECHNIQUES, VAPOR FIXATION, AND AUTORADIOGRAPHY AS GENERALLY APPLICABLE TOOLS TO VISUALIZE DRUG TRANSPORT ACROSS HUMAN STRATUM CORNEUM*

Autoradiography seems to be a generally applicable technique to visualize drug transport across membranes because most of the diffusible compounds can be labeled with tritium in an appropriate manner. However, this type of research is usually hampered by difficulties encountered in localizing diffusible substances at the electron microscopic level. These problems are concerned mainly with dislocation and/or extraction of the drug during sample preparation.

In the very few papers on the topic of visualizing drug transport across the stratum corneum [e.g., 25,32,33,35,40], the problems regarding sample preparation are still not circumvented completely. The diffusible substances were localized by chemical precipitation, and in some of these studies x-ray microanalysis (transmission electron microscopy mode) was employed in conjunction with ultrastructural studies to determine the elemental composition of localized regions of the tissue. In this way Sharata and Burnette [35] obtained a spatial resolution of 0.5–0.75 μm. As already stated by these authors, localization of diffusible compounds by freezing techniques is preferable to chemical precipitation. Several studies [e.g., 41–43] employed "cryo" techniques in conjunction with x-ray microanalysis for localization of native electrolytes within the epidermis or for localization of topically applied ions. Although satisfactory results were obtained, most of these studies employed x-ray microanalysis in the scanning electron microscopy mode using thick specimens, which resulted in poor spatial resolution; for example, Grundin et al. [43] reported a spatial resolution of 10–12 μm.

However, x-ray microanalysis is applicable for only a small range of compounds. At the present stage of technical development, the method of choice for visualization of compounds diffusing across the stratum corneum is most likely electron microscopic autoradiography, since (almost) all drugs and penetration enhancers can be tritiated. The combination of cryo techniques (for excluding extraction during sample preparation) and autoradiography seems a rational approach.

At the light microscopic level, several reliable techniques for the autoradiographic localization of diffusible substances are available. In these techniques a photographic emulsion is brought into contact with a frozen hydrated or freeze-dried cryosection; for review, see Stumpf [44]. However, at the electron microscopic level (our aim) severe practical problems exist [45,46]. Although some

*From Ref. 39.

authors have described the analysis of such ultrathin sections by autoradiography [47–49], still the risk of rehydration (and consequently dislocation of diffusible compounds) is substantial (e.g., during transfer to the electron microscope, during application of a photographic emulsion, during transfer to the carbon coating equipment).

A promising method for avoiding dislocation and/or extraction during sample preparation for electron microscopic autoradiography can be derived from the work of Stirling and Kinter [50]. As starting material, these authors used rapidly frozen unfixed tissue (rings of hamster intestine), which was subsequently freeze-dried, fixed with osmium tetroxide vapor, and embedded in Epon. Frederik and Klepper [51] and Frederik et al. [52] used essentially the same technique for localizing tritiated steroids in testes at the electron microscopic level.

The aim of the research described in this section is to investigate whether the combination of electron microscopic autoradiography and "dry" sample preparation (rapid freezing, freeze-drying, osmium tetroxide vapor fixation, Epon embedment under vacuum) is suited for the localization of diffusible substances in the stratum corneum. Tritiated hydrocortisone is used as a model drug. Essential items to be considered are preservation of the ultrastructure of the stratum corneum, possible extraction/dislocation, and the detection limit.

A. Materials and Methods

1. Chemicals

Only distilled water was used. Sodium bromide used for separation of the epidermis from the dermis, alcohol, dimethyl sulfoxide, and all buffer salts were analytical grade. Freon 22 was purchased from Hoek Loos (Schiedam, The Netherlands). For tissue fixation, osmium tetroxide (Merck, Darmstadt, F.R.G.), glutaraldehyde (Taab, Aldermaston, U.K.), and potassium ferrocyanide (analytical grade) were used. The epoxy resin components necessary for Epon embedment were supplied as an LX-112 resin kit by Ladd Research Industries (Burlington, VT). Propylene oxide (99.6%) was obtained from Janssen (Beerse, Belgium). All chemicals used in the development and fixation of the autoradiographs and the post-staining reagents were analytical grade. Hydrocortisone (European Pharmacopoeia) was supplied by OPG (Utrecht, The Netherlands).

[1,2-^{3}H]Hydrocortisone with a specific activity of 51.9×10^3 Ci/mol was obtained from New England Nuclear Corporation (Boston, MA) in solution in ethanol 10% (v/v) and benzene 90% (v/v). Before use, the radiochemical purity was tested by thin-layer chromatography.

2. Conventional "Wet" Sample Preparation

Skin samples 2 mm in diameter were punched. Chemical fixation was performed in a 1.5% (w/v) glutaraldehyde solution in 0.1 M cacodylate buffer (pH 7.2) for 4 hr at 4°C. After rinsing these samples two times (5 min each) in 0.1 M cacodylate buffer (pH 7.2), postfixation was performed for 4 hr at 4°C in a 1% (w/v) osmium tetroxide solution in 0.1 M cacodylate buffer (pH 7.2) containing 0.05 M potassium ferrocyanide. After two more rinses in the buffer, dehydration was carried out in graded ethanol series at room temperature. Then the specimens were immersed in propylene oxide for 30 min, followed by immersion in a mixture of propylene oxide and nonaccelerated Epon (1:1 v/v) for 30 min. Further embedment was carried out with an Epon mixture according to standard procedures. Polymerization took place for 48 hr at 60°C.

3. "Dry" Sample Preparation

The method described by Frederik and Klepper [51] was slightly adapted in the following manner. Skin samples of 2 mm diameter were punched and then rapidly frozen by plunging into solid/liquid Freon 22. These samples were transferred under liquid nitrogen into a specially designed sample holder, which subsequently was mounted in a Balzers Freeze Etching system BAF 400 d (Balzers, Liechtenstein). The stage for the sample holder was thermostated at −80°C, and the lid of the sample holder was hung on a pin that was attached to the knife of the Balzers, which was kept at < −150°C and served as a cold trap. After evacuation of the Balzers and positioning of the cold knife just above the sample holder, the freeze-dry run was started. This run took 15 hr under the following conditions: sample temperature −80°C, cold trap temperature < −150°C, vacuum < 10^{-6} torr. Drying was completed by slowly increasing the sample temperature to 30°C. Finally the sample holder was covered with the lid by manipulation of the knife, and dry nitrogen was admitted to the chamber.

The sample holder containing the dry samples in vacuo was dismounted and transferred to a specially designed desiccator, where it was mounted again (see 6 in Fig. 8). The desiccator (see Fig. 8) was covered with a lid, and the working chamber was evacuated (with vacuum valve 2 opened and using a vacuum pump). By using a manipulator (5), the lid of the sample holder was lifted and removed. Osmium tetroxide vapor was admitted to the working chamber by opening a side port (7) between a chamber under a screw containing osmium tetroxide crystals (3) and the working chamber (4). Vapor fixation was carried out for 20 hr at room temperature. Fixation was terminated by pumping away the osmium tetroxide vapor, and the working chamber was evacuated again.

Using a syringe, nonaccelerated Epon was injected through a septum in the desiccator lid onto the samples in the sample holder. This vacuum impregnation took 4 hr. Subsequently the working chamber was flushed with dry air (vacuum valve 1 in Fig. 8 opened) and re-evacuated several times to improve impregnation. Further embedment and polymerization were carried out in the same way as described for the conventional sample preparation after the propylene oxide/ Epon immersion.

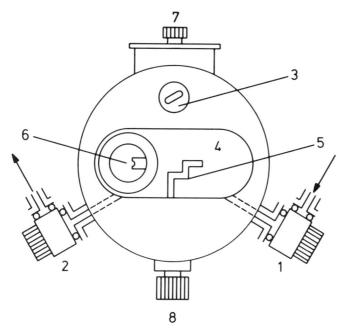

Figure 8 Desiccator for vapor fixation and embedment under vacuum (schematic diagram). *1, 2,* vacuum valves; *3,* osmium chamber under screw; *4,* working chamber; *5,* mechanism for lifting lid of sample holder; *6,* mounting place for sample holder; *7,* handle for controlling osmium inlet; *8,* handle for controlling lifting of sample holder lid.

4. Essential Backgrounds of the "Dry" Sample Preparation

Plunging small tissue blocks into solid/liquid Freon 22 causes vitrification of the samples over a range of about 10–20 μm [53], meaning that in this region water solidifies as an amorphous glass and the formation of ice crystals is avoided. During ice crystal formation, solutes are separated from ice, causing dislocation of all solutes including diffusing drugs. Ice crystal formation may also cause ultrastructural artifacts. During freeze-drying the sample temperature is maintained at −80°C; at higher temperatures the growth of ice crystals may obscure the results, whereas at lower temperatures the freeze-drying is too slow. At −80°C the vapor pressure of water is 4×10^{-4} torr.

In the manipulations following a freeze-dry run, extreme care is taken to prevent rehydration of the hygroscopic tissue and resulting artifacts (ultrastructure, dislocations). The subsequent dry osmium tetroxide vapor fixation fixes

Table 1 Relevant Steps in "Dry" and Conventional "Wet" Sample Preparation

"Dry" method	Conventional method
Rapid freezing (physical fixation)	Fixation in aqueous glutaraldehyde solution
Freeze-drying (physical dehydration)	Postfixation in aqueous osmium tetroxide solution
Osmium tetroxide vapor fixation	Dehydration in graded alcohol series
In vacuo impregnation in Epon	Impregnation in propylene oxide and propylene oxide/Epon
Embedment in Epon	Embedment in Epon

the tissue, renders contrast for microscopy in the specimen, and anchors some diffusible substances (e.g., steroids) to the tissue.

During sample preparation, liquids may act as solvents and cause extraction or dislocation of the diffusing drug. From Table 1 it is evident that there are several "wet" steps in conventional sample preparation, including the use of various excellent solvents. In "dry" sample preparation, the only remaining "wet" step, and therefore the only possible extractive step, is the embedment in Epon. Compounds soluble in Epon (a poor solvent) and not anchored to the tissue by osmium tetroxide vapor, may be extracted to some extent. Two alternatives exist for reducing or preventing extraction of such compounds: the use of another embedding agent (nonextractive or less extractive for the compound under study) and/or the use of another vapor fixative.

5. Electron Microscopy

All sections were cut about 100 nm thick on a Reichert Om U_2 microtome using dry glass knives. They were examined in a Philips EM 201 electron microscope.

6. Autoradiography

For electron microscopic autoradiography the sections were collected on collodion-coated copper grids and covered with a light gray layer of carbon. The emulsion layer was applied using the loop method [54]; the wire loop enclosed a fully gelled film of Ilford L4 (Ilford, Mobberley, Cheshire, U.K.) prepared at a dilution of Ilford L4:water 1:2 (v/v). Exposure took place at 4°C in lighttight boxes containing silica gel. Development and fixation for autoradiography were performed at 20°C as follows: developing in D19 developer (3 min), rinsing in water, fixation in sodium thiosulfate 24% (w/v), and rinsing three times in water.

The background grain density and the possible occurrence of negative chemography (latent image fading) and/or positive chemography were determined according to standard procedures [55].

7. Experiments for Determining Effects of "Dry" Sample Preparation on Stratum Corneum Ultrastructure

Fresh human abdomen skin (female, 56 years of age), received from the hospital, was split with a dermatome (Padgett Electro Dermatome, Model B) set at 200 μm and prepared for electron microscopy using both the described conventional "wet" method and our "dry" method. The sections were post-stained for 10 min in 7% aqueous uranyl acetate solution after washing with water 5 min in lead hydroxide (0.2% w/v lead citrate in 0.1 N NaOH).

8. In Vitro Diffusion Experiment (Autoradiography)

Fresh human abdomen skin was immersed in a 2 N aqueous sodium bromide solution for 2 hr at 37°C in order to separate the epidermis from the underlying tissue. The epidermis was then sandwiched between two cellulose acetate 0.8 μm filters (Millipore, Molsheim, France), which served as support. This sandwich was clamped between the two halves of a polytetrafluoroethylene diffusion cell. The stratum corneum side faced the donor solution (above the sandwich), which was 1.35 mL of a 5.4×10^{-4} M hydrocortisone solution in phosphate-buffered saline (pH 7.4) containing 36 μCi/mL of [1,2-^{3}H]hydrocortisone (determined with liquid scintillation counting). The acceptor compartment (beneath the sandwich) contained 1.35 mL of phosphate-buffered saline. The diffusion area was a circle with a radius of 0.8 cm. Stationary diffusion was allowed to take place for 48 hr at 32°C.

Subsequently the epidermis was prepared for microscopy using the "dry" method. The nonaccelerated Epon used for the immersion and impregnation under vacuum of the rapidly frozen, freeze-dried, and osmium tetroxide vapor fixed tissue was collected, and the possible presence of extracted [1,2-^{3}H]hydrocortisone was determined by liquid scintillation counting, after adding Dynagel scintillation fluid (Baker, Deventer, The Netherlands) using a Packard Tricarb 4640 liquid scintillation counter. Quenching was corrected for by the external standard method.

Finally, autoradiography was performed as described.

B. Results and Discussion

1. Experiments for Determining Effects of "Dry" Sample Preparation on Stratum Corneum Ultrastructure

Figure 9 shows an electron micrograph of the skin following conventional sample preparation, while Figure 10 shows the equivalent for our "dry" sample preparation. In comparing the effects of the two sample preparations on the stratum corneum ultrastructure relative to the questions to be answered by using autoradiography, the most striking features were the following.

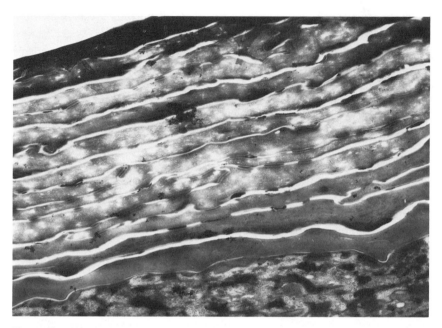

Figure 9 Electron micrograph of human stratum corneum and some of the underlying viable epidermis obtained after the conventional sample preparation and post-staining with uranyl acetate and lead hydroxide. Magnification 13,500 ×.

Both methods allowed clear discrimination between inter- and intracellular domains. This is an absolute requirement for discriminating between intercellular and transcellular pathways for drug transport across the stratum corneum.

The "dry" method preserved more intercellular material than the conventional sample preparation. Lipids are very relevant constituents of the intercellular materials and are probably essential to drug transport across the stratum corneum [3,7]. From the literature it is known that conventional procedures for fixation, dehydration, and embedment cause significant extraction of lipids and lipidlike substances.

The "dry" sample preparation preserved more layers of intact stratum corneum (average of 20) than did the conventional method (average of 13). The most logical explanation is that the "wet" steps in the conventional method extract intercellular material and loosen the stratum corneum layers.

The "dry" sample preparation completely disrupted the ultrastructure of the viable epidermis, which was left virtually intact by the conventional

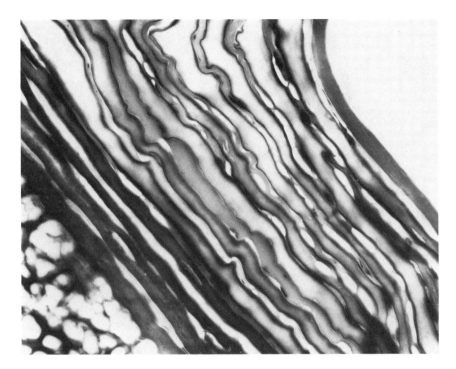

Figure 10 Electron micrograph of human stratum corneum and some of the underlying viable epidermis obtained after the "dry" sample preparation. Magnification 15,500 ×.

method. Plunging into solid/liquid Freon 22 causes vitrification to occur only over a range of 10–20 μm [53]; the stratum corneum thickness is within this region. The stratum corneum has only a low water content, making it less vulnerable to the formation of ice crystals and other freezing artifacts than other tissue. In future experiments, alternative (and better) methods for rapid freezing will be tested for improving the ultrastructural preservation of the viable epidermis.

From these results it can be concluded that the "dry" sample preparation preserved the ultrastructural features of the stratum corneum relevant to the questions to be answered by electron microscopic autoradiography better than conventional sample preparation but had damaging effects on the viable epidermis.

2. *In Vitro Diffusion Experiment (Autoradiography)*

Liquid scintillation counting of the nonaccelerated Epon used for the impregnation of the [1,2-^{3}H]hydrocortisone-loaded, rapidly frozen, freeze-dried, and

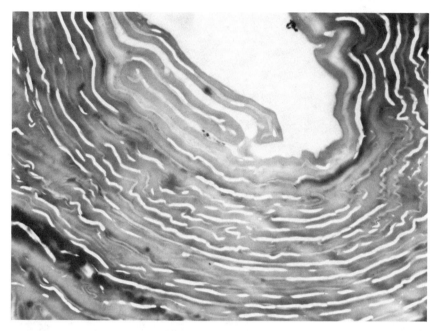

Figure 11 Electron microscopic autoradiograph obtained after a blank diffusion experiment. "Dry" sample preparation using Ilford L4 emulsion, 10 weeks of exposure, and D19b developer. Magnification 7000 ×.

osmium tetroxide vapor fixed tissue showed that no detectable amount of radioactivity was present in the Epon. Following osmium tetroxide vapor fixation, apparently hydrocortisone is not extracted during vacuum embedment in Epon. Osmium tetroxide vapor anchors steroids to the tissue and in this way prevents diffusion of hydrocortisone into the lipophilic Epon. Several other workers studied the extraction of steroids from rapidly frozen, freeze-dried, and osmium tetroxide vapor fixed tissue during Epon embedment. Attramadal [57] found for [^{3}H]estradiol 0.25% extraction of label from liver tissue after 24 hr infiltration in Epon at 50°C and 1.53% extraction from uterus tissue after 48 hr infiltration. In the same paper, for [^{3}H]testosterone, 0.19–0.35% extraction of label from liver tissue after 48 hr infiltration in nonaccelerated Epon was reported. Frederik and Klepper [51] reported that the loss of labeled steroids in Epon was lower than 1%; in their study they used testis tissue, estradiol, testosterone, and dehydroepiandrosterone.

Figure 11 shows an electron microscopic autoradiograph obtained after a blank diffusion experiment (in the absence of tritiated hydrocortisone). It can

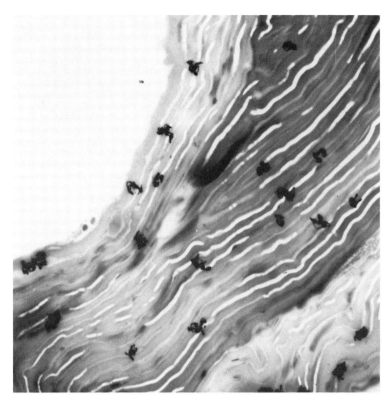

Figure 12 Electron microscopic autoradiograph obtained after the diffusion experiment with tritiated hydrocortisone. "Dry" sample preparation using Ilford L4 emulsion, 10 weeks of exposure, and D19b developer. Magnification 5600 ×.

be seen that the background grain density was extremely low and that positive chemography did not occur. Separate experiments indicated that negative chemography did not occur either.

Figure 12 shows an electron microscopic autoradiography developed after 10 weeks of exposure at 4°C. It can be seen that the ultrastructure of the stratum corneum is clearly recognizable and that the developed grains are clearly projected on the underlying tissue. This indicates that from this point of view the combination of the "dry" sample preparation and electron microscopic autoradiography is feasible.

Figures 11 and 12 confirm the findings described earlier regarding the influences of the "dry" sample preparation on the ultrastructure of the stratum corneum. Inter- and intracellular domains can clearly be discriminated, intercellular material can be detected, and many intact layers of the stratum corneum are preserved.

Figure 12 shows that a sufficient number of grains had developed, that is, no problems exist regarding the detection limit. The donor solution contained only 36 μCi/mL of [1,2-^{3}H]hydrocortisone in phosphate-buffered saline. This latter concentration can easily be increased, as the specific activity of the labeled compound is 51.9×10^3 Ci/mol.

In the electron microscopic autoradiographs the grain density over the Epon is identical to the background grain density, indicating that diffusion of labeled compound into the photographic emulsion had not occurred. Furthermore, these autoradiographs show that (almost) no grains had developed over the Epon at the margins of the tissue (i.e., in close vicinity to the stratum corneum), suggesting that the drug had not diffused from tissue into Epon.

The only setback in the obtained electron microscopic autoradiographs can be clearly recognized in Figure 12; the developed silver grains are too large, and hence resolution is not satisfactory. Ilford L4 and D19 developer were used because in our laboratory for electron microscopy this is the routine procedure for autoradiography. Alternatives in future experiments are the use of another nuclear emulsion and/or the use of another developer. For the combination of Ilford L4 emulsion and a gold latensification-elon ascorbic acid developer, Ginsel et al. [58] empirically determined the half-distance of resolution (HD) to be 115 nm (for 62-nm sections). Kopriwa et al. [59] determined that the HD value for sections of pale gold interference color was 76 nm for Ilford L4 emulsion and Agfa-Gevaert solution physical developer (SP) preceded by latensification in gold thiocyanate. Salpeter and Szabo [60] described even better results for the combination of Kodak NTE-2 emulsion and Dektol developer.

Preliminary results for the combination of Ilford L4 emulsion and a gold latensification-elon ascorbic acid developer are shown in Figure 13. These results are obtained after a diffusion experiment with tritiated testosterone. In Figure 13 the intercellular material is darker than the intracellular material. The larger black (more electron-dense) grains are the grains that should be produced and are indicated by arrows. The location of these grains would suggest that testosterone follows intercellular pathways through the stratum corneum. However, the presence of the many smaller particles (probably gold) indicates that the latensification and development steps still have to be optimized and that a definite conclusion about the diffusion pathway of testosterone through the human stratum corneum cannot be drawn at this moment.

The electron micrographs indicate that the intracellular and intercellular domains have thicknesses of 0.3–0.6 μm and 0.10–0.15 μm, respectively. These dimensions are also obtained when the electron micrographs and the corresponding magnifications in the standard work of Odland and Reed [61] are considered. Furthermore, these data are in good agreement with those of Elias [3], who

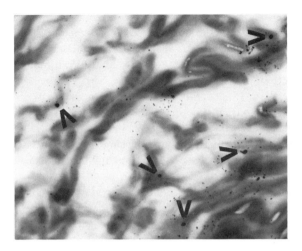

Figure 13 Electron microscopic autoradiograph obtained after a diffusion experiment with tritiated testosterone. "Dry" sample preparation using Ilford L4 emulsion, 10 weeks of exposure, a gold latensification-elon ascorbic developer. The arrows indicate the appropriate silver grains. Magnification 16,000 ×.

indicated the volume fractions of the intracellular and intercellular domains to be 79% and 21%, respectively. Considering these dimensions and the resolution attainable for electron microscopic autoradiography, it should be possible to discriminate between intercellular and transcellular drug transport across the stratum corneum.

3. Conclusion

The results suggest that the combination of "dry" sample preparation and electron microscopic autoradiography promises to be an excellent method for visualizing drug transport across the stratum corneum:

The described combination is feasible.
There is little or no extraction during sample preparation.
Preservation of the ultrastructure of the stratum corneum is excellent.
No problems arise regarding detection limits.
Almost all drugs can be visualized using tritium labeling.

IV. FUTURE PERSPECTIVES

In recent years immunogold techniques for visualization at the electron microscopic level have developed enormously. In general these techniques are used for visualization of cellular antigens. The method involves immunostaining with antibodies specific for a given antigen and then labeling the antibodies with gold-conjugated anti-immunoglobulin. Currently a broad range of gold-conjugated anti-immunoglobulins are available, and since conjugates of gold with goat anti-mouse immunoglobulin, for instance, can be used for all mouse antibodies, a very wide variety of antigens can be visualized. The gold marker sizes commonly available are 5, 10, 15, 20, and 30 nm; even 1-nm gold markers are currently available. The 1-nm gold must be silver-enhanced before it can be seen. Although small 5-nm markers will give a high labeling efficiency (relatively good penetration), they have the disadvantage of being difficult to see. The described immunogold technique can be used even on light microscopic sections by applying silver enhancement techniques.

For our research item of interest, visualization of drug transport across human skin (especially the stratum corneum) and of the effects of penetration enhancers on this process, the described immunogold techniques are promising tools because an improvement of resolution over that of autoradiography seems feasible. Antibodies against a broad range of drugs (e.g., androgens, corticosteroids, mineralocorticoids, estrogens, progestins, prostaglandins, peptides, peptide hormones, methotrexate, and morphine) are currently commercially available, implying that many drugs can be visualized using immunogold labeling.

It is important that immunolabeling not be obtained at the expense of morphology, and the many methods developed for ultrastructural immunocytochemistry illustrate the difficult balance between morphology and antigenicity. For visualization of drug transport across skin, pre-embedment techniques (immunocytochemical procedures undertaken on unfixed tissues) seem inappropriate, for during the "wet" immunocytochemical steps the diffusing drug may be extracted. For postembedment techniques (i.e., on sections) it should be realized that routine processing methods of glutaraldehyde and osmium fixation will render the majority of antigens unrecognizable by their antibody; furthermore, the choice of embedment agent also influences the antigenicity. The so-called dry method, described in Section III, involves a heavy osmium tetroxide vapor fixation step and hence seems inappropriate. Several more sensitive methods of tissue processing have proved successful with a wide variety of antigens. The two most promising techniques are the use of ultrathin frozen sections (cryo sections) and freeze substitution. The use of frozen sections is described by Tokuyasu [62]. After minimal fixation, tissues are cryopreserved in high concentrations of sucrose and frozen in liquid nitrogen. These initial steps seem to be extractive and probably make this technique less suited for our research purpose. The frozen tissues are sectioned at around −100°C, and the sections are collected and thawed. Also during thawing there is the risk of extraction or dislocation.

The most promising method seems to be that of freeze substitution. Freeze substitution relies upon the rapid freezing of samples (compare to the first step of the ''dry'' sample preparation), followed by the removal of the ice from the sample at about −80°C by either acetone or methanol. The acetone or methanol may contain very low concentrations of glutaraldehyde, formaldehyde, or osmium tetroxide. Subsequently the samples are embedded in Lowicryl resin at low temperature and polymerized with ultraviolet light. Monaghan and Robertson [63] obtained tissue blocks that had not been fixed at all with aldehyde or osmium fixatives. The morphology of tissues thus prepared is remarkably similar to that produced by conventional techniques, and the immunocytochemical possibilities are considerable.

Several critical factors have to be investigated when freeze substitution in combination with immunogoldlabeling is to be used for visualizing drug transport across human skin. The three major factors are:

1. How significant is the extraction of drug during the actual freeze substitution? When this would be significant, how can this extraction be decreased without decreasing the antigenicity?
2. What is the extent of extraction during the embedment in Lowicryl?
3. Is there any extraction of the antigen–antibody (i.e., drug–antibody) complex during the rinsing of the section for removing the excess of antibody, and is there any extraction of the antigen–antibody–gold-anti-immunoglobulin during the rinsing of the section for removing the excess of the gold–anti-immunoglobulin conjugate?

Research using the combination of immunogold labeling and freeze substitution for visualizing drug transport across human skin will be started within our research group in the very near future.

A very elegant and promising technique that is operable only at the light microscopic level is confocal laser microscopy in combination with fluorescence detection and computerized image-analysis techniques such as video-enhanced fluorescence microscopy. Using this technique it is possible to follow the diffusion of a fluorescent drug (or a drug that is labeled with, e.g., fluorescein isothiocyanate, which is relatively easy for peptides) through untreated and unprocessed tissue (i.e., no chemical fixation, dehydration, or other processing) as a function of time. The depth resolution is about $0.5-1.0 \ \mu m$. The obvious advantages of this method are that all tissue-processing steps are circumvented and the complete diffusion process can be followed as a function of time in a single run without introducing artifacts like extraction. The drawbacks are the relatively poor resolution (at the light microscopic level) and the limited range of compounds that can be investigated—fluorescent compounds or compounds marked with a fluorescent label. This technique will also be used within our research group in the near future to visualize the diffusion of compounds across the skin and the possible effects of penetration enhancers on it.

REFERENCES

1. R. J. Scheuplein, *J. Invest. Dermatol. 45*, 334 (1965).
2. R. J. Scheuplein, *J. Invest. Dermatol. 48*, 79 (1967).
3. P. M. Elias, *Int. J. Dermatol. 20*, 1 (1981).
4. M. L. Williams and P. M. Elias, *Crit. Rev. Ther. Drug Carrier Syst. 3*, 95 (1987).
5. B. W. Barry, in *Delivery Systems for Peptide Drugs*, S. S. Davis, L. Illum, and E. Tomlinson, Eds., Plenum, New York, 1986, p. 265.
6. I. Brody, *Nature 209*, 472 (1966).
7. P. A. Bowser and R. J. White, *Br. J. Dermatol. 112*, 1 (1985).
8. S. E. Friberg and D. W. Osborne, *J. Soc. Cosmet. Chem. 36*, 349 (1985).
9. W. Curatolo, *Pharm. Res. 4*, 271 (1987).
10. B. W. Barry, *Int. J. Cosmet. Sci. 10*, 281 (1988).
11. J. W. Wiechers, *Pharm. Weekbl. (Sci.) 11*, 185 (1989).
12. J. Hadgraft, *Pharm. Int. 5*, 252 (1984).
13. B. W. Barry, *J. Controlled Release 6*, 85 (1987).
14. J. W. Wiechers, R. A. de Zeeuw, B. F. H. Drenth, and J. H. G. Jonkman, *Pharm. Weekbl. (Sci.) 8*, 329 (1986).
15. J. C. Beastall, J. Hadgraft, and C. Washington, *Int. J. Pharm. 43*, 207 (1988).
16. H. E. Boddé, J. Verhoeven, and L. M. J. van Driel, *Crit. Rev. Ther. Drug Carrier Syst. 6*, 87 (1989).
17. K. Knutson, R. O. Potts, D. B. Guzek, G. M. Golden, J. E. McKie, W. J. Lambert, and W. I. Higuchi, *J. Controlled Release 2*, 67 (1985).
18. K. Knutson, S. L. Krill, W. J. Lambert, and W. I. Higuchi, *Int. Conf. Controlled Release Bioact. Mat. 13*, 199 (1986).
19. T. Kurihara-Bergstrom, G. L. Flynn, and W. I. Higuchi, *J. Pharm. Sci. 75*, 479 (1986).
20. Y. Morimoto, K. Sugibayashi, K. Hosoya, and W. I. Higuchi, *Int. J. Pharm. 32*, 31 (1986).
21. B. W. Barry and S. L. Bennett, *J. Pharm. Pharmcol. 39*, 535 (1987).
22. G. M. Golden, J. E. McKie, and R. O. Potts, *J. Pharm. Sci. 76*, 25 (1987).
23. A. Hoelgaard, B. Mollgaard, and E. Baker, *Int. J. Pharm. 43*, 233 (1988).
24. K. Sato, K. Sugibayashi, and Y. Morimoto, *Int. J. Pharm. 43*, 31 (1988).
25. H. E. Boddé, M. A. M. Kruithof, J. Brussee, and H. K. Koerten, *Int. J. Pharm. 53*, 13 (1989).
26. K. Fukuyama, Autoradiography, in *Methods in Skin Research*, D. Skerrow and C. J. Skerrow, Eds., Wiley, Chichester, 1985, p. 71.
27. H. Elling, *Drug Res. 36*, 1525 (1986).
28. H. Heine, *Med. Welt 34*, 2 (1983).
29. A. Lopp, I. Shevchuck, and U. Kirso, *Cancer Biochem. Biophys. 8*, 185 (1986).
30. R. Rick, A. Dörge, and K. Thurau, in *Microbeam Analysis*, A. D. Romig, Jr. and W. F. Chambers, Eds., San Francisco, Inc., San Francisco, 1986, p. 209.
31. K. G. Malmqvist, B. Forslind, K. Themmer, G. Hyltén, T. Grundin, and G. M. Roomans, *Biol. Trace Elem. Res. 12*, 279 (1987).
32. I. Silberberg, *J. Invest. Dermatol. 50*, 323 (1968).
33. M. K. Nemanic and P. M. Elias, *J. Histochem. Cytochem. 28*, 573 (1980).

34. H. H. Sharata and R. R. Burnette, *29th Annu. Ind. Pharm. Res. Conf.*, Merrimac, WI, 1987.

35. H. H. Sharata and R. R. Burnette, *J. Pharm. Sci.* 77, 27 (1988).

36. B. W. Barry, *Pharmacol. Skin 1*, 121 (1987).

37. J. A. Bouwstra, L. J. C. Peschier, J. Brussee, and H. E. Boddé, *Int. J. Pharm.* 52, 47 (1989).

38. E. R. Cooper, *J. Pharm. Sci.* 73, 1153 (1984).

39. F. H. N. de Haan, H. E. Boddé, W. C. de Bruijn, L. A. Ginsel, and H. E. Junginger, *Int. J. Pharm.* 56, 75 (1989).

40. I. Silberg, *J. Invest. Dermatol.* 56, 147 (1971).

41. B. Forslind, *Scanning Electron Microsc. 1*, 183 (1984).

42. B. Forslind, T. G. Grundin, M. Lindberg, G. M. Roomans, and Y. Werner, *Scanning Electron Microsc.* 2, 687 (1985).

43. T. G. Grundin, G. M. Roomans, B. Forslind, M. Lindberg, and Y. Werner, *J. Invest. Dermatol.* 85, 378 (1985).

44. W. E. Stumpf, in *Methods in Cell Physiology,* Vol. 13, D. M. Prescott, Ed., Academic, New York, 1976, p. 171.

45. K. T. Tokuyasu, *Histochem. J.* 12, 381 (1980).

46. A. W. Robards and U. B. Sleytr, in *Low Temperature Methods in Biological Electron Microscopy*, A. W. Robards and U. B. Sleytr, Eds., Elsevier, New York, 1985, p. 201.

47. A. K. Christensen and L. G. Paavola, *J. Microsc. 13*, 148 (1972).

48. J. R. J. Baker and T. C. Appleton, *J. Microsc. 108*, 307 (1976).

49. I. T. Johnson and J. R. Bronk, *J. Microsc. 115*, 187 (1979).

50. C. E. Stirling and W. B. Kinter, *J. Cell. Biol. 35*, 585 (1967).

51. P. M. Frederik and D. Klepper, *J. Microsc. 106*, 209 (1976).

52. P. M. Frederik, H. J. van der Molen, D. Klepper, and H. Galjaard, *J. Cell Sci. 26*, 339 (1977).

53. H. Y. Elder, C. C. Gray, A. G. Jardine, J. N. Chapman, and W. H. Biddlecomb, *J. Microsc. 126*, 45 (1981).

54. L. G. Caro and R. P. van Tubergen, *J. Cell Biol. 15*, 173 (1962).

55. M. A. Williams, in *Practical Methods in Electron Microscopy*, Vol. 6, Part I, A. M. Glauert, Ed., Elsevier, New York, 1977, pp. 1–219.

56. O. Stein and Y. Stein, *Lipid Res. 9*, 1 (1971).

57. A. Attramadal, *Histochemie 19*, 75 (1969).

58. L. A. Ginsel, J. J. M. Onderwater, and W. Th. Daems, *Histochemistry 61*, 343 (1979).

59. B. M. Kopriwa, G. M. Levine, and N. J. Nadler, *Histochemistry 80*, 519 (1984).

60. M. M. Salpeter and M. Szabo, *J. Histochem. Cytochem. 24*, 1204 (1976).

61. G. F. Odland and H. Reed, in *Ultrastructure of Normal and Abnormal Skin*, A. S. Zelickson, Ed., Lea and Febiger, Philadelphia, 1967, p. 54.

62. K. Y. Tokuyasu, *Histochem. J. 12*, 381 (1980).

63. P. Monaghan and D. Robertson, *J. Microsc. 158*, 355 (1990).

6

Compatibility and Synergy of Permeation Enhancers with Solvents, Excipients, and Drugs

Shirley M. Ng
The R. W. Johnson Pharmaceutical Research Institute, Raritan, New Jersey

I. INTRODUCTION

In the past decade, there has been a continuous increase in the pharmaceutical industry's interest in the development of transdermal drug delivery systems, which offer an effective way to deliver many drugs topically into the systemic circulation. This type of delivery system offers many advantages, such as by-passing the "first pass" effect and ease of self-administration. However, it also has its limitations. The advantages and disadvantages of transdermal delivery systems have been thoroughly reviewed elsewhere [1–4] and will not be further discussed in this chapter. Several transdermal therapeutic systems have recently been developed for topical application to achieve systemic medication. These are Transderm Scop, Estraderm, Catapres-TTS, Frandol tape (isosorbide dinitrate), Duragesic and various nitroglycerin transdermal systems (Deponit, Nitrodisc, Nitro-Dur, Minitran Transderm-Nitro, and Nitroglycerin Transdermal System-NTS).

New technologies are still evolving in the industry for developing various transdermal delivery systems for potential candidates. These upcoming transdermal therapeutic systems include those for contraception (estrogen and progestin), nicotine (Habitrol, Prostep, Nicoderm, and Nicotrel have been recently approved by the FDA), and many others.

II. TYPES OF TRANSDERMAL DELIVERY SYSTEMS

The various types of transdermal systems that are currently marketed can be simply classified into two basic categories:

1. Drug reservoir with rate-controlling membrane: Transderm-Nitro, Catapres-TTS, Transderm Scop, and Estraderm.
2. Drug reservoir without rate-controlling membrane: Nitrodisc, Nitro-Dur, Deponit, Frandol, and Nitroglycerin Transdermal System-NTS.

In many of these systems, for example, Catapres-TTS, Transderm Scop, Deponit, and Nitro-Dur, the active ingredients are incorporated directly into an adhesive matrix. In the case of Estraderm, estradiol is incorporated in an alcohol medium gelled with hydroxypropyl cellulose. However, in Nitrodisc and the generic Nitroglycerin Transdermal Systems-NTS, the drug is incorporated in a polymeric matrix. The release mechanism of drugs from these various systems has been thoroughly discussed [2,3,5] and will not be reviewed in this chapter.

III. BASIC COMPONENTS OF TRANSDERMAL DELIVERY SYSTEMS

The major components of a transdermal delivery system are an impervious backing, a drug reservoir, a pressure-sensitive adhesive, and a release liner. The drug reservoir is usually composed of polymer, plasticizer, the active ingredient, and other excipients such as solvents and enhancers. The pressure-sensitive adhesive can also act as the drug reservoir, with the active ingredient directly dispersed and/or dissolved within the adhesive.

A. Polymer Matrix

Polymer selection is important in considering the various design criteria that must be met for a particular delivery system. The molecular weight, glass transition temperature, and chemical functionality of the polymer must allow proper diffusion and release of a specific drug. The polymer must be compatible, nontoxic, and chemically stable during storage. It should also allow the incorporation of an appropriate amount of active ingredient without destroying its polymeric properties. The various polymers that have been used successfully in transdermal systems are silicone polymers, polyethylene, polypropylene, polyvinyl chloride, polyvinylpyrrolidone, polyvinyl alcohol, polyurethane, polyesters, ethylene vinyl acetate, hydrogels, and many others. With the advances of new technologies, many new polymers can be synthesized and tailor-made for each controlled release system.

B. Plasticizers

The use of an appropriate plasticizer is important in any given polymer system. A plasticizer, as defined by the Council of the International Union of Pure and Applied Chemistry (IUPAC), is a substance or material incorporated in a plastic or elastomer material to increase its flexibility, workability, or distensibility [6]. A plasticizer may reduce the melt viscosity, lower the temperature of the second-order transition, or lower the elastic modulus of the melt. A plasticizer must be compatible with the resin, nonvolatile, nonflammable, stable to heat and light, and nontoxic. Plasticizers can be classified as primary or secondary depending upon their compatibility with the resins. Primary plasticizers are highly compatible with polymer resins, whereas secondary plasticizers are less compatible. Secondary plasticizers are generally used in mixtures with a primary plasticizer in order to confer some special balance of properties.

C. Pressure-Sensitive Adhesives

A pressure-sensitive adhesive (PSA) is generally defined as a material that will adhere to a substrate when a light pressure is applied and will leave no residue upon removal [7]. Selection of the pressure-sensitive adhesive plays an important role in the development of a successful transdermal drug delivery system by ensuring intimate contact between the delivery system and the skin surface, thus allowing the delivery of drugs to the skin. Failure to ensure adequate contact of the entire surface area of the transdermal delivery system with the skin will result in only partial delivery of the drug substance to patients. An adhesive should be nonirritating and nonsensitizing to the skin, physically and chemically compatible with drugs and excipients, and moisture-resistant. It must adhere to all types of skin, leave no residue upon removal, and, most important, allow the adhesion of the system to the skin throughout its full intended period of use.

Commonly used pressure-sensitive adhesives are polyisobutylene (PIB), acrylics, and silicones. Technologies for assessment and selection of various types of adhesives are thoroughly reviewed in the *Handbook of Pressure Sensitive Adhesive Technology* [8]. Tackifiers, plasticizers, stabilizers, solvents, and other additives are often added during the manufacture of adhesives. The residual solvents, unreacted monomers, and additives can interact with the drug substances and cause problems that should not be overlooked by the formulator.

D. Enhancers

Enhancers or solvents are other widely used excipients in transdermal drug delivery systems. In many instances, the use of an enhancer is important to the success of transdermal drug delivery because it enhances the permeation of the drug through the skin. In other cases, solvents are used to increase the solubility

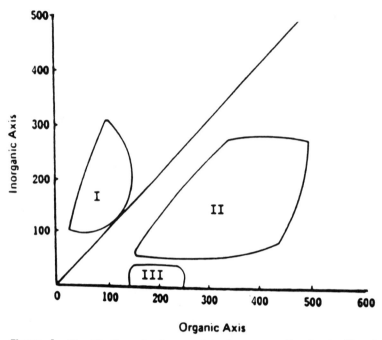

Figure 1 Classification of enhancers into three areas: I, solvents; II, enhancers for hydrophilic compounds; III, enhancers for hydrophobic compounds. (Adapted from Ref. 14.)

or miscibility of the drug with the elastomer. Numerous articles have been published that describe the mechanisms and uses of various enhancers [9–15]. Also, many patents have been issued describing the various types of enhancers used in a particular transdermal drug delivery system. The commonly used enhancers are ethanol, isopropanol, butanol, propylene glycol, ethylene glycol, Azone (1-dodecylazacycloheptane-2-one), dimethyl sulfoxide (DMSO), oleic acid, oleyl alcohol, and surfactants. Hori et al. [14] classified enhancers on a conceptional diagram, which separates enhancers into three distinct areas (Fig. 1).

Area I contains DMSO, 2-pyrrolidone, and propylene glycol, which are called solvents. Compounds like Azone, oleic acid, and lauryl alcohol, which are included in area II, appear to increase the absorption of hydrophilic compounds. Finally, area III contains enhancers such as oleyl alcohol and mineral oil, which enhances the permeation of lipophilic compounds. In general, these compounds do not contain any polar groups. Compounds in areas I and II are also referred to as polar and nonpolar solvents, respectively, by other authors [15]. It has also been shown that a binary mixture of enhancers from areas I (polar) and II (nonpolar) enhances the permeation of drugs much more than either one alone [9,12].

IV. COMPATIBILITY AND SYNERGY OF COMPONENTS

Numerous articles, books, and patents have been published during the past decade on the design, development, and enhancement of transdermal drug delivery systems. However, not enough has been said with regard to potential stabilization resulting from the selection and compatibility of the various formulation components. In this section, some examples of potential formulation component compatibility and synergy are discussed.

A. Compatibility with Drugs

The basic theory of the effect of penetration enhancers on the percutaneous absorption of drugs has been described in detail by various authors [9, 11, 15]. In general, the flux, J, of a drug across a skin membrane can be written as

$$J = -D \frac{\partial c}{\partial x}$$

where D is the diffusion coefficient, c is the drug concentration, and x is the distance. The concentration gradient is the rate of change of concentration with distance within the skin membrane. Therefore, to enhance the flux of a drug, one must increase D or c or a combination of the two. D is an important parameter in transdermal drug delivery because it can be affected by many formulation parameters. It is a function of molecular size, shape, and flexibility of the diffusing molecule as well as the membrane resistance.

Since the drug concentration in the skin is limited by its physicochemical properties, it is not expected that the drug concentration within the skin membrane can be increased tremendously by the use of enhancers. It has been postulated that the effect of penetration enhancer on flux is more likely to be greater on the diffusion coefficient of the drug substance in the skin layers than on the drug concentration [9]. The physicochemical properties of the penetrant must be considered in choosing the appropriate penetration enhancers. The behavior of an enhancer or a solvent depends upon the penetrant. When formulated with a drug in an elastomer or adhesive polymer matrix, an enhancer may alter the drug solubility, polymorphism, stability, and degree of ionization, which may further result in affecting the drug partitioning from the device [16].

It has been recommended that an enhancer should have a solubility parameter (δ) similar to that of the skin, which is estimated to be around 10 $(\text{cal/cm}^3)^{1/2}$. The Hildebrand solubility parameter is directly related to the compound's co-

Table 1 Solubility Parameters of Some Common Solvents,
Enhancers, and Plasticizers

Solvent, enhancer, plasticizer	Solubility parameter (δ) $(cal/cm^3)^{1/2}$
Ethanol	12.7
Isopropanol	11.5
n-Butanol	11.4
Propylene glycol	12.6
Ethylene glycol	14.6
Oleic acid	7.91[a]
Oleyl alcohol	8.94[a]
Lauryl alcohol	8.1
Dimethyl formamide	12.1
Dimethyl sulfoxide	12.0
Mineral oil	7.09[a]
Benzyl alcohol	12.1
Dioctyl adipate	8.7
Dioctyl phthalate	7.9
Dioctyl sebacate	8.6
Di-n-hexyl phthalate	8.9

[a]These values are from Ref. 15; all others are from Ref. 17.

hesive energy density and is a constant for any given compound. The solubility parameter, which describes the attractive strength between molecules of the material, has been defined as the square root of the cohesive energy density [17],

$$\delta_i = \left(\frac{\Delta E_i^v}{V_i}\right)^{1/2}$$

where ΔE_i^v is the energy of vaporization of species i and V_i is the molar volume of i in the mixture. The solubility parameter can be easily calculated from the structural formula and density of the compound or determined experimentally. Grulke [17] lists the solubility parameters for many solvents, plasticizers, and polymers. Others have described the use of solubility parameters to predict the permeation of drugs through the skin [15,18]. Table 1 lists some of the commonly used enhancers/solvents and their solubility parameters.

B. Compatibility with Polymers and Plasticizers

The common polymeric drug matrix systems that are used are those of polyvinyl chloride, silicone polymers, polyvinylpyrrolidone, and polyurethane. For example, the Nitroglycerin Transdermal System-NTS employs polyvinyl chloride (PVC) as the drug matrix in which the drug is dissolved and/or dispersed. The PVC resins used in transdermal systems must be modified by the incorporation of appropriate additives for satisfactory processing and end-use performance [19]. These additives are a plasticizer, a stabilizer, and a lubricant. The function of a plasticizer is to convert the hard, inherently brittle PVC resin into compositions of varying degrees of softness and flexibility for proper adherence to the skin. Stabilizers are also added to improve the heat and light stability of PVC resins. The functions of a lubricant in PVC resins are to reduce the friction at and adhesion to various surfaces during processing. The additive properties of lubricants are to lower the interparticle and intermolecular friction. In certain instances, some stabilizers also have a lubricant action and/or benefit from synergy with certain lubricants; some lubricants also exert a stabilizing effect.

PVC polymers and copolymers are known to be susceptible to degradation by heat and light, with degradation being more rapid and severe in the presence of oxygen. Titow [20] discusses in depth the degradation mechanism of PVC polymers, modes of action of various stabilizers, physical testing, and mechanisms of evaluation of PVC stability. The primary manifestations of thermal degradation of PVC polymers are the evolution of hydrogen chloride, the deterioration of physical and chemical properties, and color changes. Dehydrochlorination can be catalyzed by evolved HCl or promoted or initiated by other strong acids. The compatibility of a drug substance with the HCl evolved from the PVC polymer can be a primary stability issue for such a transdermal delivery system.

Besides their primary functions, plasticizers, stabilizers, and lubricants can potentially interact with each other. A formulator should take into account the potential secondary interactions of all these components. The compatibility and synergistic effects of plasticizers and various formulation components for PVC polymers are discussed by Titow [19]. The theoretical aspects can be applicable to other types of polymer systems and other components such as enhancers. Titow also discusses the importance of the Hildebrand solubility parameter (δ) in choosing the appropriate plasticizer. In general, complete miscibility is expected to occur if the solubility parameters of a solvent and a solute are similar and the degree of hydrogen bonding is similar between the components [16]. The same theory can apply in choosing appropriate enhancers or solvents. Therefore, when the incorporation of permeation enhancers or solvents into the polymeric drug reservoir is deemed necessary, it is advisable to compare their solubility parameters to those of the polymers in order to predict their compatibility and miscibility with the system. The solubility parameters of some commonly used polymers are listed in Table 2.

If an enhancer is not completely miscible with the PVC resin, it may result in unsatisfactory formation of a gelled PVC polymer as a drug reservoir. The

Table 2 Solubility Parameters of Some Common Polymers

Polymer	Solubility parameter (δ) $(cal/cm^3)^{1/2}$
Polyvinyl alcohol	12.6
Polyvinyl chloride	9.4–10.8
Polybutadiene	8.1–8.6
Polyisoprene	7.4–10.0
Polyisobutene	7.1–8.3
Polymethyl methacrylate	8.5–13.3
Polyethylene	7.7–8.8
Polypropylene	9.2–9.4
Polymethylene	7.0
Polyoxyethylene	8.9–10.9
Silicone rubber	7.0–11.4
Cellulose	15.7
Cellulose acetate	13.3–13.6
Ethyl cellulose	10.3
Polybutyl acrylate	7.0–12.7
Polyurethane	10.0
Polyisobutylene	7.7–8.1
Natural rubber	8.0–8.4

Source: Adapted from Ref. 17.

total amount of enhancer used in a given polymer system is also critical. In general, no more than 15% (w/w) enhancer can be incorporated in the PVC resin without causing syneresis. For example, the incorporation of 20% propylene glycol in PVC resin for the delivery of estradiol resulted in syneresis of solvent on the surface of the polymeric drug reservoir after several days at room temperature [unpublished results]. With the loss of available enhancer from the system, the flux was also decreased with time. Also, depending upon the manufacturing process of a polymeric drug reservoir, a volatile solvent or enhancer will not be able to be incorporated in the system. For example, ethanol is not capable of being incorporated into a PVC polymeric drug reservoir, which requires heat for gelation.

The action of some plasticizers can be synergistically enhanced by other enhancers or solvents. For example, polyethylene glycol and *N,N*-diethyl-*m*-toluamide (DEET), which are common solvents and enhancers, can act as secondary plasticizers when used in combination with dioctyl phthalate. Azone, in excess concentration of 35% in the formula, can also act as a primary plasticizer for the PVC resins [unpublished results]. In this case, a PVC plasticizer can

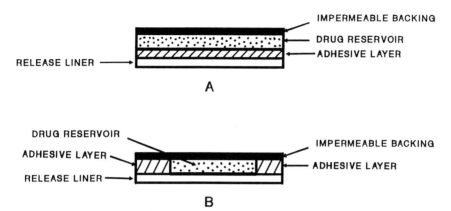

Figure 2 Schematic diagram of a face adhesive design (A) and a peripheral adhesive design (B).

easily be eliminated from the formulation. An example of this is the transdermal delivery of isosorbide dinitrate containing Azone as enhancer/plasticizer [21].

C. Compatibility with Pressure-Sensitive Adhesives

Pressure-sensitive adhesive (PSA) is one of the most important components in transdermal delivery systems because it acts to promote sufficient contact and adhesion between the patch and the skin. Basically, there are two types of adhesive design: peripheral adhesive design and face adhesive design (Fig. 2). In a peripheral adhesive design, the adhesive film is located around the drug reservoir and does not come into direct contact with the drug or enhancer. In the face adhesive case, the adhesive will have direct contact with the drug and enhancers whether the adhesive layer is applied on top of a drug reservoir matrix with or without an overlaid rate-controlling membrane or when the drug is directly incorporated into the adhesive. In either case, both the drug and the enhancer must be able to diffuse through the adhesive without adversely affecting the adhesive properties of the PSA. The PSA should be physically and chemically compatible with both the diffusing drug and the enhancer, and it should not affect the overall delivery rate of the drug. Chemical compatibility between the PSA, drug, enhancer, and other excipients must be established during the initial phase of patch development. Early assessment of the effects of an enhancer on the adhesive must be established initially and under conditions of accelerated aging.

Two important parameters that can be used to measure chemical compatibility between PSA, drug, enhancer, and other excipients are tack and cohesive strength. The cohesive strength of most PSAs has a tendency to decrease upon aging, thus resulting in softening of the pressure-sensitive adhesive [22]. The loss of cohesive strength may also result in adhesive residue being left on the skin upon removal of the patch, and a loss of adhesive tackiness. Besides the effect on cohesive strength, enhancers and solvents can also adversely affect the viscoelastic properties of the adhesive as well as the end-use properties such as peel force and skin adhesion [16].

The types of enhancers and their maximum acceptable levels in the various types of adhesives are also critical. Pfister and Hsieh [16] studied the effects of some enhancers on the tack, peel strength, and adhesion of silicone adhesives. They reported that relatively hydrophilic enhancers such as urea and propylene glycol are compatible with silicone adhesive at a level of 10% (w/w). However, hydrophobic enhancers like Azone and isopropyl palmitate reduce the cohesive strength of the silicone adhesive at a level of 5% (w/w). In general, the maximum allowable percentage of enhancer or solvent that can be incorporated in any adhesive system is 10% (w/w). Ethanol, which is a commonly used solvent and enhancer, can easily destroy the cohesive strength of a PSA. Other researchers have also reported that amine-containing compounds can react and destroy silicone adhesive properties [23].

Depending upon the solubility of the drug in the particular adhesive, a PSA is capable of storing a loading dose. This is especially important when PSA is applied on top of a rate-controlling membrane, which is laminated on top of a drug-loaded matrix to control the release of the drug substance. In some cases, it is beneficial to have an immediate release of an initial amount of loading dose. An example of this is the Transderm Scop, which contains the scopolamine drug reservoir, a polypropylene controlling membrane, and a face adhesive of polyisobutylene, mineral oil, and scopolamine. It is claimed that the initial priming dose, released from the face adhesive layer of the patch, saturates the skin binding sites and rapidly brings the plasma concentration of scopolamine to the required steady-state level. Subsequently, a continuous release of scopolamine from the drug reservoir, controlled by the rate-controlling membrane, maintains a constant plasma level [24]. In other cases, this may cause an alarming release of a large amount of drug if the drug substance has a high solubility in the adhesive layer. Therefore, extreme care must be taken in developing a face adhesive patch where the rate-controlling membrane is also used intentionally to control the release of drug substance. The saturated solubility of a drug substance in PSA, and the total amount of loading dose, which depends upon the thickness of an adhesive layer, must be determined. For example, mineral oil is a common plasticizer for polyisobutylene (PIB) adhesives and may favor partition of a hydrophobic drug out of the drug reservoir into a PIB face adhesive.

V. STABILITY OF TRANSDERMAL DRUG DELIVERY SYSTEMS

Because of the complexity of this type of delivery system, a careful choice of various appropriate components is important for the successful development of a transdermal delivery system for its intended use. The challenge of developing an acceptable adhesive type of transdermal delivery system with the desired adhesive and cohesive strengths is that of meeting the regulatory requirements of various worldwide health authorities. Above all, a successful transdermal delivery system must be stable both physically and chemically, and the drug release profile must not change upon aging. The criteria for developing a stable transdermal delivery system is not much different than the criteria for the development of other dosage forms. The physicochemical properties of a drug such as its solubility, stability, partition coefficient, melting point, and molecular size are important for choosing components for the final patch design. Bova et al. [25] discuss some of the basic approaches and considerations necessary for the successful development of transdermal delivery systems. Some of the basic steps in developing a transdermal dosage form are as follows:

Choice of the candidate drug
Feasibility study of transdermal delivery of the candidate drug
Determination of initial skin flux from saturated solutions
Determination of the need for enhancement
Test for skin irritation and sensitization
Choice of components
Design of the system
Optimization of final formulation
Evaluation of wearability of the final formulation

Stability studies must be conducted under various conditions, and the final patch design should meet the stability guidelines set forth by the appropriate agencies. The formulator must develop a set of criteria or product specifications for stability studies of the final delivery system. A proposed set of finished product specifications of a typical transdermal drug delivery system comprises

1. Patch size
2. Appearance
3. Color
4. Odor
5. Drug content

6. In vitro drug release profile
7. Degradation products and impurities
8. Residual monomers and solvents
9. Adhesive properties: tack, peel strength, adhesion
10. Condition of package

A. Physical Stability

A transdermal drug delivery system, including the package, must be physically stable throughout its intended shelf life. Criteria such as dissolution or drug release profile, drug crystallization, syneresis of enhancer, and adhesive properties should be identified. Color change may be an indication of incompatibility between components such as the polymer matrix, drug, and enhancers. Others have reported that a severe color change from yellow to black was observed when nitroglycerin was incorporated into natural rubber adhesives [26]. The generation of hydrogen chloride as a result of polyvinyl chloride decomposition may also result in unacceptable color change, even though the drug is chemically stable.

An excess of drug substance is generally used in the drug matrix to facilitate passive diffusion, and the drug is usually incorporated as a solid dispersion or has only limited solubility in various elastomers. Crystal growth within the drug matrix or crystallization of drug substance on the surface of the drug reservoir is also a common phenomenon observed during aging. Adhesives are known to absorb moisture from the atmosphere. The uptake of water into the polymer matrix can adversely affect drug solubility in the elastomers. It may also cause the bleeding of highly hydrophobic solvents or enhancers from the matrix. Thus, crystallization could be a sign of inadequate packaging, and the drug release profile and adhesive properties of the system may be affected. Therefore, packaging is important to prevent moisture permeation.

Adhesive properties such as tack and cohesive strength can easily be monitored by methods such as the peel strength measurements specially developed for the evaluation of adhesive properties. Fukuzawa [22] reported the effects of various additives on the aging properties of pressure-sensitive adhesives at various temperatures and conditions. However, stability studies must include all the packaging components that are in direct contact with the drug matrix and adhesives. Sometimes, depending upon the backing used, the drug reservoir layer may become delaminated from its backing as a result of the interaction between the adhesive–drug matrix and the backing. Similarly, as a result of a change in the adhesive/cohesive strength of the adhesive, the release liner may fail to be removed from the patch. All these are important to the physical stability of a transdermal system.

B. Chemical Stability

The drug intended for transdermal delivery must be chemically stable in the final system. Any components are capable of affecting the chemical stability of a drug substance. It has been reported that the presence of mineral oil reduces the chemical stability of tulobuterol in a polyisobutylene (PIB) adhesive reservoir [27]. Mineral oil has to be eliminated from this particular PIB layer. Stability-indicating methods must be developed to monitor the stability of the drug substance. Drug degradation may occur as a result of interaction with residual solvents and/or monomers. Therefore, degradation products and impurities must also be monitored during stability studies.

C. In Vitro Drug Release Studies

A major challenge to the pharmaceutical scientists and manufacturers is the development of control methods to accurately monitor the reproducibility of drug delivery through intact skin. In order to monitor the batch-to-batch or lot-to-lot reproducibility of transdermal drug delivery systems, various in vitro drug release methods have been developed to evaluate the drug release profile of a transdermal system [28,29]. Those methods have also been used during stability studies to monitor the drug release characteristics of stability samples. Drug release studies should be monitored initially and again at various time intervals after storage at reasonable temperatures.

Patches that contain both a rate-controlling membrane and a face adhesive must be allowed to equilibrate for at least a week at room temperature before initial drug release characteristics can be established. If drug release studies are conducted prior to equilibration, an inaccurate amount of loading dose will be determined. A change in drug release profile, measured under identical experimental conditions, may indicate potential instability of the drug substance or incompatibility of the drug with various components.

In some cases, in vitro skin permeation studies using human cadaver skin are also used to monitor the bioavailability of stability samples. Assuming that the drug release profile was unchanged and that there was no variation from skin samples, the in vitro skin permeation data should also be reproducible throughout the stability studies. Wester and Maibach [30] present some basic experimental designs to generate meaningful in vitro skin permeation data. In vitro permeation studies are best conducted with human cadaver skin. Due to skin source variability, a minimum of three skin sources is recommended to generate meaningful data. In vitro skin permeation studies are needed during the initial phase of formulation development. In general, it is not required to use this method during the stability studies, assuming that valid in vitro drug release characteristics have been developed. However, such studies will provide additional information to guarantee the consistent bioavailability of a drug substance delivered transdermally.

Finally, once the final system with adequate stability and in vitro drug release profiles has been developed, a wear test on human subjects must also be conducted. Even before the system has been finalized, wear tests conducted with placebo patches are also recommended. The results from such studies can provide a great deal of information on the feasibility of certain components under consideration for transdermal systems.

VI. SUMMARY

Many transdermal drug delivery systems have been successfully developed and marketed during the past decade from the earliest nitroglycerin patches to the most recently approved nicotine patch. However, this type of dosage form presents tremendous challenges to the development scientists and engineers. Choice of appropriate components, compatibility of these components, identification of acceptable and compatible enhancers, patch design, packaging, and manufacturing requirements are all important for the successful development of an aesthetically acceptable and physically and chemically stable transdermal product.

Physical and chemical compatibility between various components must be determined during the initial phase of patch development. New technologies are still evolving for identifying compatible adhesive polymers such as those newly developed silicone adhesives or cross-linked acrylic adhesives that are tailor-made for each system. More novel manufacturing technologies, such as those developed by Cygnus [31], are still evolving in an attempt to minimize the most challenging compatibility issues. Compatibility is always a challenge for formulators during dosage form development. However, if the basic physicochemical properties of each of the individual components and their possible interactions are well understood, the development of a successful transdermal system will be much easier.

REFERENCES

1. Y. W. Chien, in *Transdermal Controlled Systemic Medications*, Y. W. Chien, Ed., Marcel Dekker, New York, 1987, p. 1.
2. Y. W. Chien, in *Transdermal Controlled Systemic Medications*, Y. W. Chien, Ed., Marcel Dekker, New York, 1987, p. 25.
3. A. F. Kydonieus, in *Transdermal Delivery of Drugs*, Vol. 1, A. F. Kydonieus and B. Brener, Eds., CRC Press, Boca Raton, FL, 1987, p. 3.
4. R. H. Guy, *J. Controlled Release 4*, 237 (1986).
5. Y. W. Chien, in *Transdermal Delivery of Drugs*, Vol. 1, A. F. Kydonieus and B. Brener, Eds., CRC Press, Boca Raton, FL, 1987, p. 81.
6. D. L. Buszard, in *PVC Technology*, 4th ed., W. V. Titow, Ed., Elsevier, New York, 1984, p. 117.
7. M. C. Musolf, in *Transdermal Controlled Systemic Medications*, Y. W. Chien, Ed., Marcel Dekker, New York, 1987, p. 93.

8. D. Satas, Ed., *Handbook of Pressure Sensitive Adhesive Technology*, 2nd ed., Van Nostrand-Reinhold, New York, 1989.

9. E. R. Cooper and B. Berner, in *Transdermal Delivery of Drugs*, Vol. 2, A. F. Kydonieus and B. Berner, Eds., CRC Press, Boca Raton, FL, 1987, p. 57.

10. M. Goodman and B. W. Barry, in *Percutaneous Absorption*, 2nd ed., R. L. Bronaugh and H. I. Maibach, Eds., Marcel Dekker, New York, 1989, p. 567.

11. E. R. Cooper, in *Transdermal Controlled Systemic Medications*, Y. W. Chien, Ed., Marcel Dekker, New York, 1987, p. 83.

12. E. R. Cooper, *J. Pharm. Sci. 73*(8), 1153 (1984).

13. D. Friend, P. Catz, and J. Heller, *J. Controlled Release 9*, 33 (1989).

14. M. Hori, S. Satoh, and H. Maibach in *Percutaneous Absorption,* 2nd ed., R. L. Bronaugh and H. I. Maibach, Eds., Marcel Dekker, New York, 1989, p. 197.

15. W. R. Pfister and D. S. T. Hsieh, *Pharm. Technol. 14*(9), 132 (1990).

16. W. R. Pfister and D. S. T. Hsieh, *Pharm. Technol. 14*(10), 54 (1990).

17. E. A. Grulke, in *Polymer Handbook*, 3rd ed., J. Brandrup and E. H. Immergut, Eds., Wiley, New York, 1989, p. VII/519.

18. K. B. Sloan, S. A. M. Koch, K. G. Siver, and F. P. Flowers, *J. Invest. Dermatol. 87*, 244 (1986).

19. W. V. Titow, in *PVC Technology*, 4th ed., W. V. Titow, Ed., Elsevier, New York, 1984, p. 79.

20. W. V. Titow, in *PVC Technology*, 4th ed., W. V. Titow, Ed., Elsevier, New York, 1984, p. 255.

21. V. Rajadhyaksha, J. Anisko, S. M. Ng, A. F. Kydonieus, et al., 12th Int. Symp. Controlled Release Bioactive Materials, Geneva, Switzerland, 1985.

22. K. Fukuzawa, in *Handbook of Pressure Sensitive Adhesive Technology*, 2nd ed., D. Satas, Ed., Van Nostrand-Reinhold, New York, 1989, p. 244.

23. L. A. Sobieski and T. J. Tangney, in *Handbook of Pressure Sensitive Adhesive Technology*, 2nd ed., D. Satas, Ed., Van Nostrand-Reinhold, 1989, p. 508.

24. *Physician's Desk Reference*, 47th ed., Medical Economics Co., New Jersey, 1993, p. 880.

25. D. J. Bova, V. N. Ahmuty, R. L. Cirrito, K. O'Toole Holmes, K. Kasper, C. LaPrade, R. LaPrade, G. A. Maag, J. A. Mantelle, J. A. McCarty, J. Miranda, F. A. Morton, and S. Sablotsky, in *Transdermal Controlled Systemic Medications*, Y. W. Chien, Ed., Marcel Dekker, New York, 1987, p. 379.

26. H.-M. Wolff, H. R. Hoffmann, and G. Cordes, in *Transdermal Controlled Systemic Medications*, Y. W. Chien, Ed., Marcel Dekker, New York, 1987, p. 365.

27. Y. Nakano, T. Horiuchi, S. Fujiwara, and S. Unozawa, Eur. Patent Appl. 374,980, June 27, 1990.

28. Y.-C. Huang, in *Transdermal Controlled Systemic Medications*, Y. W. Chien, Ed., Marcel Dekker, New York, 1987, p. 159.

29. V. P. Shah and J. P. Skelly, in *Transdermal Controlled Systemic Medications* Y. W. Chien, Ed., Marcel Dekker, New York, 1987, p. 399.

30. R. C. Wester and H. I. Maibach, in *Percutaneous Absorption*, 2nd ed., R. L. Bronaugh and H. I. Maibach, Eds., Marcel Dekker, New York, 1989, p. 653.

31. J. Miranda and G. W. Cleary, U.S. Patent 4,915,950, April 10, 1990.

7

A General Method for Assessing Skin Permeation Enhancement Mechanisms and Optimization

Charan R. Behl
Pharmaceutical Research and Development, Hoffmann–La Roche, Inc., Nutley, New Jersey

Nancy J. Harper
Pharmaceutical Research and Development, Pfizer Central Research, Groton, Connecticut

Joyce Y. Pei
Bristol–Myers Squibb, Princeton, New Jersey

Saran Kumar, Deepak Mehta, Hing Char, Sunil B. Patel, David Piemontese, Giuseppe Ciccone, and Waseem Malick
Pharmaceutical Research and Development, Hoffmann–La Roche, Inc., Nutley, New Jersey

I. INTRODUCTION

With the development of the first transdermal patch, scopolamine [1], interest in using the skin as an alternative route for systemic drug delivery increased tremendously. A large number of drug candidates have been and are being evaluated for administration via this route [2–15]. Transdermal delivery systems of six more drugs have been developed and are on the market. These products contain nitroglycerin, clonidine, estradiol, testosterone, fentanyl, and nicotine [1]. Several additional drugs are currently under development. Were it not for the skin's extraordinary barrier properties, one would see many more drugs on the market available for transdermal administration. The fact is that most drugs lack sufficiently high permeability through the skin to produce therapeutic effects. This has led to numerous studies evaluating a large number of chemicals for their potential to enhance skin permeability. These chemicals include water

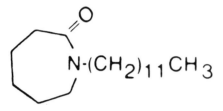

1-DODECYLAZACYCLOHEPTAN-2-ONE

Figure 1 Schematic structure of Azone. (From [19].)

[16], dimethyl sulfoxide [17], ethanol [18], oleic acid [19], propylene glycol [19], pyrrolidones [19], various surfactants [15,19], urea [19], *N,N*-diethyl-*m*-toluamide [19], and isopropyl myristate [13]. In addition to these enhancers, Azone, 1-dodecylazacycloheptan-2-one (Fig. 1), produced by Nelson Research, Irvine, California, has been extensively evaluated for its permeation-enhancing properties [20].

In most studies reported to date, enhancer effects are typically examined with individual drugs, using a variety of vehicles and experimental conditions. In studies of this nature, it is often difficult to make predictions regarding (1) the general types of substances that would benefit from a given enhancer's effects, (2) the suitability of any given formulative covehicle, or (3) enhancer concentrations necessary to induce maximum delivery enhancement. Moreover, it is difficult to factor out the biological versus physicochemical (thermodynamic) effects. In this chapter, a unique approach will be presented where the effects of a given enhancer (Azone) are studied in a systematic manner, specifically addressing the issues mentioned above.

II. CHARACTERISTICS OF AN IDEAL ENHANCER

The principal characteristics of an ideal enhancer are [21,22]:

1. The enhancer should be pharmacologically inert and should possess no action of itself at receptor sites in the skin or in the body in the amount or concentration used.
2. The enhancer should not be toxic, irritating, or allergenic.
3. On application, the onset of action should be immediate, and the duration of the effect should be predictable and suitable.
4. When the enhancer is removed from the skin, the exposed tissue should immediately and fully recover its normal barrier properties.

5. The barrier function of the skin should reduce in one direction only, so as to promote penetration into the skin. Body fluids, electrolytes, or other endogenous materials should not be lost to the environment.
6. The enhancer should have a good enhancement efficacy and be chemically and physically compatible with a wide range of drugs and pharmaceutical adjuvants.
7. The enhancer should be an excellent solvent for drugs, so that only minimal quantities of drug are required.
8. The enhancer should spread well on the skin and possess a suitable skin "feel."
9. The enhancer should be able to be formulated readily into lotions, suspensions, ointments, creams, gels, aerosols, and skin adhesives.
10. The enhancer should be inexpensive, odorless, tasteless, and colorless so as to be cosmetically acceptable.

III. PROPERTIES OF AZONE

Azone is a colorless, odorless liquid possessing what is described as an oily yet nongreasy feel. It is one of a series of N-alkylated cyclic amides specifically developed as a permeation enhancer. Azone is generally considered to be pharmacologically inert, although this appears to be a controversial issue [21]. It is reportedly devoid of adverse effects (e.g., irritancy, sensitization, and phototoxicity) when applied to human skin, although vehicle influences and concentration effects may not have been fully examined [20]. The physical properties of Azone include:

Boiling point 160°C (0.05 mmHg)
Viscosity 45.2 cps
Refractive index 1.470 np
Specific gravity 0.912
Surface tension 32.65 dynes/cm
Flash point 100°C
LD_{50} 9 g/kg (rat)
Miscible with most organic solvents
Immiscible with water

In terms of its enhancement effects, Azone is claimed to be a potential enhancer of a wide variety of drugs, lipophilic as well as hydrophilic [20,23–25]. Its reported effectiveness at relatively low concentrations has been promoted as an attractive feature. As will be shown later in this chapter, these claims are not always true, and optimum effects involve an interrelationship among permeant, enhancer concentration, and vehicle lipophilicity.

IV. DRUGS EXHIBITING PERMEATION ENHANCEMENT INDUCED BY AZONE

Table 1 documents the wide range of drug substances that have demonstrated Azone-induced skin permeation enhancement [20,27–39].

V. THE PRESENT APPROACH

A. Use of Homologous Series as Test Permeants and Test Vehicles

In the present study, ^{14}C-labeled n-alkanols, methanol, butanol, and octanol were used as test permeant, [40,41]. The test vehicles were methanol, ethanol, butanol, hexanol, octanol, and decanol, each containing Azone in concentrations of 0.0%, 2.5%, 5.0%, 10%, 25%, 50%, and 100%. The rationale behind this approach is that the partition coefficients of the permeants can be varied substantially without significantly altering other properties. The use of a homologous series, n-alkanols in this case, as test vehicles provides an option of varying the vehicle lipophilicity in a systematic and easily defined manner.

A substantial amount of work has been carried out by using alkanols and alkanoic acids as model permeants. These studies were aimed at investigating effects of various parameters on skin permeability: hydration effects [42–44]; burn-induced effects [45–49]; age-related effects [50]; solvent/vehicle effects [51]; surfactant effects [52,53]; and iontophoretic effects [54,55]. These test permeants have also been used in the evaluation of new animal models for skin permeation [56–58] and the effects of skin sectioning [59,60]. They are useful because they delineate three major mechanisms of skin transport of drugs as depicted in Figure 2 [61]. It is shown in this chapter that the enhancement effect of Azone is mostly a "membrane effect." It must be considered differently from one class or enhancers to another [62]. Thus, a series of permeants that cover these major pathways is most likely to give insight into the mechanistic aspects of drug permeation enhancement.

B. Use of Synthetic Membrane

A synthetic membrane, Silastic sheeting (polydimethylsiloxane; Dow Corning, Midland, MI) of 250-μm thickness and nonreinforced type, was used to further understand the mechanistic aspects of Azone-induced permeation enhancement effects. This particular membrane was selected for this study because it has been shown previously that the skin's lipoidal pathway is closely paralleled by chemical permeation across Silastic membrane and thus permeation profiles can be altered by changing the compositions of the formulations applied on the skin (i.e., by changing partitioning; Figs. 2–4 [11,44,61,63,64]). The sharp rise in

Table 1 Drugs That Exhibit Azone-Induced Permeation Enhancement

Class	Compound	Ref.
Antibiotics	Clindamycin phosphate	20
	Erythromycin base	20
	Sodium fusidate	20
Antifungals	Griseofulvin	20
	Metronidazole	26
	Tolnaftate	20
Antivirals	Cytarabine	20
	Trifluorothymidine	20
	Idoxuridine	27
Anthelminthics	Thiabendazole	20
Antimetabolites	5-Fluorouracil	27, 28
Depigmenting agents	Hydroquinone	20
Corticosteroids	Amcinonide	20
	Desonide	20
	Desoximethasone	20
	Diflorasone diacetate	20
	Fluocinoline acetonide	20
	Fluocinonide	20
	Triamcinolone acetonide	20
Nonsteroidal anti-inflammatory drugs	Ibuprofen	20, 29
	Indomethacin	20, 29
Narcotic antagonists	Naloxone	30
Cardiovasculars	Amlodipine	31
	Isosorbide dinitrate	20
	Nitroglycerin	32
	Propranolol	33
Alkaloids	Dihydroergotamine	34
	Morphine	35
Sympathomimetics	Isoproterenol	36, 37
Benzodiazepines	Midazolam maleate	38
	Diazepam	38, 39

the plot of the logarithm of permeability coefficient versus alkyl chain length (see Fig. 2) is attributed to a partitioning-dependent pathway, and its slope is called the pi value. This pi value in Silastic membrane is comparable to that obtained in various skins. Therefore, enhancer effects that are related to partitioning-dependent lipoidal pathways can be better understood by comparisons of Silastic membrane data to data obtained from skin membranes.

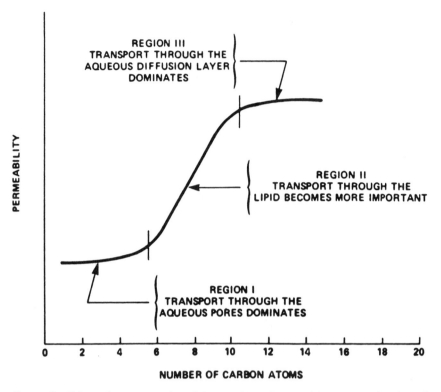

Figure 2 Schematic representation of three major pathways of drug permeation through the skin. (From [61].)

VI. PROTOCOL OF THE PRESENT STUDY

A. *Using Hairless Mouse Skin*

Permeation of [^{14}C]methanol from the following vehicles: methanol, ethanol, butanol, hexanol, octanol, and decanol, each containing Azone in 0%, 2.5%, 5.0%, 10%, 25%, and 100% concentrations.

Permeation of [^{14}C]butanol from the following vehicles: ethanol, butanol, and octanol, each containing Azone in 0%, 2.5%, 5.0%, 10%, 25%, 50%, and 100% concentrations.

Permeation of [^{14}C]octanol from the following vehicles: methanol, butanol, and octanol, each containing Azone in 0%, 2.5%, 5.0%, 10%, 25%, 50%, and 100% concentrations.

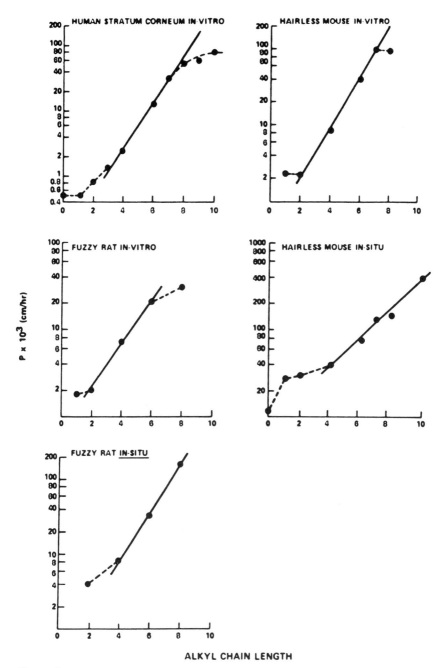

Figure 3 Plots of logarithm of permeability coefficients (*P* values) versus alkyl chain length of alkanol permeants for human (in vitro), hairless mouse (in vitro), fuzzy rat (in vitro), hairless mouse (in situ), and fuzzy rat (in situ) skins. (From [11].)

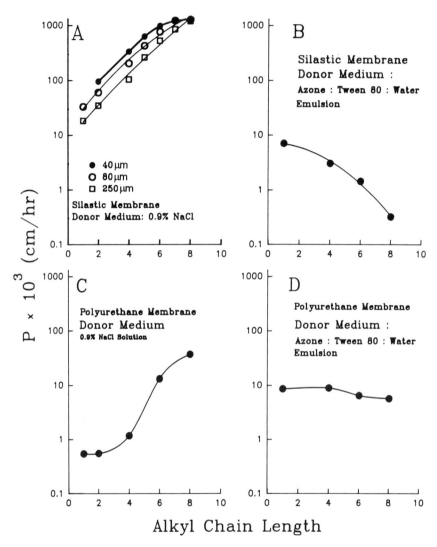

Figure 4 Plots of logarithm of permeability coefficients (*P* values) versus the alkyl chain length of alkanol permeants for (A) Silastic membrane of different thicknesses and using 0.9% NaCl aqueous solution in donor compartment, (B) Silastic membrane using Azone/Tween 80/water emulsion in donor compartment, (C) polyurethane membrane using 0.9% NaCl aqueous solution in donor compartment, and (D) polyurethane membrane using Azone/Tween 80/water emulsion in donor compartment.

B. *Using Silastic Membrane*

Permeation of [^{14}C]methanol from the following vehicles: ethanol, butanol, and octanol, each containing Azone in 0%, 2.5%, 5.0%, 10%, 25%, and 100% concentrations.

Permeation of [^{14}C]octanol from the following vehicles: methanol, butanol, and octanol, each containing Azone in 0%, 2.5%, 5.0%, 10%, 25%, 50%, and 100% concentrations.

VII. EXPERIMENTAL

All experiments were carried out in vitro. Two-compartment horizontal permeation cells were used in these studies. The membranes used were full-thickness hairless mouse skin excised from the dorsal surface of freshly killed mouse (SKH-hr-1 strain). The membrane (skin or Silastic sheeting) was sandwiched between the two identical halves of the permeation cell, and the assembled cell was placed in a constant-temperature water bath maintained at 37°C. The receptor compartment contained saline solution (0.9% NaCl), and the donor compartment contained a vehicle combination. The permeation process was monitored by sampling the receptor side and assaying it radioisotopically for the permeant concentration. The permeability coefficients were computed by plotting the receptor concentration versus time and obtaining the slopes of the apparent steady-state portions of the plots. The following equation was used for this purpose:

$$P = J/A\Delta C$$

where P is the permeability coefficient (cm/hr), J is the apparent steady-state flux (mg/hr), A is the area of the membrane (cm^2), and C is the concentration difference between the two compartments (mg/mL). Sink conditions were maintained; therefore, ΔC was taken to be equal to the permeant concentration in the donor compartment.

VIII. RESULTS

A. Hairless Mouse Skin Data

Tables 2–4 contain the experimental data on the permeability coefficients of methanol, butanol, and octanol, respectively, for hairless mouse skin studies. Data are arranged according to Azone concentration used. Azone-induced enhancement effects were calculated from these data according to the formula

Percent Azone effect =

$$\frac{\text{permeability with Azone} - \text{permeability without Azone}}{\text{permeability without Azone}} \times 100$$

Table 2 In Vitro Permeability Coefficients (*P* Values) of [^{14}C]Methanol Through Hairless Mouse Skin from Alkanol Vehicles Containing Varying Concentrations of Azone

% Azone in vehicle	*P* Values × 10³ (cm/hr) of [^{14}C]Methanol					
	Methanol	Ethanol	Butanol	Hexanol	Octanol	Decanol
0.0	45.4	4.80	79.1	245	275	132
2.5	47.0	5.01	97.6	301	295	—
5.0	69.8	7.23	109	331	283	—
10	104	13.2	114	317	232	—
25	269	261	426	306	161	101
100	379	379	379	379	379	379

This computation served to normalize the data with respect to intrinsic permeability from each of the alkanol vehicles. Tables 5–7 contain the computed Azone effect values for the permeation of methanol, butanol, and octanol, respectively.

Figure 5 is a graphical representation of methanol permeability values versus Azone concentration. Each subplot corresponds to a specific covehicle, ranging from methanol to decanol. The permeability coefficient of methanol increased with elevations in Azone concentration when methanol and ethanol were used as vehicles. A maximum was observed at 25% Azone concentration with butanol used as the vehicle. Much less of an effect was observed for permeation from hexanol where an apparent maximum at 5% Azone concentration was observed. In cases where octanol and decanol were used as covehicles, the methanol per-

Table 3 In Vitro Permeability Coefficients (*P* Values) of [^{14}C]Butanol Through Hairless Mouse Skin from Alkanol Vehicles Containing Varying Concentrations of Azone

% Azone in vehicle	*P* Value × 10³ (cm/hr) of [^{14}C]Butanol		
	Ethanol	Butanol	Octanol
0.0	0.360	2.12	20.3
2.5	0.721	2.28	29.6
5.0	2.17	2.05	28.4
10	4.17	2.06	32.3
25	20.3	3.94	34.1
50	29.6	25.4	34.3
100	28.9	28.9	28.9

Table 4 In Vitro Permeability Coefficients (P Values) of $[^{14}C]$Octanol Through Hairless Mouse Skin from Alkanol Vehicles Containing Varying Concentrations of Azone

% Azone in vehicle	P Value $\times$ 10^3 (cm/hr) of $[^{14}C]$Octanol		
	Methanol	Butanol	Octanol
0.0	0.76	0.331	0.930
2.5	1.08	0.320	—
5.0	1.48	0.210	0.960
10	3.29	0.210	0.930
25	5.04	0.160	0.901
50	3.92	0.200	0.702
100	0.862	0.862	0.862

meability values actually decreased with Azone concentration in the mixed vehicles (i.e., less than 100% Azone). When 100% Azone was used as the vehicle, methanol permeability was greater than that from any of the pure alkanol vehicles (i.e., vehicles containing 0% Azone). Figure 6 shows that the percent Azone effect was the most striking with ethanol used as a vehicle (note that the axes are *not* scaled similarly). This is due in part to the low intrinsic methanol permeability observed from pure ethanol (recall that the Azone effect calculation normalizes the data with respect to the pure alkanol vehicle). The Azone effect at any given Azone concentration generally increased with increasing covehicle lipophilicity up to a maximum alkyl chain length, with subsequent reductions thereafter. This point is graphically illustrated in Figure 7 for methanol. A

Table 5 Summary of Percent Azone Effects on the In Vitro Permeability Coefficients of $[^{14}C]$Methanol Through Hairless Mouse Skin from Alkanol Vehicles Containing Varying Concentrations of Azone

Percent Azone	Percent Azone effect with alkanol vehicles					
	Methanol	Ethanol	Butanol	Hexanol	Octanol	Decanol
0.0	0	0	0	0	0	0
2.5	3.52	4.2	23.4	23.1	7.30	—
5.0	53.7	50.0	38.2	35.4	2.69	—
10	130	175	44.3	29.7	−15.7	—
25	493	5346	438	25.1	−41.6	−23.7
100	734	7790	379	54.9	37.6	186

Table 6 Summary of Percent Azone Effects on the In Vitro Permeability Coefficients of [^{14}C]Butanol Through Hairless Mouse Skin from Alkanol Vehicles Containing Varying Concentrations of Azone

	% Azone effect with alkanol vehicle		
% Azone	Ethanol	Butanol	Octanol
0.0	0	0	0
2.5	100	7.5	45.8
5.0	503	−3.3	39.9
10	1058	−3.3	58.9
25	5700	85.4	67.8
50	8117	1099	68.9
100	7928	1264	42.4

change in lipophilicity of the vehicles brings about a substantial change in the enhancement profiles of methanol.

The permeability coefficients of butanol also increased with Azone concentration. This increase was most pronounced from ethanol vehicles, less from butanol vehicle, and much smaller from octanol vehicle (Tables 3 and 6). This observation is graphically illustrated in Figure 8. Again, as the lipophilicity of the vehicle increased, both qualitative and quantitative Azone-induced changes were observed. A substantial increase in the permeability of butanol was obtained from ethanol and butanol with Azone concentrations extending to 50%. This observation is in contrast with earlier beliefs that Azone is maximally effective at low concentrations.

Table 7 Summary of Percent Azone Effects on the In Vitro Permeability Coefficients of [^{14}C]Octanol Through Hairless Mouse Skin from Alkanol Vehicles Containing Varying Concentrations of Azone

	% Azone effect from alkanol vehicle		
% Azone	Methanol	Butanol	Octanol
0.0	0	0	0
2.5	42.4	−3.00	—
5.0	94.7	−36.4	3.2
10	333	−36.4	0
25	563	−51.5	−3.2
50	416	−39.4	−24.7
100	13.4	161	−7.31

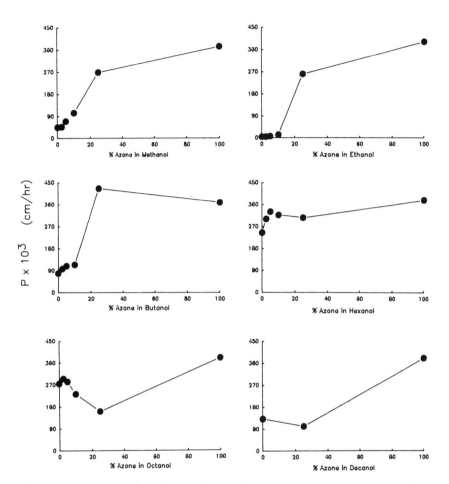

Figure 5 Plots of permeability coefficients (*P* values) versus Azone concentration in alkanol vehicles for the permeation of [^{14}C]methanol through hairless mouse skin from alkanol vehicles.

The permeability of octanol was affected by Azone in a different way (Tables 4 and 7). In the polar covehicle (methanol), one observes a significant permeation enhancement up to 25% Azone concentration and then a subsequent decrease back to baseline values at 100% Azone concentration. Azone influences in the two less polar covehicles (butanol and octanol) were almost negligible for this permeant. These effects are graphically shown in Figures 9–11. With increasing alkyl chain length of the vehicle, octanol permeation was altered much less than that observed for the permeation of methanol and butanol (Figs. 6 and 8).

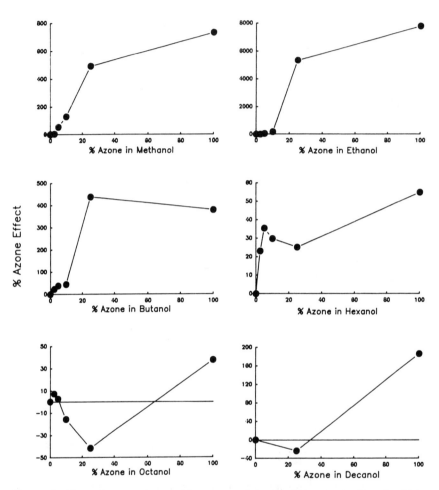

Figure 6 Plots of percent Azone effects versus Azone concentration in alkanol vehicles for the permeation of [^{14}C]methanol through hairless mouse skin from alkanol vehicles.

B. Silastic Data

Table 8 contains a summary of the permeability coefficient of [^{14}C]methanol through Silastic membrane of 250-μm thickness from ethanol, butanol, and octanol, each vehicle containing varying concentrations of Azone. The corresponding Azone effect data are tabulated in Table 9. Similar data on the permeability coefficient and Azone effects for [^{14}C]octanol are presented in Tables 10 and 11, respectively.

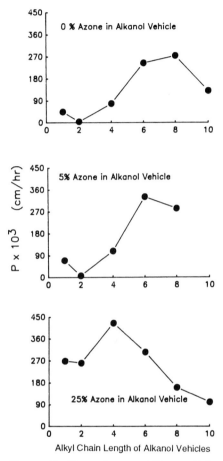

Figure 7   Plots of permeability coefficients (P values) versus alkyl chain length of alkanol vehicles for the permeation of [^{14}C]methanol through hairless mouse skin from alkanol vehicles containing varying concentration of Azone.

The data show slight enhancement of methanol permeation through Silastic membrane when ethanol was used as a vehicle (Fig. 12,13). There was a reduction in methanol permeation with Azone concentration from butanol and octanol with comparable effects observed for the two vehicles studied. The modest increase in methanol permeability with increasing covehicle lipophilicity (Fig. 14) demonstrates partitioning changes as a function of vehicle polarity for this polar permeant.

The data of octanol permeation are plotted in Figs. 15–17 in a manner similar to that used for the permeation of methanol shown in Figs. 12–14. No enhance-

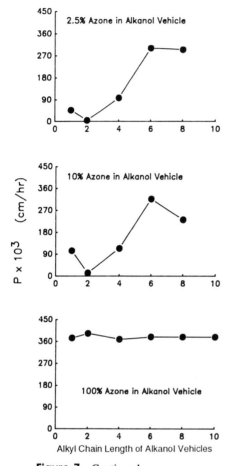

Figure 7 Continued

ment in the permeation of lipophilic permeant octanol was observed at any Azone concentration in any of the three vehicles used: methanol, butanol and octanol. Actually, the permeation of octanol decreased with increasing concentrations of Azone.

DISCUSSION

A. Polar Permeant (Methanol)

It is readily evident that the nature and magnitude of Azone-induced permeability changes observed in the skin are not reflected in the Silastic transport data

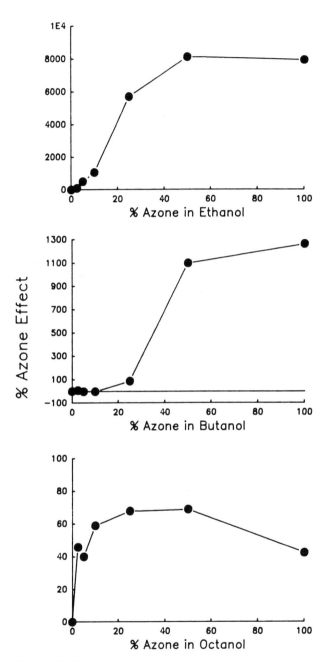

Figure 8 Plots of percent Azone effects versus Azone concentration in alkanol vehicles for the permeation of [^{14}C]butanol through hairless mouse skin from alkanol vehicles.

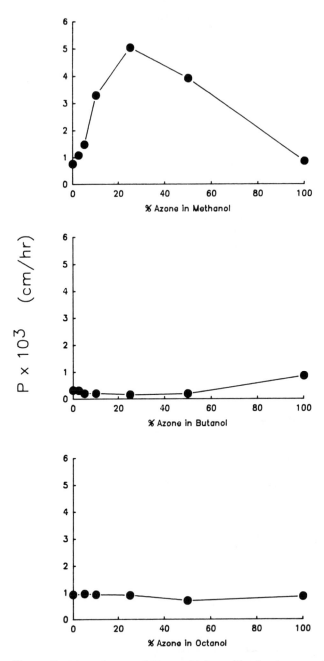

Figure 9 Plots of permeability coefficients (*P* values) versus Azone concentration in alkanol vehicles for the permeation of [^{14}C]octanol through hairless mouse skin from alkanol vehicles.

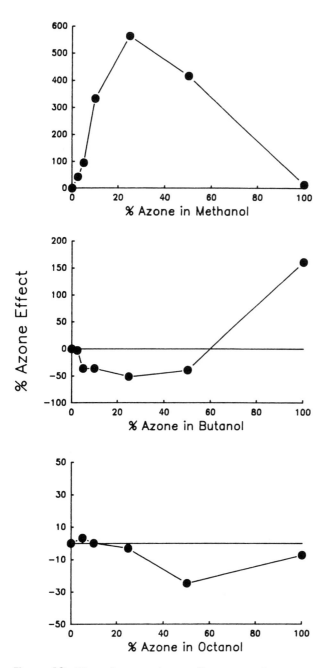

Figure 10 Plots of percent Azone effects versus Azone concentration in Alkanol vehicles for the permeation of [^{14}C]octanol through hairless mouse skin from alkanol vehicles.

Table 8 Permeability Coefficients (*P* Values) of [^{14}C]Methanol Through Silastic Membrane of 250-μm Thickness from Alkanol Vehicles Containing Varying Concentrations of Azone

% Azone in vehicle	*P* Values × 10^3 (cm/hr) of [^{14}C]Methanol		
	Ethanol	Butanol	Octanol
0.0	19.0	50.8	75.9
2.5	24.3	52.4	72.9
5.0	21.8	48.8	71.0
10	18.8	34.8	62.7
25	28.0	27.4	57.2
100	39.2	39.2	39.2

Table 9 Summary of Percent Azone Effects on the Permeability Coefficients of [^{14}C]Methanol Through Silastic Membrane of 250-μm Thickness from Alkanol Vehicles Containing Varying Concentrations of Azone

% Azone	% Azone effect; vehicle		
	Ethanol	Butanol	Octanol
0.0	0	0	0
2.5	27.9	3.14	−3.95
5.0	14.7	−3.94	−6.46
10	−1.05	−31.5	−17.4
25	47.4	−46.1	−24.6
100	106	−22.8	−48.4

Table 10 Permeability Coefficients (*P* Values) of [^{14}C]Octanol Through Silastic Membrane of 250-μm Thickness from Alkanol Vehicles Containing Varying Concentrations of Azone

% Azone in vehicle	*P* Values × 10^3 (cm/hr) of [^{14}C]Octanol		
	Methanol	Butanol	Octanol
0.0	2.39	1.61	0.961
2.5	1.91	1.53	1.03
5.0	1.75	1.21	0.831
10	1.94	1.34	0.810
25	1.37	1.15	0.694
50	1.22	0.991	0.600
100	0.551	0.551	0.551

Table 11 Summary of Percent Azone Effects on the Permeability Coefficients of [^{14}C]Octanol Through Silastic Membrane of 250-μm Thickness from Alkanol Vehicles Containing Varying Concentrations of Azone

	% Azone effect; vehicle		
% Azone	Methanol	Butanol	Octanol
0.0	0	0	0
2.5	−20.1	−5.0	7.3
5.0	−26.8	−24.8	−13.5
10	−18.8	−16.8	−15.6
25	−42.7	−28.6	−28.1
50	−49.0	−38.5	−37.5
100	−76.9	−65.8	−42.7

for this permeant. In the Silastic membrane, permeation enhancement is observed only with the most polar vehicle. This is consistent with an assumption of increasing vehicle lipophilicity as Azone is added to the covehicle, making it less favorable for the polar permeant, thus increasing its partitioning into the membrane. This effect is quite modest, with at most a doubling of the permeability coefficient. Since this influence was so slight in the most polar vehicle studied, ethanol, it is not surprising that permeability is actually reduced when Azone is added to the two less polar covehicles, butanol and octanol, where one may assume that methanol partitions to a greater extent from these neat vehicles than from pure methanol.

In contrast to Silastic data, hairless mouse skin permeability increases very dramatically with the inclusion of the enhancer in the three most polar covehicles (methanol, ethanol, and butanol). Up to 80-fold enhancement is observed, with the highest permeability coefficient occurring with relatively high Azone concentration (greater than 25%). The observation that permeation is enhanced *at all* from the butanol covehicle is indicative of a change in the membrane barrier property that greatly overshadows any vehicle-related partitioning alterations.

Considering the overall covehicle alkyl chain length effects, one observes an increase in permeability coefficient with increasing alkyl chain length up to a particular maximum n followed by a drop in permeability as n further increases (Fig. 7). The slightly elevated permeability coefficients in methanol vehicle relative to ethanol can most likely be explained by considering a skin delipidization effect caused by the methanol covehicle. This would be expected to increase the flux of a polar permeant. If Azone were acting as an inert solvent, simply altering vehicle lipophilicity (i.e., thermodynamic activity of the permeant in the vehicle), one would not expect to see reductions in the permeability coefficients

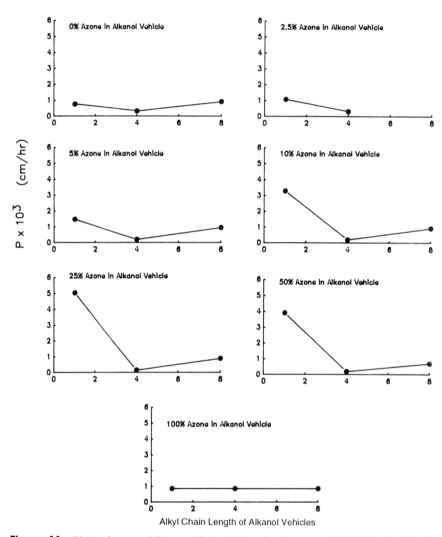

Figure 11 Plots of permeability coefficients (P values) versus alkyl chain length of alkanol vehicles for the permeation of [^{14}C]octanol through hairless mouse skin from alkanol vehicles containing varying concentrations of Azone.

with increasing covehicle chain length at any Azone concentration. One may visualize this by considering that the partition coefficient reflects methanol's affinity for the stratum corneum relative to the donor vehicle. If it is assumed that methanol's affinity for the stratum corneum is constant in these experiments (i.e., if the membrane is an inert barrier), then any change in partition coefficient

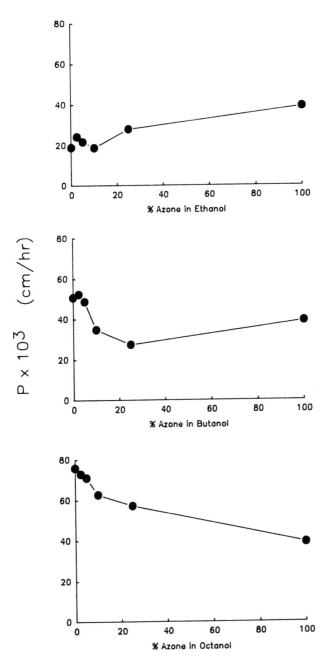

Figure 12 Plots of permeability coefficients (*P* values) versus Azone concentration in alkanol vehicles for the permeation of [^{14}C]methanol through Silastic membrane of 250-μm thickness from alkanol vehicles.

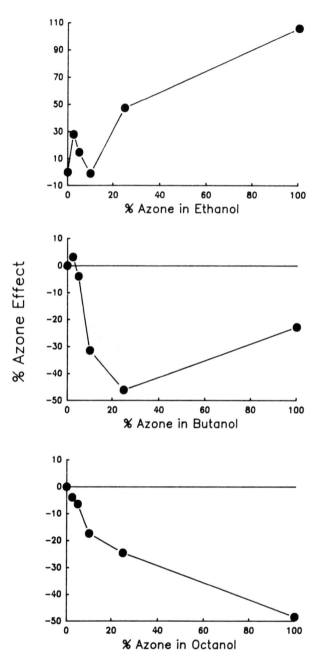

Figure 13 Plots of percent Azone effects versus Azone concentration in alkanol vehicles for the permeation of [^{14}C]methanol through Silastic membrane of 250-μm thickness from alkanol vehicles.

will be a direct result of changes in methanol's affinity for the vehicle. As the vehicle varies from polar to lipophilic (i.e., as the alkyl chain length increases), one has to assume that methanol (being quite polar) will experience a progressively reduced affinity for the vehicle with increasing alkyl chain length and thus the membrane-to-vehicle partition coefficient will steadily increase. The Silastic data in Figure 14 show the expected continuous increase in permeability with increased covehicle alkyl chain length, with the magnitude of chain length effect diminishing slightly in systems containing greater Azone concentrations.

Additionally, one sees that these enhancement maxima observed in skin occur at progressively smaller alkyl chain lengths as Azone concentration in the vehicle increases. Furthermore, for a given alkanol covehicle, the enhancement maxima generally occur at progressively lower Azone concentrations as covehicle lipophilicity increases. The permeability coefficients at these enhancement maxima tend to increase with increasing Azone concentration for a given covehicle and decreasing covehicle lipophilicity for a given enhancer concentration.

All of these observations are consistent with the concept of partitioning maximization, not only with respect to the permeant, but also considering the enhancer. Maximum methanol permeability is observed from polar vehicles at high Azone concentration, because Azone is lipophilic and increases methanol's "leaving tendency." Azone has an optimum effect at progressively lower concentrations as the vehicle's lipophilicity increases because the more nonpolar vehicles progressively reduce Azone's leaving tendency.

B. Permeant of Intermediate Polarity (Butanol)

Many of the general trends discussed above for methanol are also observed with butanol as a permeant, including

Azone-induced permeability enhancement, predominantly in more polar vehicles, and

A general increase in the permeability with alkyl chain length, with the magnitude of the effects diminishing as Azone concentration increases.

Thus, based on the data in hand, one might conclude that partitioning-related changes described for methanol similarly affect butanol permeation.

C. Lipophilic Permeant (Octanol)

Theoretical arguments concerning partition coefficient alterations with octanol are essentially the reverse of those just given for the polar permeants. That is, one expects an increasing permeant affinity for the vehicle upon either addition of Azone or increased alkyl chain length of the covehicle.

Again, assuming an inert barrier, either of these effects will reduce partitioning and therefore permeability. This behavior is, in fact, demonstrated by the

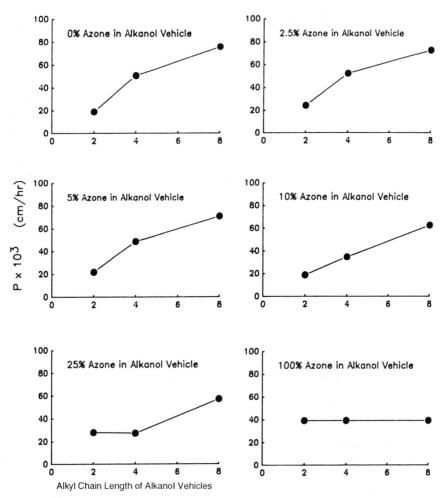

Figure 14 Plots of permeability coefficients (*P* values) versus alkyl chain length of alkanol vehicles for the permeation of [14C]methanol through Silastic membrane of 250-μm thickness from alkanol vehicles containing varying concentrations of Azone.

Silastic data. In mouse skin, comparable (albeit modest) results were obtained in butanol and octanol covehicles, whereas the methanolic solvent system shows a unique trend. The increase in permeability with Azone concentration (up to 25%) may be related to improved Azone partitioning into the barrier, thus over-shadowing slight permeant partitioning alterations. These latter thermodynamic effects may then become significant enough as Azone concentration is further increased, to negate any favorable membrane augmentations.

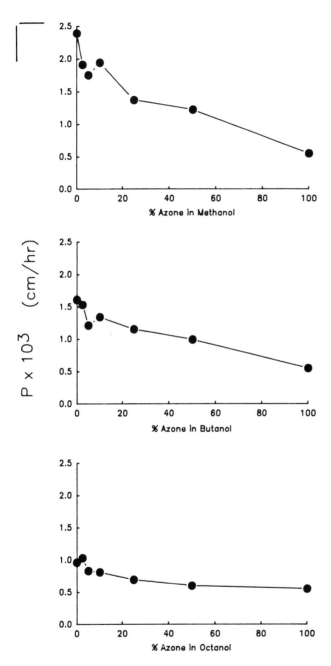

Figure 15 Plots of permeability coefficients (*P* values) versus Azone concentration in alkanol vehicles for the permeation of [^{14}C]octanol through Silastic membrane of 250-μm thickness from alkanol vehicles.

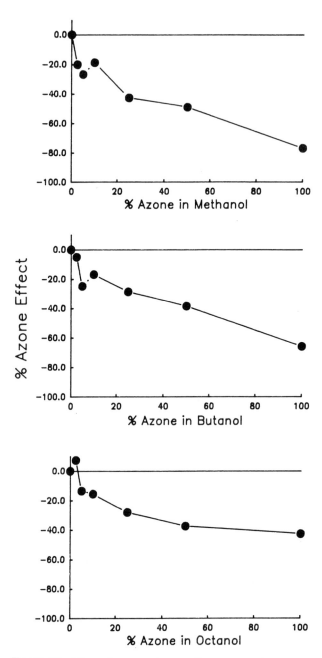

Figure 16 Plots of percent Azone effects versus Azone concentration in alkanol vehicles for the permeation of [^{14}C]octanol through Silastic membrane of 250-μm thickness from alkanol vehicles.

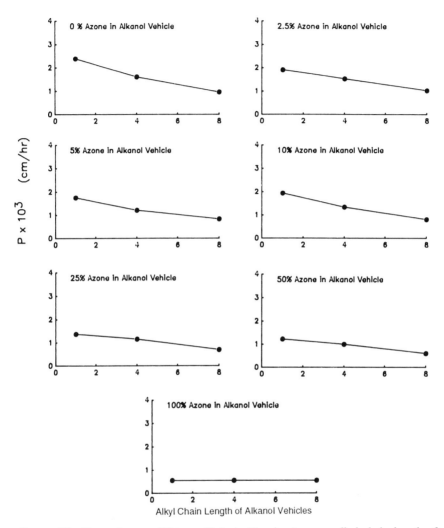

Figure 17 Plots of permeability coefficients (*P* values) versus alkyl chain length of alkanol vehicles for the permeation of [¹⁴C]octanol through Silastic membrane of 250-μm thickness from alkanol vehicles containing varying concentrations of Azone.

SUMMARY AND CONCLUSIONS

All three permeants tested in the present studies, representing a broad range of lipophilicities, showed significant Azone-induced permeation enhancement in hairless mouse skin. Maximum enhancements ranged from fivefold for the lipophilic permeant octanol to 80-fold for the more polar permeants methanol and butanol. The magnitudes of these effects were far in excess of effects observed using the synthetic membrane Silastic sheeting. The fact that enhancement maxima occurred only when more polar covehicles were used substantiates the formulation guidelines suggested by Vaidyanathan et al. [20]. These authors suggested that lipophilic formulation vehicles appear to bind Azone, thereby suppressing its enhancing ability. The data presented herein suggest a relatively straightforward partitioning alteration of both permeant and enhancer, the latter of which is presumed to directly affect Azone's ability to exert its effect on the biological barrier. While it is evident that Azone exerts a significant enhancement effect—for example, on methanol permeability in polar vehicle—it should be borne in mind that the magnitude of the maximum permeability coefficient is really not that much greater than methanol permeability from a pure lipophilic vehicle such as octanol. Perhaps, when evaluating the enhancement potential of new agents (or even old ones!) one should make comparisons not with enhancer-free controls but with vehicles that intrinsically induce maximal permeant partitioning into the barrier.

Quantitatively, enhancement effects typically increase with increases in Azone concentration, except that plateaus in permeability are not always seen. Several investigators have suggested or implied [20,33] that enhancement is a saturable process, with maximum enhancement associated with a particular optimum enhancer concentration, after which no further changes occur. It is apparent from the current study that this is not universally true and that vehicle selection plays a major role in

1. Whether or not an enhancement plateau will occur at all and
2. Producing a maximal enhancer concentration after which permeation becomes hindered.

In conclusion, the approaches presented in this study provide a useful starting point for the evaluation of the nature and extent of enhancement potential of almost any skin permeation enhancer provided it is suitably compatible (miscible or soluble) with the vehicle utilized. Many, if not most, of the currently known penetration enhancers would, in fact, be suitable for studies of this type.

REFERENCES

1. G. W. Cleary, Transdermal drug delivery, *Cosmet. Toiletries 106*, 97 (1991).
2. J. E. Shaw, W. Bayne, and L. Schmidt, Clinical pharmacology of scopolamine, *Clin. Pharmacol. Ther. 19*, 115 (1976).
3. J. E. Shaw, Pharmacokinetics of nitroglycerin and clonidine delivered by the transdermal route, *J. Am. Heart 108*, 217 (1984).
4. J. C. Findlay, V. A. Place, and P. J. Snyder, Transdermal delivery of testosterone, *J. Clin. Endocrin. Metab. 64*, 266 (1987).

5. J. P. Dubois, A. Sioufi, D. Mauli, and P. R. Imhof, Pharmacokinetics and bioavailability of nicotine in healthy volunteers following single and repeated administration of different doses of transdermal nicotine systems, *Methods Findings 11*, 187 (1989).

6. J. B. McCrea, P. H. Vlasses, T. J. Franz, and L. Zeoli, Transdermal timolol: beta blockade and plasma concentrations after application for 48 hours and 7 days, *Pharmacotherapy 10*, 289 (1990).

7. M. V. Miles, R. Balasubramanian, A. W. Pittman, S. H. Grossman, K. A. Pappa, M. F. Smith, W. A. Wargin, and M. F. Frosolono, Pharmacokinetics of oral and transdermal triprolidine, *J. Clin. Pharmacol. 30*, 572 (1990).

8. M. S. Powers, P. Campbell, and L. Schenkel, A new transdermal delivery system for estradiol, *J. Controlled Release 2*, 89 (1985).

9. S. K. Chandrasekaran, A. S. Michaels, and J. E. Shaw, Scopolamine permeation through human skin in vitro, *AIChE J. 22*, 828 (1976).

10. Y. Chien, P. Keshary, Y. Huang, and P. Sarpotdar, Comparative controlled skin permeation of nitroglycerin from marketed transdermal delivery systems, *J. Pharm. Sci. 72*, 968 (1983).

11. B. H. Idson and C. R. Behl, in *Transdermal Delivery of Drugs*, A. F. Kydonieus and B. Berner, Eds., CRC Press, Boca Raton, FL, 1987, p. 85.

12. E. Cooper in *Percutaneous Absorption: Mechanisms—Methodology—Drug Delivery*, R. L. Bronaugh and H. I. Maibach, Eds., Marcel Dekker, New York, 1985, Chapter 39.

13. R. L. Bronaugh, E. R. Congolon, and R. J. Scheuplein, The effect of cosmetic vehicles on the penetration of *N*-nitrodiethanolamine through excised human skin, *J. Invest. Dermatol. 76*, 94 (1981).

14. G. L. Flynn, W. M. Smith, and T. A. Hagen, in *Transdermal Delivery of Drugs*, A. F. Kydonieus and B. Berner, Eds., CRC Press, Boca Raton, FL, 1987, Chapter 4.

15. Y. W. Chien, in *Transdermal Delivery of Drugs*, A. F. Kydonieus and B. Berner, Eds., CRC Press, Boca Raton, FL, 1987, Chapter 7.

16. C. R. Behl, G. L. Flynn, T. Kurihara, N. Harper, W. Smith, W. I. Higuchi, N. F. H. Ho, and C. L. Pierson, Hydration and percutaneous absorption. I. Influence of hydration on alkanol permeation through hairless mouse skin, *J. Invest. Dermatol. 75*, 346 (1980).

17. M. F. Coldman, T. Kalinovsky, and B. J. Poulsen, The in vitro penetration of fluocinonide through human skin from different volumes of DMSO, *Br. J. Dermatol. 85*, 457 (1971).

18. V. Srinivasan, M. Su, W. I. Higuchi, and C. R. Behl, Iontophoresis of polypeptides: effect of ethanol pretreatment of human skin, *J. Pharm. Sci. 79*, 588 (1990).

19. B. W. Barry, in *Percutaneous Absorption: Mechanisms—Methodology—Drug Delivery*, R. L. Bronaugh and H. I. Maibach, Eds., Marcel Dekker, New York, 1985, Chapter 37.

20. R. Vaidyanathan, V. J. Rajadhyaksha, B. K. Kim, and J. J. Anisko, in *Transdermal Delivery of Drugs* A. F. Kydonieus and B. Berner, Eds., CRC Press, Boca Raton, FL, 1987, Chapter 5.

21. J. W. Wiecher, Absorption, distribution, metabolism and excretion of the cutaneous penetration enhancer azone, Ph.D. Thesis, Groningen Center for Drug Research, Bioanalysis and Toxicology Group, Univ. Center for Pharmacy, Groningen, The Netherlands, September 1989.

22. M. Katz and B. J. Poulsen, in *Handbook of Experimental Pharmacology*, B. B. Brodie and J. Gillette, Eds., Springer-Verlag, New York, 1971, p. 103.

23. R. B. Stoughton and W. O. McClure, Azone enhances percutaneous absorption, Presented at the 41st Annual Meeting of American Academy of Dermatology, New Orleans, LA, Dec. 4–9, 1982.

24. J. W. Wiechers and R. A. DeZeeuw, Transdermal drug delivery: efficacy and potential applications of the penetration enhancer Azone, *Drug Discovery Delivery 6*, 87 (1990).

25. B. W. Barry, Effect of penetration enhancers on the permeation of mannitol, hydrocortisone and progesterone through human skin, *J. Pharm. Pharmacol. 39*, 535 (1987).

26. P. K. Wotton, B. Mollgaard, J. Hadgraft, and A. Hoelgaard, Vehicle effect on topical drug delivery, III. Effect of Azone on the cutaneous permeation of metronidazole and propylene glycol, *Int. J. Pharm. 24*, 19 (1985).

27. E. Tuitou, Sink permeation enhancement by *n*-decyl methyl sulfoxide: effect of solvent systems and insights on mechanisms of action, *Int. J. Pharm. 43*, 1 (1988).

28. Y. Adachi, K. Hosoya, K. Sugibayashi, and Y. Morimoto, Duration and reversibility of the penetration-enhancing effect of Azone, *Chem. Pharm. Bull. 36*, 3702 (1988).

29. K. Sugubayashi, M. Nemoto, and Y. Morimoto, Effect of several penetration enhancers on the percutaneous absorption of indomethacin in hairless rats, *Chem. Pharm. Bull. 36*, 1519 (1988).

30. B. J. Aungst, N. J. Rogers, and E. Shefter, Enhancement of naloxone penetration through human skin in vitro using fatty acids, fatty alcohols, surfactants, sulfoxides and amides, *Int. J. Pharm. 33*, 225 (1986).

31. M. L. Francoeur and R. O. Potts, Transdermal flux-enhancing pharmaceutical compositions, U.S. Patent 86-925641, 1986.

32. H. L. G. M. Tiemessen, H. E. Bodde, H. Mollee, and H. E. Junginger, A human stratum corneum–silicone membrane sandwich to simulate drug transport under occlusion, *Int. J. Pharm. 53*, 119 (1989).

33. J. Hori, Linewar-Burk analysis of skin penetration enhancement, *J. Controlled Release 16*, 263 (1991).

34. E. M. Niazi, A. M. Molokhia, and A. S. El-Gorashi, Effect of Azone and other penetration enhancers on the percutaneous absorption of dihydroergotamine, *Int. J. Pharm. 56*, 181 (1989).

35. K. Sugibayashi, C. Sakanoue, and Y. Moromoto, Utility of topical formulations of morphine hydrochloride containing Azone and *N*-methyl-2-pyrrolidone, *Sel. Cancer Ther. 5*, 119 (1989).

36. R. C. Vasavada and R. A. Patel, Investigation of physicochemical and formulation parameters for transdermal delivery of isoproterenol hydrochloride, Proceedings of Third European Congress of Biochemistry and Pharmacokinetics, Vol. 1, 1987, p. 218.

37. R. A. Patel and R. C. Vasavada, Transdermal delivery of isoproterenol hydrochloride: an investigation of stability, solubility, partition coefficients and vehicle effects, *Pharm. Res. 5*, 116 (1988).

38. E. Touitou, Transdermal delivery of anxiolytics: in vitro skin permeation of midazolam maleate and diazepam, *Int. J. Pharm. 33*, 37 (1986).

39. C. R. Behl, J. Pei, and A. W. Malick, Sin permeation profiles of diazepam, Presented at 133rd Annual Meeting Am. Pharm. Assoc., San Francisco, CA, March 1986, Basic Pharm. Abstr. 2.

40. C. R. Behl, N. H. Bellantone, and J. Pei, Azone altered skin permeability of model compounds. Part I, Presented at 130th Annual Meeting Am. Pharm. Assoc., New Orleans, LA, April 1983, Basic Pharm. Abstr. 31.

41. N. H. Bellantone and C. R. Behl, Azone altered skin permeability of model compounds II, Presented at 31st National Meeting Acad. Pharm. Sci., Miami Beach, FL, November 1983, Basic Pharm. Abstr. 68.

42. C. R. Behl, G. L. Flynn, and M. Barrett, Hydration and percutaneous absorption. II. Influences of hydration on *n*-alkanol permeation through Swiss mouse skin: comparison with hairless mouse data, *J. Pharm. Sci. 70*, 1212 (1981).

43. C. R. Behl, M. Barrett, G. L. Flynn, T. Kurihara, K. A. Walters, N. Harper, W. I. Higuchi, and N. F. H. Ho, Hydration and percutaneous absorption. III. Influences of stripping and scalding (60 C; 60 sec) on hydration induced changes in the permeability of hairless mouse skin to water and *n*-alkanols, *J. Pharm. Sci. 71*, 229 (1982).

44. R. J. Scheuplein and I. H. Blank, Permeability of the skin, *Physiol. Rev. 51*, 702 (1971).

45. C. R. Behl, G. L. Flynn, T. Kurihara, W. Smith, O. Gatmaitan, W. I. Higuchi, N. F. H. Ho, and C. L. Pierson, Permeability of thermally damaged skin. I. Immediate influences of 60 C scalding on hairless mouse skin, *J. Invest. Dermatol. 75*, 340 (1980).

46. C. R. Behl, G. L. Flynn, K. A. Walters, E. E. Linn, Z. Mohamed, T. Kurihara, and C. L. Pierson, Permeability of thermally damaged skin. II. Immediate influences of branding at 60 C on hairless mouse skin permeability, *Burns 7*, 389 (1981).

47. G. L. Flynn, C. R. Behl, K. A. Walters, O. Gatmaitan, A. Wittkowsky, T. Kurihara, N. F. H. Ho, and W. I. Higuchi, Permeability of thermally damaged skin. III. Influences of scalding temperature on mass transfer of water and *n*-alkanols across hairless mouse skin, *Burns 8*, 47 (1981).

48. C. R. Behl, G. L. Flynn, M. Barrett, E. E. Linn, C. L. Pierson, W. I. Higuchi, and N. F. H. Ho, Permeability of thermally damaged skin. IV. Influences of branding iron temperature on the mass transfer of water and *n*-alkanols across hairless mouse skin, *Burns 8*, 86 (1981).

49. G. L. Flynn, C. R. Behl, E. E. Linn, W. I. Higuchi, N. F. H. Ho, and C. L. Pierson, Permeability of thermally damaged skin. V. Permeability over the course of maturation of a deep partial thickness wound, *Burns 8*, 196 (1981).

50. C. R. Behl, G. L. Flynn, T. Kurihara, W. Smith, N. Harper, O. Gatmaitan, W. I. Higuchi, and N. F. H. Ho, Aging and anatomical site influences on the permeation

of water and *n*-alkanols through hairless mouse skin, *J. Soc. Cosmet. 35*, 237 (1984).

51. C. R. Behl, K. A. Walters, G. L. Flynn, and W. I. Higuchi, Mechanisms of solvent effects on percutaneous absorption. I. Effects of methanol and acetone on the permeation of *n*-alkanols through hairless mouse skin, Presented at 127th Annual Meeting Am. Pharm. Assoc., Washington, DC, April 1980, Basic Pharm Abstr. 101.

52. C. R. Behl, J. Krueter, G. L. Flynn, K. A. Walters, and W. I. Higuchi, Mechanisms of surfactant effects on percutaneous absorption. I. Effects of Polysorbate 80 on permeation of methanol and *n*-octanol through hairless mouse skin, Presented at 127th Annual Meeting Am. Pharm. Assoc., Washington, DC, April 1980, Basic Pharm. Abstr. 102.

53. K. A. Walters, Penetration enhancers and their use in transdermal therapeutic systems, in *Transdermal Drug Delivery*, J. Hadgraft and R. H. Guy, Eds., Marcel Dekker, New York, 1989, pp. 197–246.

54. S. DelTerzo, C. R. Behl, and R. A. Nash, Iontophoretic transport of a homologous series of ionized and nonionized model compounds. Influence of hydrophobicity and mechanistic interpretation, *Pharm. Res. 6*, 85 (1989).

55. C. R. Behl, S. Kumar, A. W. Malick, S. DelTerzo, W. I. Higuchi, and R. A. Nash, Iontophoretic drug delivery: effects of physiocochemical factors on the skin uptake of nonpeptide drugs, *J. Pharm. Sci. 78*, 355 (1989).

56. C. R. Behl, N. H. Bellantone, and J. Pei, Effects of alkyl chain length and anatomical site on the alkanol permeability through fuzzy rat skins, Presented at 130th Annual Meeting Am. Pharm. Assoc., New Orleans, LA, April 1983, Basic Pharm. Abstr. 32.

57. C. R. Behl and N. H. Bellantone, Influence of the alkyl chain length on the in situ permeation of *n*-alkanols through fuzzy rat skins and comparisons of the fuzzy rat and the hairless mouse skin results, Presented at 31st Natl., Meeting Acad. Pharm. Sci., Miami Beach, FL, November 1983, Basic Pharm. Abstr. 38.

58. C. R Behl, S. Kumar, and A. W. Malick, Skin uptake studies: considerations and criteria for selecting an appropriate animal model, methodologies and data treatment, Presented at 1st Eastern Regional Meeting Am. Assoc. Pharm. Sci., Atlantic City, NJ, Abstr. PD 20.

59. G. L. Flynn, H. Durrheim, and W. I. Higuchi, Permeation of hairless mouse skin, II. Membrane sectioning techniques and influence on alkanol permeabilities, *J. Pharm. Sci. 70*, 52 (1981).

60. C. R. Behl, G. L. Flynn, E. E. Linn, and W. M. Smith, Influence of age, anatomical site and skin sectioning on permeation of hydrocortisone through hairless mouse skin, Presented at 127th Annual Meeting Am. Pharm. Assoc., Washington, DC, April 1980, Basic Pharm. Abstr. 100.

61. C. R. Behl, Systems approach to the study of vaginal drug absorption in the rhesus monkey, Ph.D. Thesis, Univ. of Michigan, Ann Arbor, MI, 1979.

62. B. W. Barry, Lipid-protein-partitioning theory of penetration, *J. Controlled Release 15*, 237 (1991).

63. G. L. Flynn, C. R. Behl, T. Kurihara, W. M. Smith, J. L. Fox, H. H. Durrheim, and W. I. Higuchi, Correlation and prediction of mass transport across membranes. III. Boundary layer and membrane resistances to diffusion of water and *n*-alkanols through polydimethylsiloxane (Silastic) membranes, Presented at 26th Nat, Meeting Acad. Pharm. Sci., Anaheim, CA, April 1979, Basic Pharm. Abstr. 30.

64. C. R. Behl, N. H. Bellantone, L. Dethlefsen, and A. H. Goldberg, Design of transdermal delivery systems, I. Characterization of permeability behaviours of rate controlling synthetic membranes. Evaluation of the Alkyl chain length and vehicle influences, Presented at 131st Annual Meeting Am. Pharm. Assoc., Montreal, Canada, May 1984, Basic Pharm. Abstr. 1.

8

Permeation Enhancement with Ethanol: Mechanism of Action Through Skin

S. Yum, E. Lee, L. Taskovich, and F. Theeuwes
ALZA Corporation, Palo Alto, California

I. INTRODUCTION

Ethanol is an inactive or active ingredient in numerous prescription and non-prescription drug products, particularly those for topical application. Its role has been primarily to solubilize drugs. Some topical products contain ethanol at concentrations of up to 90% [1].

Ethanol is used to enhance the permeation of drugs from products such as creams, gels, and ointments, as well as controlled-release transdermal products. For example, Percutacrine Androgenique forte, a topical solution manufactured in France for systemic testosterone therapy, contains ethanol, which appears to act as a permeation enhancer [2]. Ethanol is also an ingredient in Estraderm, a controlled-release transdermal system [3], where it substantially increases the rate of estradiol delivery through skin [4–6]. Another ethanol-containing transdermal system, which delivers fentanyl, is available for the treatment of chronic pain [7].

Ethanol has a relatively low incidence of topical reactions such as contact dermatitis [8]; even under occlusion, levels of skin irritation (mainly erythema) on human subjects are acceptable when the duration of application is short and the ethanol concentration in the formulation is low. With Estraderm applied twice weekly to different parts of the trunk, skin irritation is minimized because the controlled rate of release maintains the low ethanol concentration at the skin–system interface.

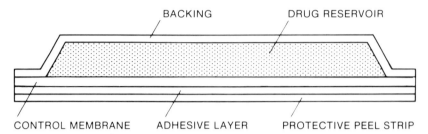

Figure 1 Schematic diagram of the form-fill-seal design of a transdermal therapeutic system.

Loss of ethanol can be nearly eliminated with a form-fill-seal design such as that used in both estradiol and fentanyl transdermal systems (Fig. 1). In this design, the drug formulation, including ethanol, is placed in a reservoir between the impermeable backing and the rate-controlling membrane, which is heat-sealed onto the periphery of the backing. The membrane is protected by a liner that is peeled off just before the system is applied to the skin.

In this chapter, we discuss the mechanism of action of ethanol as a permeation enhancer. We first provide some background, then review the literature, and finally present our own experiments that determined the effects of ethanol on the transdermal permeation of solutes having widely different ionization characteristics.

II. BACKGROUND

Skin permeation enhancers can be classified into several categories based on their physicochemical properties: (1) ionic surfactants, (2) nonionic surfactants, (3) lipid solvents, and (4) hydrogen-bonding solvents. Examples of anionic and cationic surfactants include sodium lauryl sulfate and cetyl trimethyl ammonium bromide, respectively. Decylmethyl sulfoxide is a typical nonionic surfactant, and a 2:1 chloroform/methanol mixture is an excellent lipid solvent. Dimethyl sulfoxide (DMSO) and primary alcohols with a small number of carbons are examples of hydrogen-bonding solvents.

The mechanism of action of these compounds as permeation enhancers must be considered in conjunction with an appropriate model of the stratum corneum, which is the rate-limiting barrier in mass transport processes across the skin [9]. The stratum corneum is the external layer of the epidermis, a heterogeneous structure composed of approximately 40% dead cells (keratinocytes), which are relatively polar; about 40% water; and about 20% lipids (triglycerides, free fatty acids, free sterols, and ceramides), which are nonpolar. Protein is present in both the inter- and intracellular phases, whereas lipid is concentrated largely in the

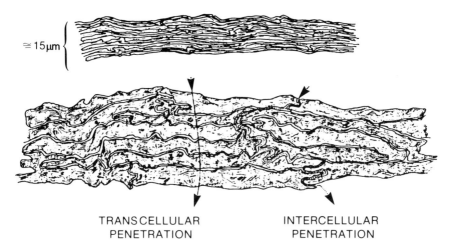

TRANSCELLULAR   INTERCELLULAR
PENETRATION   PENETRATION

Figure 2   Schematic illustration of the stratum corneum membrane. Two anatomically distinct routes of penetration are indicated. (From Ref. 10. Copyright © 1972, Appleton-Century-Crofts, Meredith Corporation, New York. Reproduced with permission from Plenum Publishing Corporation.)

intercellular phase, particularly in the continuous membranes surrounding the keratinocytes.

Elias [10] proposed a ''brick-and-mortar'' model for the normal stratum corneum in which the intercellular lipids are the mortar and the keratinized cells are the bricks. In this model, the fatty acid and other lipids surrounding the keratinocytes are the major barrier to permeation of solutes through the stratum corneum. Keratinocytes represent a minor barrier to most compounds. Elias supported his proposal with clinical evidence, such as an abnormally high transepidermal water loss when there was an essential fatty acid deficiency and abnormal cohesion of keratinocytes when there were abnormal lipids in the stratum corneum.

Molecules penetrate the stratum corneum via two distinct paths, both governed by Fickian solution–diffusion processes. One route of penetration is through the two phases in series—that is, transcellular penetration. The other pathway consists of transport solely through the lipid phase. Both routes are shown in Figure 2 [9]. Permeation enhancers could affect either or both of these routes; in other words, both intracellular protein and intercellular lipids may be physically or chemically altered by permeation enhancers.

It is generally recognized that protein denaturation or conformational changes in the keratin may contribute to enhanced permeability of the stratum corneum [11–14]. Epidermal protein can be denatured by ionic surfactants; however, the denaturation does not quantitatively correlate with changes in epidermal permeability, as demonstrated by Wood and Bettley [12], who evaluated various ionic surfactants for their ability to denature keratin of the human stratum corneum and later the barrier function of the tissue. They measured denaturation by titrating thiol groups and measured rate changes in epidermal permeation by using both sodium and potassium ions as permeants in in vitro tests. The correlation between the degree of keratin denaturation, as expressed by total thiol groups, and the increase in permeability was only qualitative and partial. Sodium lauryl sarcosinate was strongly denaturing but had minimal effect on ionic permeability in the epidermis; conversely, sodium sulfosuccinate lauric monoethanolamide had little effect on the protein but caused a major increase in ion permeability.

It was Bettley [11] who first speculated that the surfactants that denature keratin, the keratinocytes, may impair the barrier properties of stratum corneum by "opening up" the proteinaceous polar pathway. These structural changes in the stratum corneum induced by surfactants may be similar to those effected by some of the hydrogen-bonding solvents. Under certain conditions DMSO, ethanol, dimethylformamide, methanol, and propanol can expand the stratum corneum and hence increase the diffusivity of permeants in the barrier [14–18]. Moreover, Cooper [18] also demonstrated experimentally that decylmethyl sulfoxide, a nonionic surfactant, increased the permeability of ionic and polar permeants across human epidermis in vitro. He concluded that it interacts with protein to open up the polar pathway.

However, Rhein and coworkers [19] found virtually no expansion above normal hydration levels of human stratum corneum when they evaluated several ethoxylated nonionic surfactants. They observed the greatest swelling of tissue with anionic surfactants (e.g., sodium lauryl sulfate) and very little with cationics (e.g., dodecyl trimethylammonium bromide). The expansion of stratum corneum caused by surfactants increased with time, was concentration-dependent, and was partially reversible. Maximum swelling appeared to occur near the critical micelle concentration of anionic surfactants such as sodium lauryl sulfate.

Chandrasekaran et al. [16] showed in vitro that when a gradient of DMSO concentration was imposed across the skin, irrespective of its direction relative to that of a solute, the permeability of the skin to the solute was greatly increased. Microscopic examination of the skin subjected to such treatment revealed marked swelling and intercellular delamination of the stratum corneum. These authors hypothesized that these effects were due to the development of very high swelling stresses (e.g., the DMSO gradients) within the stratum corneum.

III. CONCENTRATED ETHANOL

It is conceivable that similar changes in the structure of the stratum corneum occurred in other cases, where primary alcohols (those with up to three carbons), as either highly concentrated aqueous solutions (>50 vol %) or neat liquids, were placed on one or both sides of the skin in in vitro tests [15,17,20]. In experiments with aqueous ethanol, the permeability of estradiol in hairless mouse skin deviated significantly from the classical lipid barrier model, leading to the conclusion that highly concentrated ethanol solutions induced new or activated latent "pores" [17,20]. Scheuplein and Blank [15] showed that when neat primary alcohols such as ethanol were placed in vitro on the stratum corneum side only, they could cause irreversible damage to the tissue, which in turn caused a significant increase in the permeability of relatively innocuous solutes such as butanol.

Even the osmotic stress damage caused by hydrogen-bonding solvents may be less effective for increasing skin permeability than partial or complete delipidization of the stratum corneum. A solvent mixture such as chloroform/methanol effectively removes the lipids, increasing stratum corneum permeability by several orders of magnitude compared to that of untreated tissue [14,21]. The increase in permeability is due predominantly to increased solute diffusivity in the delipidized stratum corneum. For example, the diffusion coefficient for scopolamine increased from 4×10^{-10} cm^2/sec in untreated tissue to 2×10^{-7} cm^2/sec in the delipidized stratum corneum, a 500-fold increase [21]. As expected, the delipidized stratum corneum was highly and equally permeable to both polar and nonpolar molecules [14]. Another consequence of delipidization was the reduced activation energy of diffusion of small molecules (water, propanol, and heptanol), from 10–20 kcal/mol to about 5 kcal/mol. The lowered activation energy suggests diffusion through water-filled pores in the delipidized tissue [14].

IV. DILUTE ETHANOL AND PARTITION INTO THE STRATUM CORNEUM

As with most hydrogen-bonding solvents, ethanol has a negative log octanol/water partition coefficient (log $P = -0.31$). As a small polar molecule at low concentrations, ethanol may preferentially partition into the protein phase of the stratum corneum [22].

This partition action of dilute ethanol may be similar to that of other polar solvents at low activity such as DMSO (log $P = -1.35$), dimethylformamide (log $P = -1.01$), N-methyl-2-pyrrolidone (log $P = -1.0$), and polypropylene (log $P = -1.4$) [22]. It is unclear whether dilute ethanol (<25–50 vol %) would significantly partition into the lipid region and increase its fluidity.

Increased lipid-phase fluidity, determined by differential scanning calorimetry or infrared spectrometry, has been associated with increased permeability of the stratum corneum [23]. Nonpolar compounds such as oleic acid have been found to increase lipid fluidity [22]. In addition, Ghanem et al. [17] found that dilute ethanol ($\leq$25 vol %) may increase lipid fluidity of hairless mouse stratum corneum and hence increase the permeability of β-estradiol and hydrocortisone but not polar molecules, mannitol, and tetraethylammonium bromide. As mentioned previously, Ghanem and associates proposed that highly polar molecules permeate through pores in the stratum corneum but that at 25% ethanol there are no significant new pores formed. However, at 50% ethanol, they found a significant amount of new pore formation and a corresponding increase in the permeation of mannitol and tetraethylammonium bromide. They ruled out partition effects of dilute ethanol for nonpolar solutes because their data indicated that estradiol and hydrocortisone had identical flux-enhancement ratios. They assumed that the flux-enhancement factor for estradiol should be greater than that for hydrocortisone, because the solubility of estradiol in 25% ethanol as compared to that in saline was increased more than the solubility of hydrocortisone. Therefore they concluded that the primary effects of dilute ethanol were to increase lipid fluidity and solute diffusivity in the stratum corneum.

Scheuplein and Blank [15] studied the transepidermal permeation of primary alcohols from dilute aqueous solutions (0.1 mol/liter) through human epidermis. They calculated diffusivity from the permeability coefficient of the solutes, stratum corneum thickness, and the solute partition coefficient. It is interesting to note that the diffusion coefficient values for methanol and ethanol were approximately the same as that for water. These authors [15] consider the major reason for an increase in permeability coefficient to be a change in partition coefficient, not diffusivity.

Using thermal perturbation and Fourier transform infrared (FTIR) techniques, Krill et al. [24] studied the effects of ethanol at the molecular level in the stratum corneum of the hairless mouse. They observed that ethanol decreases the transition temperature of the gel-to-liquid crystalline phase; they did not observe any changes in lipid alkyl chain structure at or below 37°C. They concluded that the flux enhancement induced by ethanol are not necessarily a result of alkyl chain fluidization, as originally suggested by Ghanem et al. [17]. These observations appear to be in agreement with the differential scanning calorimetry and infrared experimental results obtained by Golden et al. [25], who observed that there were no changes in the IR spectra and transition temperatures in porcine stratum corneum after ethanol treatment.

Several published studies strongly suggest that the enhanced partition of solutes into the stratum corneum is the primary mode of action of dilute ethanol as a permeation enhancer [26–29]. Observations common to the results of many of these studies were

1. The solubility of solutes appeared to be an exponential function of ethanol concentration in the vehicle.

2. The transdermal flux of solutes and ethanol concentration in the donor vehicle appeared to have the same relationship as solubility and ethanol concentration.
3. The increased flux of solute across the epidermis or stratum corneum seemed to be directly proportional to its concentration in the tissues, which was also increased by ethanol.
4. These linearities between solutes and ethanol or ethanol-induced solubilities ceased to exist when ethanol concentrations exceeded approximately 50 vol %, beyond which solute and concomitant ethanol fluxes started to decrease, probably due to ethanol's dehydrating effect on skin tissues.
5. The calculated diffusivities of solutes in the stratum corneum did not change appreciably in the presence of dilute ethanolic solutions.

Both nonionizable and ionizable drugs (solutes) were evaluated in these studies: estradiol [29], nitroglycerin [28], nicardipine hydrochloride [26], and an unidentified ionizable compound [27]. It seems that the linear correlations are independent of polarity or ionizability of solutes and are dependent primarily on the solubility and copartitioning of solutes in ethanolic solutions, in vehicles, and in the stratum corneum.

V. SKIN PERMEATION AND SORPTION EXPERIMENTS

We conducted a series of experiments to establish the relationship between drug solubility, both in aqueous ethanolic solutions and in human skin tissues, and drug permeation kinetics through skin. Our goals were to define the relative contributions of increased drug solubility and diffusivity for enhancing drug flux across the skin. The experiments and results are presented here along with our interpretation of the experimental data.

A. Materials

1. Human Epidermis and Stratum Corneum

Nonhairy skin sections were excised from cadavers with an electric dermatome and stored in sealed polyethylene bags at 4°C until used. The epidermis was separated from the dermis by stirring the piece of skin for 60 sec in distilled water at 60°C, after which the epidermis was gently removed with the edge of a spatula and punched out in an appropriate size. Stratum corneum samples were prepared using the trypsin digestion method, described elsewhere [16].

2. Chemicals

^{3}H[6,7-^{3}H(N)]Estradiol (NET 013), L-[4-^{3}H]propranolol (NET 515), and [1-^{14}C]ethanol (NEC-029) were obtained from Dupont New England Nuclear, as were Aquassure, 2-5-diphenyloxazole (PPO), and 2,2-p-phenylenebis(5-phenyl-oxazole) (POPOP). [N-Phenyl-U-^{14}C]fentanyl was obtained from Amersham. The purity of all radiolabeled compounds was >99%. Estradiol was obtained from Searle, propranolol from Ayerst, and fentanyl from Johnson Matthey Inc. Glass containers of neat ethanol were supplied by Gold Shield Chemical Co. Bovine serum albumin was obtained from Sigma Chemicals. Sodium phosphate monobasic and toluene (Scintillar grade) were obtained from Mallinckrodt Inc.

3. Equipment

An epidermis specimen was placed vertically in each custom-made glass permeation cell with a permeation area of 1.13 cm^2, donor compartment volume of 2 mL, and receptor compartment volume of 10 mL. Other equipment included custom-made wide-mouth Teflon screw-cap vials of 2-mL capacity, a Dubnoff metabolic shaking incubator (Precision Scientific), a thickness gauge (Teclock), a pyromagnetic hot plate stirrer (Lab Industries) with an Omega controller, an incubator, and a Nuclear Chicago scintillation counter.

B. Methods

All experiments were conducted using radioactive drugs and ethanol as tracers. Radioactive drug donors were prepared in water or nonradioactive ethanolic solutions. Nonradioactive drugs were used to prepare donors in radioactive ethanolic solutions. All samples and the corresponding specific activity standards were counted in scintillation counters. The counts were corrected to disintegrations per minute by means of established quench curve programs.

1. Drug Solubility and Preparation of Donor Solutions

Excess amounts of the solid drugs were equilibrated with the corresponding vehicle (water; 10, 20, and 30 wt % ethanol) by stirring the mixtures (in tightly sealed vials) for 48 hr at 32°C. After equilibration, aliquots of the various solutions were filtered at 32°C using custom-made microfilters. Aliquots of the weighed and diluted filtrate were counted in Aquassure fluor in a scintillation counter to determine drug solubility or ethanol concentration.

2. Determination of Ethanol and Drug Concentrations in Epidermis and Stratum Corneum

Circular pieces of human epidermis and stratum corneum (1.63 cm^2) were blotted between pieces of filter paper and transferred to a flat-bottom vial (capacity 2 mL) containing a small dialysis tubing cup. Each vial was filled with saturated drug donor solutions at different ethanol concentrations (without excess drug), and the dialysis tubing cup was filled with the drug donor solution containing a large excess of solid drug (to avoid depletion of the drug in the solution in contact with the tissue). The tightly capped vials were placed in an incubator at

32°C for 48 hr and carefully swirled three or four times each day. After equilibration, the drug or ethanol concentration in the donor solution was determined as described previously; the tissue specimens were removed and processed for the determination of ethanol or drug content.

The content of ethanol or drug in the epidermis was determined by quickly rinsing it in the corresponding nonradioactive vehicle (1–2 sec) and blotting it between two pieces of filter paper; it was then transferred to a tared scintillation vial, sealed, and weighed. To eliminate evaporation of [^{14}C]ethanol, we froze the tissues by covering the vials with dry ice; NCS tissue solubilizer was added to the frozen tissue.

3. In Vitro Permeation Experiment

Circular specimens of human epidermis were mounted on vertical permeation cells with the stratum corneum facing the donor compartment of the cell. Receptor solution (10.0 mL) was pipetted into the receptor compartment (for estradiol, 0.6% BSA in water; for propranolol and fentanyl, 0.05 M sodium phosphate monobasic). The cells were placed in the water-bath shaker at 32°C. After temperature equilibration, the donor solution (2 mL at saturation and containing excess drug) was transferred to the donor compartment. At given time intervals, all the receptor solutions were removed and replaced with equal volumes of fresh receptor solution previously equilibrated at 32°C. Aliquots of the receptor solutions were weighed in scintillation vials and counted in Aquassure fluor for drug concentrations. As in the equilibrium sorption experiments, epidermis was used from three skin donors in duplicate.

C. Results and Discussion

1. Solubility of Drugs in Aqueous Ethanolic Solution

The solubilities in aqueous ethanolic solutions of estradiol, fentanyl, and propranolol are plotted in Figures 3–5 as a function of ethanol weight percent. Regardless of drug polarity, the solubility–ethanol concentration profiles deviate from the classic log-linear relationship, a deviation that seems to become larger at ethanol concentrations of approximately 20 wt % for all three drugs evaluated. It is interesting to note that as the ethanol concentrations increased from 0 to 20 wt %, drug solubility increased by a factor of about 3–5, accelerating after concentrations of 20 wt %. The overall increase in drug solubility at 30% ethanol was approximately 20 times the value in a pure aqueous vehicle at 32°C and does not seem to depend on the drugs tested.

The increase in the slope of solubility curves may be at least partly due to an increase in the activity coefficient of drugs in concentrated ethanolic solutions [30]. The theory developed by Yalkowsky and Roseman [30], which is based on the ideal solution theory, also predicts that the slope of the semilog relation-

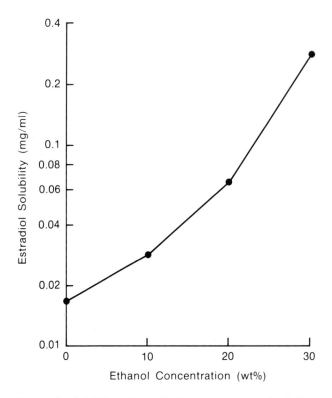

Figure 3 Solubility of estradiol in aqueous ethanol solutions versus ethanol concentration (32°C).

ship is primarily determined by the octanol/water partition coefficient of the solutes. The calculated values of log (octanol/water) partition coefficients using the fragment method [31] for estradiol, fentanyl base, and propranolol base are 4.3, 4.0, and 3.6, respectively. Therefore, it might have been predicted that the solubilization slopes for the three seemingly different drugs would be approximately the same, as shown in Figures 3–5.

The same conclusion regarding the effect of drug octanol/water partition coefficient on solubilization slopes can be obtained without invoking regular solution theory and attendant assumptions other than the linearity of the semilogarithmic relations between drug solubility and weight fraction of cosolvent. Let C_m, C_E, and C_w be the solubilities of drugs in the mixed solvents, cosolvents, and a basic vehicle such as water, and let f be the weight fraction of cosolvents. Then, because of the linearity of semilogarithmic relationships, we can define the following equation:

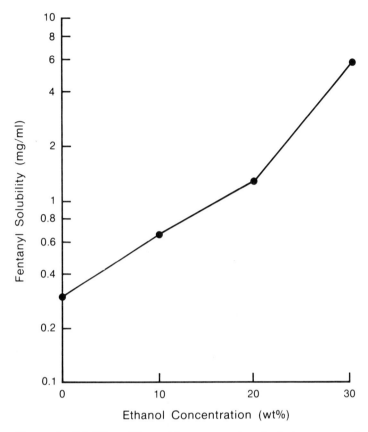

Figure 4   Solubility of fentanyl in aqueous ethanol solutions versus ethanol concentration (32°C).

$$\log C_m = f(\log C_E - \log C_w) + \log C_w \tag{1}$$

or

$$\log C_m = f \log (C_E/C_w) + \log C_w \tag{2}$$

because

$$C_E/C_w = (C_{oct}/C_w)(C_E/C_{oct}) \tag{3}$$

we get

$$C_E/C_w = P_{oct/w} (\mathbf{P}_{oct/E})^{-1} \tag{4}$$

where $P_{oct/w}$ and $P_{oct/E}$ are the octanol/water and octanol/cosolvent partition coefficients.

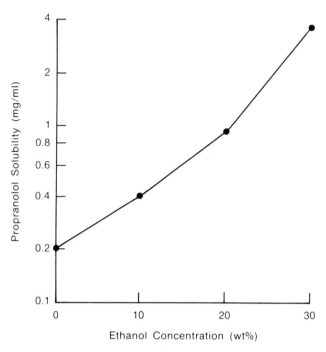

Figure 5 Solubility of propranolol in aqueous ethanol solutions versus ethanol concentration (32°C).

By substituting Equation (4) into Equation (2) for C_E/C_w, we obtain

$$\log C_m = f[\log P_{oct/w} - \log P_{oct/E}] + \log C_w \tag{5}$$

Therefore, from Equation (5), it is concluded that for given cosolvents, the slope of the semilog relationship for a group of drugs is constant if $P_{oct/w}$ of the drugs is identical, since in general $P_{oct/w}$ and $P_{oct/E}$ are directly proportional to each other [30].

In addition, for given drugs and different cosolvents, the solubilization slope is proportional to the ratio $P_{oct/w}/P_{oct/E}$; therefore the slope will be large and positive if $P_{oct/w}$ is much greater than $P_{oct/E}$. That is, for relatively lipophilic drugs such as those studied, a more hydrophobic cosolvent (such as ethanol, compared with octanol) should be more effective. Equation (5) indicates that other situations are possible, depending on the relative magnitudes of the two terms in the brackets, such as zero slope and negative slope.

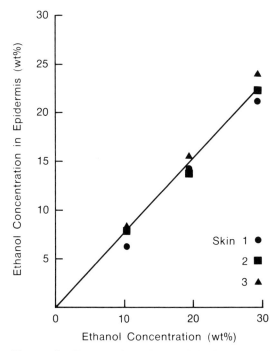

Figure 6 Concentration of ethanol in human epidermis versus its concentration in equilibration solutions containing estradiol at saturation (32°C, in vitro).

2. Equilibrium Sorption of Ethanol in Human Epidermis

In Figures 6–8, concentrations of ethanol in human epidermis are plotted against the concentration in external equilibrium solutions. The straight lines represent a regression of the data points, and the slopes do not appear to be significantly different from each other in spite of the fact that the aqueous ethanol solutions were near or at saturation with different drugs. In Figure 6, the external equilibrating solution contained estradiol; in Figure 7, fentanyl base; and in Figure 8, propranolol base. The apparent partition coefficient of ethanol between the epidermis and ethanolic solution is about 0.6–0.8, as calculated form the slopes of the lines. The partition (or slope) appears to be slightly lower at room temperature (Figure 7) than at 32°C.

3. Equilibrium Sorption of Drugs in Skin

It might be expected that drug sorption into the epidermis would follow certain patterns common to the drug solubility profile in ethanolic solutions and ethanol partitioning in human epidermis. In epidermis, the equilibrium drug concentra-

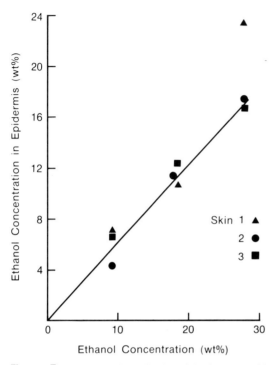

Figure 7 Concentration of ethanol in human epidermis versus its concentration in equilibration solutions containing fentanyl at 80% saturation (room temperature, in vitro).

tion for estradiol seems to be a nonlinear function of external ethanol concentration (Fig. 9). Although there are large variations in these sorption data, in one series of experiments (Fig. 9) the rate of increase in estradiol sorption with ethanol concentration appeared to follow closely the ethanol solubilization (Fig. 3). That is, sorption increased slowly up to an ethanol concentration of about 20 wt %, beyond which it accelerated. Figure 10 shows a similar equilibrium drug sorption profile for fentanyl base. However, fentanyl sorption was an order of magnitude greater than that for estradiol over the entire range of external ethanol concentrations. This was also true of estradiol and fentanyl solubilities in ethanolic solutions, as shown in Figures 3 and 4, respectively.

Figure 11 shows the equilibrium concentrations of propranolol in human epidermis at different concentrations of external ethanol. The overall profile seems to be identical to those of estradiol and fentanyl except that the concentrations of propranolol in the tissue appear to be greater than with the other two drugs.

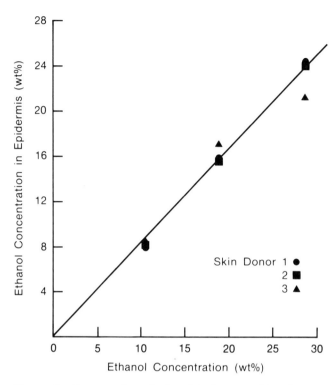

Figure 8 Concentration of ethanol in human epidermis versus its concentration in equilibration solutions containing propranolol at saturation (32°C, in vitro).

In Figures 12–14, the equilibrium drug concentrations in human epidermis and stratum corneum are compared at different concentrations of external ethanol for estradiol, fentanyl, and propranolol. The two curves are either parallel, as for estradiol, or indistinguishable from each other, as for fentanyl and propranolol. The estradiol content in the epidermis may be 50–70% higher than in the stratum corneum, which is half as thick. Because epidermis and stratum corneum samples were obtained from the same skin specimen, one would assume that their characteristics are identical. Therefore it can be said that the differences in estradiol sorption between the two tissues are due mainly to the epidermal layers. Note that the drug sorption profiles for fentanyl and propranolol in epidermis and stratum corneum are the same. It appears that for these two drugs the stratum corneum is the major drug depot and that drug sorption by the epidermal layer is not significant.

It is also interesting to note that for these drugs the slopes of the logarithm of drug sorption versus external ethanol concentrations in epidermis and/or stra-

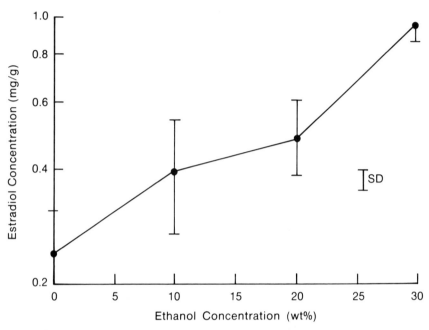

Figure 9   Equilibrium sorption of estradiol in human epidermis versus concentration of ethanol in equilibration solutions (32°C, in vitro, $n = 3$).

tus corneum appear to be of the same order of magnitude. Average slopes between 0 and 20% ethanol are about 0.03 for estradiol, 0.02 for fentanyl, and 0.01 for propranolol and are not different from the drug solubilization slopes shown in Figures 1–3 for the same ethanol concentration range.

4.   Permeation of Drugs through Human Epidermis In Vitro

The time-lag diffusion coefficient may be determined from the cumulative amount of solute permeated versus time plots, as shown in Figures 15–17 for estradiol, fentanyl base, and propranolol base, respectively. As expected, the cumulative amounts of drugs permeated through the epidermis increase with increasing concentration of ethanol in the drug donor solutions. The time-lag values for all three drugs, which are estimated by extrapolating the steady-state portions of each line to the time axes, do not appear to depend on ethanol concentrations.

The average time-lag values are about 2.1 hr for estradiol, 3.2 hr for fentanyl base, and 2.0 hr for propranolol base. Assuming that the thickness of fully hydrated stratum corneum is 30 μm and remains constant regardless of donor

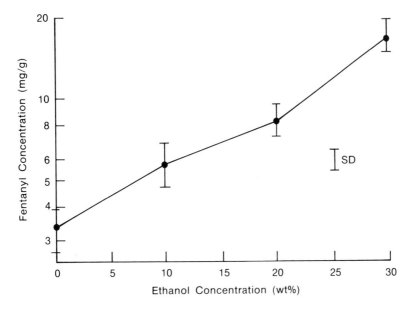

Figure 10 Equilibrium sorption of fentanyl in human epidermis versus concentration of ethanol in equilibration solutions (32°C, in vitro, $n = 3$).

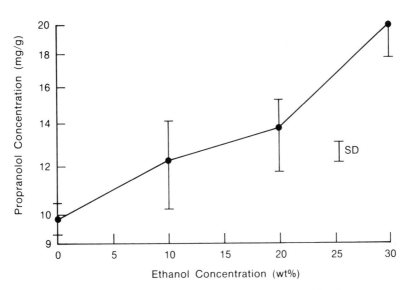

Figure 11 Equilibrium sorption of propranolol in human epidermis versus concentration of ethanol in equilibration solutions (32°C, in vitro, $n = 3$).

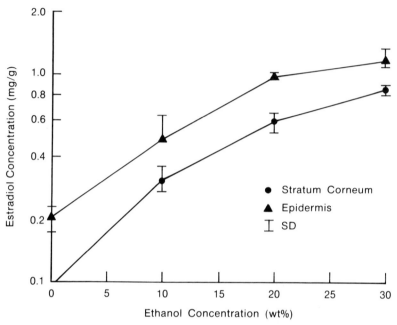

Figure 12 Equilibrium sorption of estradiol in human epidermis and stratum corneum versus concentration of ethanol in equilibration solutions (32°C, in vitro, $n = 3$).

solution, the diffusion coefficient (D) of the three drugs can be calculated using the equation

$$D = l^2/6\tau \tag{6}$$

where τ is the time lag and l the thickness.

The values of D are approximately the same—2.0×10^{-10} cm^2/sec for estradiol, 1.3×10^{-10} cm^2/sec for fentanyl base, and 2.1×10^{-10} cm^2/sec for propranolol base—reflecting the fact that these drugs have similar molecular weights. It is also possible that those properties of the stratum corneum relevant to the diffusion process of these drugs might also be identical between the epidermis specimens used. The diffusion coefficient values for the three drugs appear to be in agreement with the values for relatively small molecules such as alkanols [32] and scopolamine [16].

From the steady-state portions of the cumulative amount of permeated drug versus time plots in Figures 15–17, we can calculate approximate steady-state drug fluxes at different ethanol concentrations. Figures 18–20 show steady-state flux through human epidermis as a function of ethanol concentration for estra-

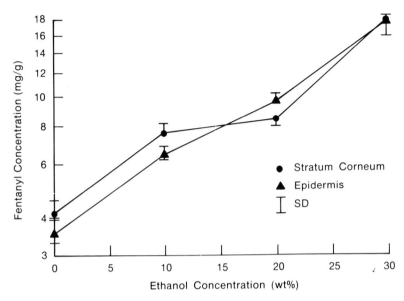

Figure 13 Equilibrium sorption of fentanyl in human epidermis and stratum corneum versus concentration of ethanol in equilibration solutions (32°C, in vitro, $n = 3$).

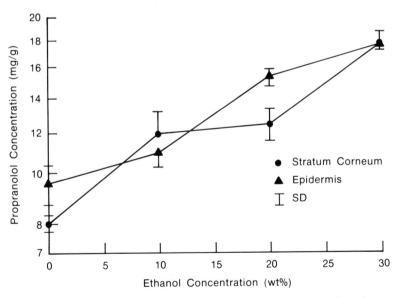

Figure 14 Equilibrium sorption of propranolol in human epidermis and stratum corneum versus concentration of ethanol in equilibration solutions (32°C, in vitro, $n = 3$).

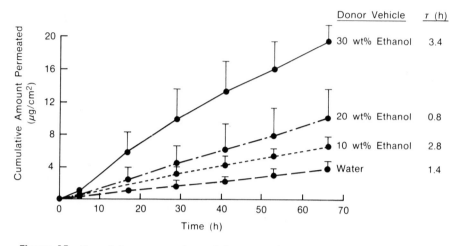

Figure 15 Cumulative amount of estradiol permeated through human epidermis (32°C, in vitro).

diol, fentanyl, and propranolol, respectively. It appears that plots of log (drug flux) versus ethanol concentration are linear over the entire range of ethanol concentrations. Approximate values of the slope are 0.02 for these drugs, and they do not change significantly with increasing ethanol as do the drug solubilities in the ethanolic solutions (Figs. 3–5).

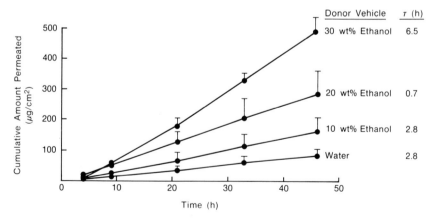

Figure 16 Cumulative amount of fentanyl permeated through human epidermis (32°C, in vitro).

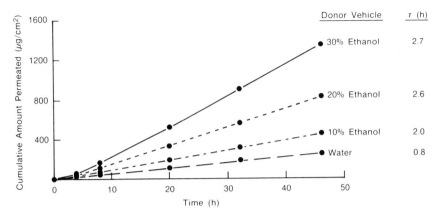

Figure 17 Cumulative amount of propranolol permeated through human epidermis (32°C, in vitro).

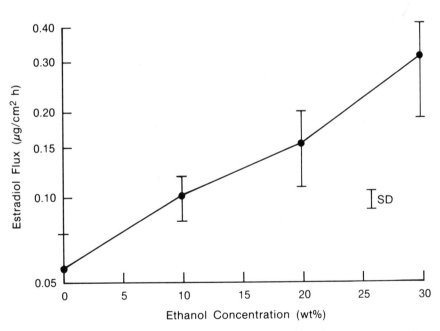

Figure 18 Steady-state flux of estradiol through human epidermis versus concentration of ethanol in donor solutions (32°C, in vitro, $n = 3$).

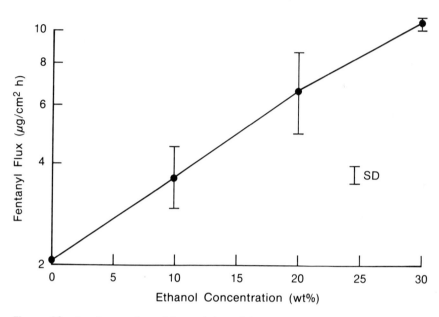

Figure 19 Steady-state flux of fentanyl through human epidermis versus concentration of ethanol in donor solutions (32°C, in vitro, $n = 3$).

The rates of flux enhancement and increased drug solubility and permeation characteristics due to dilute ethanol seem to be essentially identical for the three drugs. The implication is that enhancement of flux may be due to increased drug solubility in the stratum corneum. If we assume that this is the case for the drugs studied, it follows from Fick's law of diffusion that

$$J/J_0 = C/C_0 \tag{7}$$

where J and J_0 are drug flux and C and C_0 are drug solubility, with and without ethanol, respectively.

Two assumptions are made for Equation (7): (1) The thickness of stratum corneum with and without dilute ethanol is constant and (2) the diffusion coefficient of drugs in the stratum corneum is also constant. These two assumptions can be replaced by a single assumption: the ratio of diffusion coefficient to stratum corneum thickness is constant. Any significant deviation from Equation (7) will mean that the diffusivity/thickness ratio has been affected by ethanol or drug or both.

C/C_0 and J/J_0 can be calculated from Figures 9–11 and Figures 18–20, respectively, at ethanol concentrations of 10, 20, and 30 wt%. Figures 21–23 are the plots of J/J_0 versus C/C_0 for estradiol, fentanyl, and propranolol, respectively.

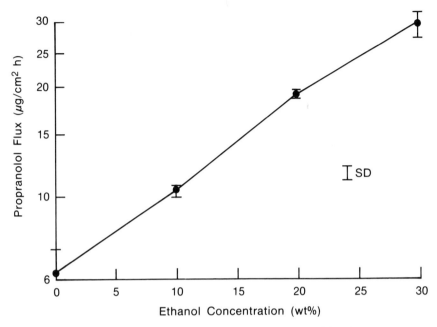

Figure 20 Steady-state flux of propranolol through human epidermis versus concentration of ethanol in donor solutions (32°C, in vitro, $n = 3$).

All the data points in these figures are positive deviations from Equation (7), indicating that the D/l ratio is not constant at all concentrations of ethanol but rather increases with ethanol concentration.

For estradiol and fentanyl (Figs. 21 and 22), the maximum deviations from Equation (7) are approximately $+40\%$, indicating that increased drug solubility in the stratum corneum (C/C_0) enhances drug flux more than expected from constant D/l. The greater deviations occurred with ethanolic solutions saturated with propranolol (Fig. 23). The magnitude of the positive deviations—about 60–70%—may result from unique properties of either propranolol or the ethanolic solution of propranolol. There is a trend toward increasing positive deviations with increasing ethanol concentration regardless of drug.

The increase in the D/l ratio may be due primarily to the increase in D, because the reduction in l due to dehydration by ethanol should entail a proportional decrease in D; thus the ratio should remain constant. It would be interesting to determine if the increase in D results from either minor expansion of the stratum corneum or delipidization or both. It is unlikely that the aqueous ethanol solutions of 10–30 wt% would significantly remove stratum corneum lipids. A factor of 40–70% change in the drug diffusion coefficient may not be

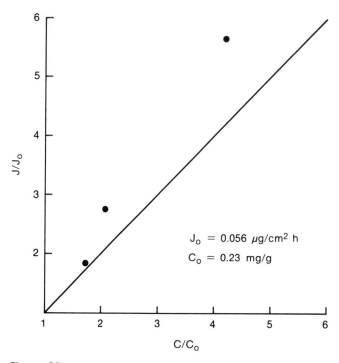

$J_o = 0.056$ $\mu g/cm^2$ h
$C_o = 0.23$ mg/g

Figure 21 Flux-enhancement ratio of estradiol versus increased drug solubility in human epidermis in the presence of ethanol (32°C, in vitro).

easily detected by the time-lag method. In Figures 15–17, the time-lag values corresponding to 30 wt% ethanol are the largest, indicating that the corresponding diffusion coefficient would be the smallest. This contradiction between the time-lag diffusivity and the apparent increase in steady-state diffusivity, which resulted in the deviation from Fick's law of diffusion, points to the difficulties involved in accurately determining time-lag diffusivities.

VI. A MATHEMATICAL MODEL FOR THE EFFECTS OF ETHANOL ON DRUG CONCENTRATION AND FLUX

As mentioned previously, the semilogarithmic plots of drug solubility versus ethanol concentration are nearly linear up to about 20 wt% ethanol. Similar relationships between drug solubility in epidermis (or stratum corneum) and ethanol concentration exist for the three drugs studied (Fig. 9–14). For example, if C_E is the solubility of drug in pure ethanol and f' is the ethanol weight fraction

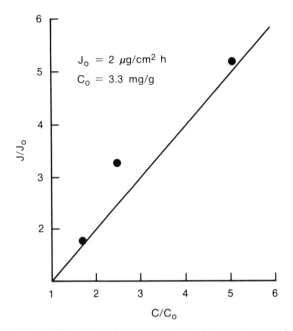

Figure 22 Flux-enhancement ratio of fentanyl versus increased drug solubility in human epidermis in the presence of ethanol (32°C, in vitro).

in skin tissue, there is a semilogarithmic relationship for drug solubility in tissue (C) in the presence of ethanol:

$$\log C = f'(\log C_E - \log C_0) + \log C_0 \qquad (8)$$

where C_0 is the drug solubility in tissue in the absence of ethanol. Equation (8) can be simplified to

$$C/C_0 = (C_E/C_0)^{f'} \qquad (9)$$

Combining Equations (7) and (9), we obtain

$$J/J_0 = (C_E/C_0)^{f'} \qquad (10)$$

From Equation (10) we can calculate the ratio of drug flux enhancement (J/J_0), which will increase by a power function of f'. The values of f' range from 0 to nearly 1, depending on the concentration of ethanol. Figures 6–8 show approximate f' values of 0, 0.08, and 0.15 at external ethanol weight fractions of 0, 0.1, and 0.20 almost regardless of the saturated drugs used in these ethanolic solutions. The drug solubilities in pure ethanol (C_E) are 30 mg/mL for estradiol, 900 mg/mL for fentanyl base, and 300 mg/mL for propranolol base. The C_0

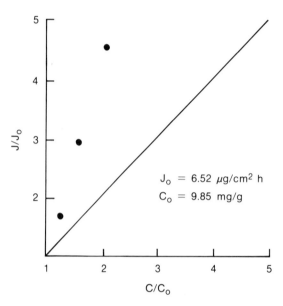

Figure 23 Flux-enhancement ratio of propranolol versus increased drug solubility in human epidermis in the presence of ethanol (32°C, in vitro).

values, as listed in Figures 21–23, are 0.23, 3.30, and 9.85 mg/g for estradiol, fentanyl, and propranolol. Therefore the values for the C_E/C_0 ratio for estradiol, fentanyl, and propranolol are 130, 273, and 30, respectively.

From Equation (10) and these values for the C_E/C_0 ratio and f', we can calculate J/J_0 values and compare them against the actual values shown in Table 1. The calculated J/J_0 values are lower than the actual values for all ethanol concentrations (X). This discrepancy resulted from two assumptions: (1) that

Table 1 Comparison of Predicted Versus Actual J/J_0

Drugs	X	f'	$(J/J_0)_{calc}$	$(J/J_0)_{act}$
Estradiol	0.1	0.08	1.5	1.8
	0.2	0.16	2.2	2.8
Fentanyl	0.1	0.08	1.6	1.6
	0.2	0.16	2.5	3.3
Propranolol	0.1	0.08	1.3	1.6
	0.2	0.16	1.7	2.9

X, external ethanol weight fraction; f', weight fraction of ethanol in tissue; $(J/J_0)_{calc}$, calculated values of J/J_0; $(J/J_0)_{act}$, actual values of J/J_0.

there was a semilogarithmic relationship between drug concentration in tissue and external ethanol concentration [Eq. (8)] and (2) that the D/l ratio in Fick's law of diffusion is constant for a given drug at all ethanol concentrations. The latter assumption appears to have weighted the outcome more than the former.

The agreement between prediction and actuality is better at 10 wt% ethanol than at 20%. At the higher concentration, the difference is greater—about 30% for estradiol and fentanyl, which is still fairly good agreement, but about 70% for propranolol, indicating a limitation of the mathematical model, which assumes a constant D/l ratio. For the propranolol-ethanol solutions this assumption appears to be invalid.

VII. CONCLUSIONS

Concentrated aqueous ethanol solutions can alter the structure of the stratum corneum in ways that appreciably increase solute diffusivity. The mechanisms by which ethanol induces damage and thereby elicits microstructural changes and increased diffusivity are not fully understood. Lipid extraction and osmotic expansions may be the most plausible explanations.

With dilute ethanolic solutions, ethanol appears primarily to increase drug solubility in the epidermis; its effect on solute diffusivity seems to be relatively small. This drug-partitioning effect may operate equally well for neutral and ionizable molecules. The octanol/water partition coefficient of solutes can be used as a measure by which ethanol's effectiveness may be estimated.

Acknowledgments We are grateful to Mrs. Jacqueline Shapiro for editorial work, to Mr. Greg Sawin for final editorial and art work, and to Ms Suanne Starner for typing this manuscript.

REFERENCES

1. W. Parker, *Am. J. Drug Alcohol Abuse 9*(2), 195–209 (1982).
2. J. C. Soufir et al., *Acta Endocrinol. 102*, 625–632 (1983).
3. *Physicians' Desk Reference*, 44th ed., Medical Economics Co., 1990, p. 853.
4. L. Laufer, J. DeFazio, J. Lu, D. Meldrum, P. Eggene, M. Sambhi, J. Hershman, and H. Judd, *Am. J. Obstet. Gynecol. 146*(5), 533–540 (1983).
5. W. Good, M. Powers, and P. Campbell, *J. Controlled Release 2*, 89–97 (1985).
6. P. Campbell and S. K. Chandrasekaran, U.S. Patent 4,379,454 (assigned to ALZA Corporation, 1983).
7. R. Caplan and M. Southam, *Adv. Pain Res. Therapy 14*, 233–40 (1990).
8. C. Drevets and P. Seebohm, *J. Allergy 32*(4), 277–282 (1961).
9. R. J. Scheuplein, in *Advances in Biology of Skin*, Vol. 12, *Pharmacology and the Skin*, S. Montagna, E. J. Van Scott, and R. B. Stoughton, Eds., Appleton-Century-Crofts, New York, 1972, p. 135.
10. P. M Elias, *J. Invest. Dermatol. 80*(6)S, 445–495 (1983).

11. F. R. Bettley, *Br. J. Dermatol.* *77*, 98–100 (1965).
12. D. C. F. Wood and F. R. Bettley, *Br. J. Dermatol.* *84*, 320–325 (1971).
13. J. Scala, D. E. McOsker, and H. H. Reller, *J. Invest. Dermatol.* *50*(5), 371–379 (1968).
14. R. Scheuplein and L. Ross, *J. Soc. Cosmet. Chem.* *21*, 853–873 (1970).
15. R. S. Scheuplein and I. H. Blank, *J. Invest. Dermatol.* *60*(5), 286–296 (1973).
16. S. D. Chandrasekaran, P. S. Campbell, and A. S. Michaels, *AIChE J.* *23*(6), 810–816 (1977).
17. A.-H. Ghanem, H. Mahmoud, W. I. Higuchi, U. D. Rohr, S. Borsadia, P. Liu, J. Fox, and W. Good, *J. Controlled Release 6*, 75–83 (1987).
18. E. Cooper, in *Solution Behavior of Surfactants: Theoretical and Applied Aspects*, Vol. 2, K. L. Mittel and E. J. Fendler, Eds., Plenum, New York, 1982.
19. C. Rhein, C. Robbins, K. Ferner, and R. Cantore, *J. Soc. Cosmet. Chem. 37*, 135–139 (1986).
20. W. Higuchi, U. D. Rohr, S. A. Burton, P. Liu, J. Fox, A. Ghanem, H. Mahmoud, S. Borsadie, and W. Good, in *Controlled-Release Technology, Pharmaceutical Applications* (ACS Symp. Ser. 348), P. Lee and W. Good, Eds., American Chemical Society, Washington, DC, 1987, pp. 232–240.
21. S. K. Chandrasekaran, P. Campbell, and T. Watanabe, *Polym. Eng. Sci. 20*(1), 36–39 (1980).
22. B. Barry, *J. Controlled Release 6*, 85–97 (1987).
23. K. Knutson, R. Pott, D. Guzele, G. Dolden, W. Lambert, J. McKie, and W. Higuchi, *J. Controlled Release 2*, 67–87 (1985).
24. S. Krill, K. Knutson, and W. Higuchi, *Pharm. Res. 5*(10), S129 (1988).
25. G. Golden, J. McKie, and R. Potts, *J. Pharm. Sci. 76*(1), 25–28 (1987).
26. T. Seki, K. Sugibayashi, and Y. Morimoto, *Chem. Pharm. Bull. 35*(7), 3054–3057 (1987).
27. S. Yum, E. Lee, L. Taskovich, and F. Theeuwes, *Proc. Int. Symp. Controlled Release Bioact. Mater. 14*, 103–104 (1987).
28. B. Berner, G. Massenga, J. Otte, and R. Steffens, *J. Pharm. Sci. 78*(5), 402–407 (1989).
29. L. Pershing, L. Lambert, and K. Knutson, *Pharm. Res. 7*(2), 170–175 (1990).
30. S. H. Yalkowsky and T. J. Roseman, in *Techniques of Solubilization of Drugs*, S. H. Yalkowsky, Ed., Marcel Dekker, New York, 1981, pp. 91–134.
31. C. Hansch and A. Leo, *Substituent Constants for Correlation Analysis in Chemistry and Biology*, Wiley, New York, 1979, Chapter 4, p. 18.
32. R. Scheuplein and I. Blank, *Physiol. Rev. 51*(4), 702–747 (1971).

9

Liposomes as Penetration Promoters and Localizers of Topically Applied Drugs

Michael Mezei
College of Pharmacy, Dalhousie University, Halifax,
Nova Scotia, Canada

I. INTRODUCTION

There are two ways to improve chemotherapy: to discover new and better drugs and/or to develop new controlled, site-specific drug delivery systems. The emphasis in pharmaceutical research efforts is on developing new drug delivery systems that enhance the efficacy and safety of existing drugs. Some of the newly developed drugs (e.g., peptides, immunotoxins) require novel delivery because of their chemical instability, potency, and inability to penetrate biological membranes. Attempts are being made to develop (1) controlled-release delivery systems and (2) selective (drug-targeting) delivery systems.

Drug targeting is one of the most exciting areas of pharmaceutical research and perhaps the most challenging. The aim is to deliver the drug to the target organ, the site of action, and minimize the distribution of the drug to nontarget tissues. Some organs (skin, eye, lungs, and body cavities) are directly accessible; consequently, if local activity is desired, one can expect to achieve drug targeting by applying the drug topically to these organs. Unfortunately, the problem is not that simple. In many cases the drug may penetrate the organs with ease, but it may be quickly removed by the blood and/or lymph systems, which may lead to systemic rather than the desired local action.

The realization of this led to a new route of drug administration, i.e., transdermal drug delivery, where the skin is viewed as a new portal of entry for drugs intended for systemic activity. Consequently, topical application of a drug may be used for both dermal and transdermal delivery to induce local or systemic activity.

In formulation of topical dosage forms, attempts are being made to design new vehicles containing penetration promoters, or to use drug carriers to ensure adequate penetration and/or localization, to prolong the residence time of the drug within the particular organ in order to enhance local effects and minimize systemic effects, or to ensure adequate percutaneous absorption to produce a desired systemic effect.

The principal factors involved in the localization or absorption of substances are (1) the properties of the drug, (2) the vehicle, and (3) the tissue of the site of application.

In biopharmaceutical terms, the rate and extent of absorption and disposition of the drug are determined by the physical and chemical nature of each of the above components and their collective interaction.

Much attention has been focused on altering these factors in an attempt to make drug delivery selective (1) to the skin surface, (2) into the epidermis and/ or dermis to induce local effects only, or (3) through the skin for the purpose of eliciting a local effect within subcutaneous tissues (such as in rheumatic joints) or producing a systemic effect in internal organs.

Penetration of the drug into or through the skin is obviously essential in both dermal and transdermal drug delivery.

II. STRUCTURE AND FUNCTION OF THE SKIN

Figure 1 shows the various layers through which a drug must pass to reach the blood vessels and thus be absorbed and possibly have a systemic effect. The first zone is a surface film of emulsified lipids (sebum, ''acid mantle''), under which lie the stratum corneum (horny layer), the viable epidermis, and finally the dermis in which the blood vessels are located.

The lipid composition of the epidermal layers is rather complex [1]. The main components of the stratum corneum lipids are ceramides and fatty acids; phospholipids cannot be found in this layer [2]. The basal layer, however, contains a high proportion of phospholipids (e.g., phosphatidylcholine, phosphatidylethanolamine, sphingomyelin). The granular layer has smaller phospholipid and higher ceramide content; it has a transient composition between the stratum corneum and the basal layer. The common feature of these epidermal layers is the presence of intercellular lipid material, which is also able to form bilayers [3]. It has been proposed that this intercellular lipid is the majority permeability barrier [4–6].

The primary function of the skin is to serve as a protective organ. It protects the underlying tissues from mechanical, chemical, and radiation-induced injuries and from invasion by pathogenic organisms. Consequently, the epidermis is an

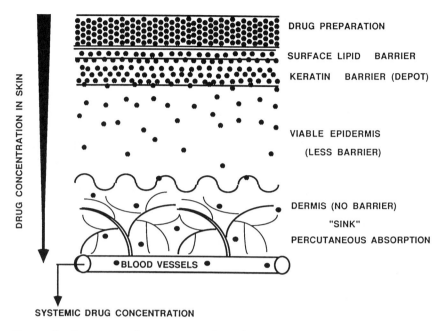

Figure 1 Cutaneous and percutaneous absorption.

effective barrier to the penetration of a whole variety of substances including drugs. The skin is also an important organ with respect to metabolism and immunology—both could serve the barrier function.

The skin has many other functions. It plays an important role in regulating body temperature and serves as an excretory organ through the sweat and sebaceous glands. Because of its sensory nerve endings it also serves as an organ of perception for touch, pain, temperature, pressure, and pleasant, sensual contact. The skin is also an organ of identity that gives rise to the hair patches, odors, and shades of color characteristic of each person and an organ of expression by way of blushing, blanching, and sweating.

The skin is therefore much more than a barrier layer. It is one of the most inhomogeneous organs of the body; it has components of many different tissues, including blood vessels, glands, nerves, smooth muscle, connective tissues, and fat. Owing to this diversity in structure and function, in vitro tests for dermal and transdermal delivery cannot provide reliable results because in vivo conditions cannot be maintained in excised or dead tissue. Moreover, human skin differs biochemically from that of test animals; and consequently even in vivo animal test results may be not relevant to clinical situations.

III. CUTANEOUS AND PERCUTANEOUS ABSORPTION

Cutaneous absorption is the penetration of a drug into various layers of the skin. *Percutaneous* or *transdermal absorption* refers to the passage of medicinal substances from the outside into and through the skin into the bloodstream.

One of the most debated areas of skin research is the mode of penetration of various substances into or through the skin. Several review articles [7–9] discuss the various theories and experimental data related to cutaneous and percutaneous absorption. The permeability barrier function of the epidermis is attributed to the basal layer, the stratum compactum [10], and the outermost layer of the skin, the stratum corneum [3,11]. The more recently accepted theory is that the polar and nonpolar lipids arranged in lamellar bilayers in the stratum corneum interstices are responsible for the barrier function [12–15].

Elias [16] proposed a pathway for percutaneous absorption through intercellular lipid-rich channels. Hadgraft [17] proposed a number of routes for transport of molecules through the skin. If one changes the physicochemical properties of a drug, one can expect different diffusion capability across the skin. The main pathway of penetration is through the epidermis, either through the cells or between them; another pathway through the hair follicles or the sweat or sebaceous glands can also exist. Although the epidermis presents a surface area 100–1000 times greater than these glands and hair follicles, we could assume that under special conditions the sweat glands or sebaceous glands may be a preferential pathway for certain drugs: for example, lipid-soluble substances may move through the sebaceous glands and polar compounds through the sweat glands. The transfollicular pathway might be an important "shunt" [18]. A more detailed review and discussion of percutaneous absorption can be found in other chapters of this book.

IV. DERMAL DRUG DELIVERY

In treating skin diseases the primary purpose of applying drugs to the skin is to induce local effects at or very close to the site of application. In such cases cutaneous absorption is desirable, but percutaneous absorption is not.

Progress in pharmaceutical technology has provided novel dermatological vehicles. Most of these new vehicles can influence the release and, to some extent, penetration of the active ingredient, but once the drug is released the vehicle no longer influences its fate. With conventional vehicles there is no effective way to limit or control percutaneous absorption. In cases of long-term and extensive treatment, with the presently available topical dosage forms (especially if penetration-promoting agents are included in the formula), percutaneous absorption may lead to unintended systemic and toxic effects with some drugs (e.g., corticosteroids, cytotoxic agents, salicylates, phenolics, and heavy metal-containing and other compounds).

For dermato-pharmacotherapy we need to develop a selective drug delivery system that enhances penetration of the active ingredient into the skin, localizes the drug at the site of action, and reduces percutaneous absorption. In the newer drug delivery systems, a special vehicle or, more often, a drug carrier controls or influences the pharmacokinetic fate of the active ingredient. Among a variety of drug carriers, liposomes seem to have the best potential.

V. LIPOSOMES AS DRUG CARRIERS

Liposomes are microscopic vesicles composed of membranelike lipid layers surrounding aqueous compartments. The lipid layers are made up mainly of phospholipids. Phospholipids are amphiphilic; they have a hydrophilic head and a lipophilic tail. In aqueous solution they are arranged in bilayers, which form closed vesicles like artificial cells. In the bilayer, the fatty acid tails, being nonpolar, are located in the membrane's interior, and the polar heads point outward.

A single bilayer enclosing an aqueous compartment is referred to as a unilamellar lipid vesicle; according to its size it is known as a small unilamellar vesicle (SUV) or a large unilamelar vesicle (LUV). If more bilayers are present, liposomes are referred to as multilamellar vesicles (MLVs) (Fig. 2).

Depending on their composition, liposomes can have positive, negative, or neutral surface charge. Depending on the lipid composition, method of preparation, and the nature of the encapsulated agent, many types of liposomal products can be formulated.

A. Liposome Constituents

The major components of liposomes are lipids (mainly phospholipids and cholesterol), water, drug, electrolytes, and possibly antioxidants, preservatives, and viscosity-inducing agents.

Most liposomes are prepared by using phosphatidylcholine, lecithin of egg or vegetable (soybean) origin. For investigatory purposes, synthetic phospholipids such as dipalmitoyl phosphatidylcholine might be used, but for large-scale production the price of synthetic lipids is prohibitive. In our biocompatibility studies [19], the hydrogenated soy lecithin provided the best results. Since liposomes are made up of substances similar to cell membranes it is assumed that they are biocompatible and biodegradable preparations. Almost any type of drug can be encapsulated into liposomes; owing to their biphasic nature (lipid and water) both lipophilic and hydrophilic ingredients are accommodated according to their solubility in the liposome components.

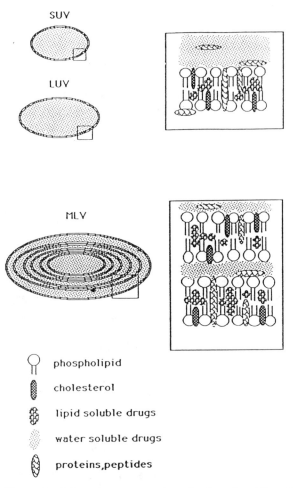

SUV

LUV

MLV

phospholipid

cholesterol

lipid soluble drugs

water soluble drugs

proteins,peptides

Figure 2 Schematic representation of uni- and multilamellar liposomes containing lipophilic and/or hydrophobic biologically active ingredients.

Cholesterol is usually included in the formula to stabilize the liposomal membrane and to minimize leaching out of the encapsulated water-soluble drug. Electrolytes are used to enhance the lipid bilayer formation and to provide isotonicity.

In the case of topically applied liposomes it is desirable to use viscosity-inducing agents to produce a consistency that makes the product easy to apply, gives it good cosmetic properties, and gains patient acceptability. Other auxiliary agents such as antioxidants and preservatives could also be included.

B. Characteristics of Liposomes

A liposomal product in physicochemical terms can be viewed as a heterogeneous liquid; lipid vesicles are dispersed in an aqueous medium. According to their size and the number of lipid bilayers present, the liposomes are classified as SUVs, LUVs, MLVs, SOVs, LOVs, or GVs.

MLVs (multilamellar vesicles) contain several lipid layers separated by aqueous layers and have a diameter of 300 nm to 15 μm.

SUVs (small unilamellar vesicles) are composed of one lipid bilayer and one aqueous compartment. Their size ranges between 20 and 200 nm.

LUVs (large unilamellar vesicles) have one lipid bilayer closing one aqueous compartment. Their size can vary between 300 and 2000 nm. They are particularly useful for entrapping water-soluble drugs owing to their high water encapsulation efficiency (20–68%).

SOVs (small oligolamellar vesicles) contain two or three lipid bilayers and are less than 200 nm in diameter.

LOVs (large oligolamellar vesicles) contain two or three lipid bilayers and are 300–2000 nm in size.

GVs (giant vesicles) are MLVs with diameters larger than 10 μm.

The net surface charge of a liposome may be neutral, negative, or positive. Lecithin can provide liposomes with a neutral surface; stearylamine and phosphatidic acid components provide positive and negative surface charge, respectively.

The ideal drug candidates for liposomal encapsulation are those that have potent pharmacological activity and are highly lipid- or water-soluble. If a drug is water-soluble it will be encapsulated within the aqueous compartment and the drug concentration in the liposomal product will depend on the volume of the entrapped water and the solubility of that drug in the encapsulated water.

The lipophilic drug is usually bound to the lipid bilayer or "dissolved" in the lipid phase. A lipophilic drug more likely will remain encapsulated longer during storage than a hydrophilic drug. Because of its partition coefficient, the lipophilic drug is associated with the lipid bilayers, rather than being leached out to the "external" water phase. Generally the encapsulation efficiency is higher for lipophilic drugs than for hydrophilic ones.

C. Advantages of Liposomal Drug Delivery Systems

The following properties make liposomes ideally suited for drug delivery.

They can accommodate both water- and oil-soluble compounds because they have both hydrophilic and lipophilic compartments.

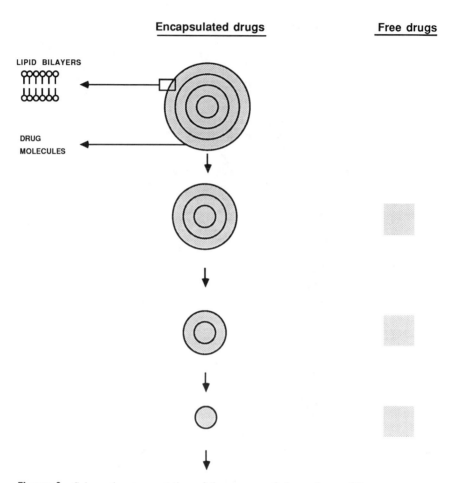

Figure 3 Schematic representation of the process of slow release of liposome-encapsulated agents.

They are composed of lipids similar to biological membranes; therefore they are biocompatible and biodegradable.
They can protect the liposome-encapsulated drug from metabolic degradation.
They can act as a depot, releasing their content slowly and gradually.

An extensive literature exists for liposomes as drug carriers (for review see Ref. 20). Liposomes can be used:

1. To target or transport the drug within the body to the site of action,

2. To localize the drug when the site of action is close to the site of administration (i.e., topical administration for local action; skin, eye, body cavities, lung), and
3. To act as slow-release vehicles.

D. Rationale of Controlled Drug Delivery with Liposomes

The principle of controlled delivery is that while the drug is encapsulated within the liposomes it cannot be metabolized, and after topical application it cannot be rapidly removed by the blood circulation; therefore the liposomes act as a depot [21,22].

If liposome preparation is formulated properly, the drug stays encapsulated; it should not leach out of the lipid vesicles during storage. The drug can be released only if the liposomal bilayer becomes permeable to the drug or is decomposed. If phospholipid molecules of the outer layer are hydrolyzed or oxidized, the micellar structure of the bilayer is changed. The bilayer eventually collapses, releasing the lipophilic drug bound or built into it. If the drug is hydrophilic, it is dissolved within the aqueous layers. If the surrounding bilayer becomes more permeable or is degraded, the hydrophilic drug in the outermost aqueous layer is released. Figure 3 illustrates the mechanism by which liposomes can act as slow-release vehicles. The rate of drug release will depend on such factors as the permeability and/or stability of the lipid bilayers in an in vivo environment. The lipid membrane stability (permeability) is determined by the type of phospholipids; amount of cholesterol in the liposomal membranes and the environment; other factors such as enzymes, pH, electrolyes, and proteins; and the possibility of lipid exchange between liposomal and biological membranes.

VI. METHODS FOR LIPOSOME ENCAPSULATION

A variety of methods have been employed for preparing liposomes. A recent literature survey indicated that there are more than 200 patents and patent applications dealing with liposome technology.

The most frequently used method, originally described by Bangham et al. [23], is the *solvent evaporation method*. The lipids or lipophilic substances are dissolved in an organic solvent, which is then removed under vacuum by rotary evaporation. The lipid residue forms a film on the wall of the container. An aqueous solution generally containing electrolytes and/or hydrophilic biologically active materials is added to the film. Agitation produces large multilamellar vesicles. Small multilamellar vesicles can be prepared by sonication or sequential filtration through filters with decreasing pore size. Small unilamellar vesicles can be prepared by more extensive sonication.

This method was improved by Mezei and Nugent [24]. To increase the surface area for the lipid film formation, inert, solid contact masses (e.g., glass beads) are placed within the vessel in which the organic solvent is evaporated. The lipid film will then be formed not only on the wall of the vessel but also on the surface of the beads. The increased surface area for film formation allows the upscaling of liposome manufacturing. With this technique 100-kg batches of liposomes can be prepared.

Solvent injection methods are suitable for preparing small or large unilamellar vesicles (SUV or LUV) without using sonication. Phospholipids (and lipophilic drugs) dissolved in organic solvents (e.g., ethanol or diethyl ether) are injected rapidly into an aqueous solution (or drug and/or electrolyte) that has been previously heated to 55–66°C, or the injection may take place at 30°C under reduced pressure [25].

An alternate method for the preparation of small unilamellar vesicles that avoids the need for sonication is the *ethanol injection technique* [26]. This method is simple, rapid, and gentle. However, it results in a relatively dilute preparation of liposomes and provides low encapsulation efficiency.

Another technique for making unilamellar vesicles is called the *detergent dialysis method* [27]. In this process the lipids and additives are solubilized with detergents by agitation or sonication, yielding defined micelles. The detergents are then removed by dialysis.

Multilamellar vesicles can be reduced both in size and in number of lamellae by extrusion through a small orifice under pressure, in a French press, for example. The French press [28] extrusion is done at pressures of 20,000 lb/in^2 at a low temperature. This is a simple, reproducible, nondestructive technique with relatively high encapsulation efficiency; however, as a starting material it requires multilamellar liposomes as point, that can be altered to oligo- or unilamellar vesicles.

Large unilamellar lipid vesicles (LUVs) can be prepared by the reversed phase evaporation method [29]. This technique consists of forming a water-in-oil emulsion of the lipid in an organic solvent and the substances to be encapsulated in an aqueous buffer solution. Removal of the organic solvent under reduced pressure produces a mixture that can then be converted to the lipid vesicles by agitation or by dispersion in an aqueous medium.

There are several patent applications for preparing liposomes by dispersion of lipid into aqueous solution. The dispersion is aided by sonication, high shear force homogenization (microfluidization), or other mechanical force such as shaking or stirring. A comprehensive review of types of liposomes and methods for preparing them can be found in Ref. 30.

Most of the methods that are suitable for large-scale manufacturing of liposomes are patented. The solvent evaporation technique was upscaled according to Mezei and Nugent [24], the detergent dialysis method by Weder et al. [31], and the reversed phase evaporation technique by Papahadjopoulos [29]. Many other patents have been granted, and more than 200 are pending.

VII. DERMAL DRUG DELIVERY BY LIPOSOMAL ENCAPSULATION

A. Topical Corticosteroids

Corticosteroids are the most frequently prescribed dermatological preparations. They are effective and relatively safe. There is, however, some risk in using potent corticosteroids, especially in children. If a large area of the body is treated for a prolonged period of time, its percutaneous absorption could lead to adrenal suppression [32,33].

It is estimated that 50% of dermatological preparations contain corticosteroids. For our first project, therefore, we selected one of the frequently prescribed corticosteroids, triamcinolone acetonide (TRMA), as a model drug for liposomal encapsulation. Several formulas were prepared, but the most stable liposomes with high efficiency of encapsulation were achieved with an optimal lipid composition of dipalmitoylphosphatidylcholine (DPPC) and cholesterol (CHOL) in 1.1:0.5 molar ratio [34,35]. The liposomal preparations, in both lotion and gel dosage forms, were applied to rabbit skin twice daily for 5 days. The control groups of rabbits were similarly treated, with the drug (0.1% TRMA) suspended (unencapsulated) in a conventional ointment (Dermabase) or in the same hydrocolloidal gel form as that in which the liposomes were incorporated. The chemical compositions of the control and liposomal gel dosage forms were similar, except that the TRMA was encapsulated in the liposomal form and "free" in the control form.

Analysis of various organs of the rabbits indicated that, compared to the ointment form, the liposomal lotion form delivered 4.5 times as much drug to the target organ (i.e., epidermis) and only one-third as much to the thalamic region, a possible site of adverse effect [34]. The gel forms delivered more "free" or "encapsulated" drug to the skin tissues than the ointment or liposomal lotion, but the liposomal gel form delivered 4.9 times as much drug to the epidermis and just slightly more than one-twelfth as much to the thalamic region as the gel form containing the free drug [35]. The blood concentration and urinary excretion of TRMA were reduced in both the above studies as a result of liposome encapsulation, indicating that the percutaneous absorption of TRMA was less if the drug was applied in liposomal form than in the ointment or gel forms.

Krowczynski and Stozek [36] compared liposomal and ointment formulations of triamcinolone by applying them on the forearm. The liposomal preparations were similar to those studied by Mezei and Gulasekharam [34], but they were incorporated in an ointment base. The free triamcinolone incorporated in the same ointment base served as control. They found that the resorption of triamcinolone from the liposome formulation was three times as much as that from the ointment. They concluded that the liposome formulation should be considered an improved delivery system for transdermal therapy.

In a series of articles, Wohlrab and Lasch [37–39] reported that the liposomal form provided a higher concentration of hydrocortisone in the human skin than the ointment form. They concluded that liposomal lecithin rapidly penetrates into the human skin. They also discussed the relevance of the lecithin penetration to the enhanced hydrocortisone penetration from the liposomal formulation.

My coworkers and I have developed two other liposomal corticosteroid products: 0.5% hydrocortisone and 0.01% betamethasone valerate. Both of these products have been evaluated by clinical studies. Results indicated better activity and patient acceptability than existing cream products (results to be published).

B. Topical Antifungals

We have formulated and evaluated several liposomal products containing econazole base or econazole nitrate. We have conducted comprehensive in vivo biodisposition studies with seven liposomal products against existing commercial products—Pevaryl Cream, gel, lotion—and also against the same formula as the liposomal one, except that the active ingredient, econazole nitrate or econazole base, was incorporated in "free" form in the conventional (suspension) dosage form. The results [40,41] indicated that most of the liposomal products produced higher drug concentrations in the skin and lower drug concentrations in the internal organs than those of conventional cream, gel, and lotion dosage forms (Fig. 4). In some cases, both dermal and transdermal penetration was increased as a result of liposomal encapsulation. This was the first indication that liposomes, depending on the formula, can be used not just to localize the drug within the skin, but also to enhance percutaneous absorption and thus be useful as a transdermal drug delivery dosage form.

To achieve adequate drug concentrations in the liposomal products and to selectively deliver the active ingredient within the skin tissue, we developed a new "multiphase liposomal drug delivery system" [41]. Clinical studies indicated that liposomal econazole is at least as active in lower concentrations (0.2% or 0.5%) as the 1% econazole in (Pevaryl) cream form. In addition, the liposomal form requires less frequent application and has higher patient acceptance, due to lack of irritation, than the cream form. As a result of these studies and

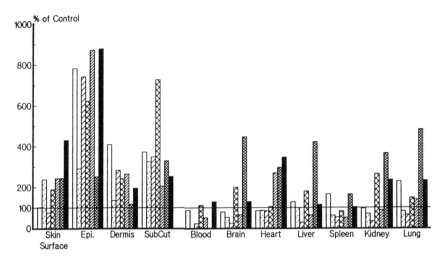

Figure 4   The effect of liposome encapsulation on the disposition of liposomal and free (control) econazole. The appropriate control (ointment, cream, or suspension form) for each liposome preparation is 100%.

others conducted by Cilag A. G., the first liposomal drug product was marketed in Switzerland in 1988 as Pevaryl Lipogel.

C. Minoxidil

In 1983, we initiated product development studies for liposomal minoxidil. Several formulas were prepared, and nine products were evaluated with respect to biodisposition in comparison to Upjohn's formulas (solutions and suspensions). The data results [22,41] indicated the superiority of the liposomal form in comparison with the conventional forms (Fig. 5). Some products have the same chemical composition in both the test (liposomal) and control (suspension) forms. The difference between the two products is that in the liposomal form minoxidil is mainly encapsulated, whereas in the conventional (suspension) form it is "free." The results clearly demonstrated that the liposomal encapsulation was responsible for the increased minoxidil concentration within the skin layers.

In some cases (products F, G, H, and particularly product I), both dermal and transdermal delivery was increased. Although transdermal delivery of minoxidil is definitely not desirable here, these products can serve as examples for the use of liposomal encapsulation for transdermal delivery of other drugs. Figures 4 and 5 clearly indicate that the in vivo fate of the liposome-encapsulated

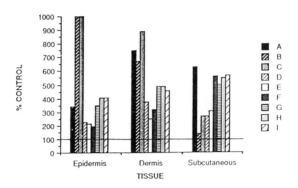

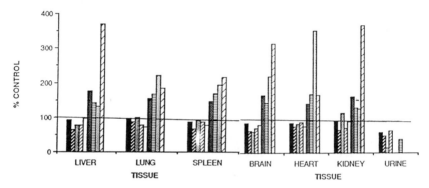

Figure 5 The effect of liposomal encapsulation on biodisposition of topically applied minoxidil in liposomal, solution, suspension, and gel dosage forms. Each liposomal product (A–F) was compared to a control (solution, gel, suspension) dosage form.

drug as far as biodisposition is concerned is dependent on the nature of the liposomal product—the lipid composition, size, and surface change of the lipid vesicles and other auxiliary agents present in the final product.

D. Local Anesthetics

Topical anesthetic agents usually have limited penetration and short residency time within the skin. Therefore, most of the available topically applied local anesthetic products are ineffective [42].

We have developed various liposomal products containing tetracaine, lidocaine, or dibucaine and tested them against existing commercial products. Experiments with normal human volunteers confirmed the superiority of the liposomal 0.5% tetracaine product compared to a product in conventional dosage form, Pontocaine cream containing 1% tetracaine [43]. In vivo biodisposition studies [44], confirmed that a direct correlation exists between the measured drug concentration at the site of action and its biological activity.

E. Retinoids

Retinoids are claimed to be the most effective agents in the treatment of acne. Retinoids are also recommended for the treatment of many types of skin disorders. Systemic retinoids, because of their teratogenic effects, are not desirable for the female population. Topical retinoids, i.e., vitamin A acid and isotretinoin, are effective but highly irritant agents. During the early weeks of therapy the symptoms of acne may worsen and inflammatory lesions may be exacerbated. The beneficial effects may be noticeable only after 2–3 weeks of therapy. Because of the irritation and lack of results during the early stage, patient compliance is not very good. In addition, may dermatologists believe that topically applied retinoids are quickly oxidized before they can penetrate to their active sites.

It was anticipated that liposomal encapsulation would reduce the local irritation and the chance of deactivation by oxidation, since a large portion of the applied dose would be enclosed within the lipid vesicles and therefore the concentration of the "free" form might be kept below the irritation level and the chance of oxidation minimized. We have developed several liposomal retinoid products. Results of preliminary investigations (Fig. 6) indicate the advantages of liposome encapsulation [45].

Masini et al. [46] also found that the liposome formulations of retinoic acid provided greater bioavailability, with higher drug concentration in the epidermis and upper dermis of hairless rats, than a conventional gel form. They also concluded that the retinoic acid release seemed to be controlled by the liposomes.

F. Interferons

Topical delivery of interferon was also more efficient from the liposomal form than from the solution, emulsion, or gel forms [47,48]. Weiner et al. [47] investigated three types of liposomal products along with a solution and an emulsion containing interferon in a cutaneous herpes guinea pig model. The topically applied liposomal products caused a reduction of lesion scores; the solution and emulsion forms were ineffective. The method of liposomal preparation influenced the efficacy; the dehydration–rehydration method was effective. They concluded that the liposomes do not appear to function as penetration enhancers but seem to provide a favorable physicochemical environment for transfer of interferon into the skin.

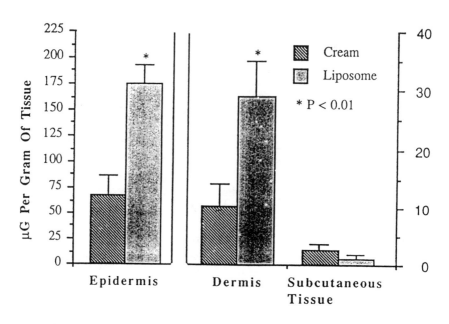

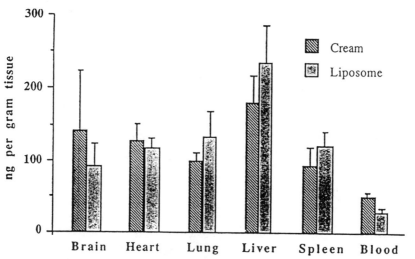

Figure 6   The effect of liposomal encapsulation on biodisposition of tretinoin in guinea pig after 5 days of treatment.

Foldvari et al. [48] investigated topical liposome-encapsulated interferon alpha for the treatment of genital papillovirus infections in human. The liposomes were manufactured by a method described by Mezei and Nugent [24] and characterized by electron microscopic and polyacrylamide gel electrophoretic techniques. Preliminary clinical studies [48] indicated that liposomes provide a suitable delivery system for interferon alpha in a dermatologically acceptable dosage form. At the end of a 12-week course of liposomal interferon treatment in a female patient the lesions were resolved, and the area showed no sign of recurrence 7 weeks after discontinuation of treatment. In the case of a male patient, several lesions on the distal foreskin and glans resolved after 2 weeks of liposomal interferon twice a day application.

G. Methotrexate

Patel [21] found that topically applied liposomes may act as sustained-release vehicles for drugs into the epidermis. He applied free and liposome-encapsulated [^{3}H]methotrexate topically onto the skin of nude mice. The entrapped methotrexate was retained in the skin two to three times as well as the free methotrexate. The pattern for blood drug concentration was the opposite—the liposomal form provided lower drug concentrations than the free form.

VIII. DRUG TARGETING WITHIN AND THROUGH THE SKIN WITH LIPOSOMAL ENCAPSULATION

The most intensive field of liposome research is related to the development of a selective drug delivery system suitable for cancer chemotherapy. The need to target the cytotoxic drug to cancer cells is obvious. Unfortunately, in spite of tremendous efforts during hundreds of investigations, liposomes have not fulfilled the expectation that they might act as a "magic bullet," transporting and targeting the drug to specific organs or cells. A more realistic view now is that liposomes require the association of a cell-recognizing molecule on the liposome surface in order to have target specificity. The latest effort in this field is to test the immunospecific targeting of liposomes with the aid of antibodies. Attempts have been made to achieve targeting by covalently binding liposomes (containing a cytotoxic drug) to tumor-specific antibodies to induce them to home in on their targets, the tumor cells [49–51].

If liposomes are injected intravenously, passive targeting can be achieved because they are "filtered out" by the reticuloendothelial system (RES), and the liposome-encapsulated drug will be concentrated in organs such as the liver, spleen, lung, and bone marrow. Consequently, when reticuloendothelial cells are infected by bacteria or parasites, liposomes can serve as efficient targeted drug delivery systems [52].

A successful targeting by liposomes can be also achieved with immunomodulators such as muramyl di- or tripeptides. The macrophages and other reticuloendothelial cells that circulate in the blood as defense against invading pathogens gobble up the liposomes; hence the drug is delivered where it is needed, activating the macrophages [53].

Most researchers have investigated the potential of liposomes for systemic drug delivery; only a few studies have been reported on the use of liposomes for topical application of drugs (for review see Refs. 54–56). Liposomes were found to be suitable for localization of topically applied drug at or near the site of application. The localizing effect is mainly due to the fact that liposomes, especially the MLV types, may act as slow-release vehicles.

Results of biodisposition studies in rabbits and guinea pigs indicate that most liposomal formulations in multiple-dose topical treatment provide higher drug concentrations of triamcinolone, progesterone, econazole, minoxidil, retinoids, and local anesthetic agents in the skin than conventional (ointment, cream, gel, or lotion) dosage forms. Certain liposomal formulations greatly enhance both dermal and transdermal drug delivery. With appropriate formulation, the drug could be targeted even within the skin.

Econazole is an antifungal agent; the site of action is within the epidermis: minoxidil is intended to increase hair growth; consequently its site of action is in the hair follicles, which are located in a deeper layer of the skin, which we designated as dermis and subcutaneous tissues when we sectioned the skin samples horizontally (a 0.2-mm slice is the epidermis, the next 0.5 mm is the dermis, and the rest of the skin sample is referred to as subcutaneous tissue).

Table 1 illustrates the results of in vivo drug disposition studies after treatment with one of the multiphase liposomal forms of each of these drugs against their appropriate control, Pevaryl cream or the Upjohn formula similar to Rogaine. It is well demonstrated that in the case of econazole the greatest difference in drug concentration is within the epidermis, where the site of action is; in the case of minoxidil, the difference in drug concentration produced by the liposomal and solution forms is the greatest within the dermis and subcutaneous tissues, where the hair follicles are located.

IX. LIPOSOME–SKIN INTERACTION

On the basis of our previous studies, including the formulation and evaluation of more than 30 liposomal preparations, we can conclude that topically applied liposomal products, in comparison to existing products, have the potential to

— Eliminate local irritation,
— Enhance local effect,
— Reduce *or* increase systemic effects,

Table 1 Effect of Liposomal Encapsulation on Drug Disposition after Topical Treatment for 3 Days

Tissue	Percent of control[a]	
	Econazole	Minoxidil
Skin surface	244.0	76.6
Epidermis	872.0	464.7
Dermis	265.0	450.5
Subcutaneous tissues	206.0	1036.0
Blood	50.0	54.8
Brain	64.6	61.3
Liver	62.9	76.4
Spleen	50.8	118.4
Lung	137.9	99.0
Heart	97.1	85.2

[a]The controls are a cream and a solution containing the same drug concentration as the liposomal products.

— Optimize dosage

— Provide prolonged release action, and

— Be cosmetically more acceptable than most of the presently available products (i.e., will not be greasy or tacky and will not stick to clothing).

While it is encapsulated within the lipid vesicles an irritant or "corrosive" drug has no direct contact with the skin tissue (cell membranes, nerve endings); therefore its irritation potential is eliminated. The concentration of the "free" form of the drug applied to the skin depends on the rate of release from the lipid vesicles. The concentration of the "free" form of the active ingredient is always lower in liposomal products than in the conventional forms. Consequently it is expected that the liposomal form causes less irritation than the cream, ointment, and lotion forms. Evidence in clinical investigations confirmed that liposomal econazole, marketed as Pevaryl Lipogel, is less irritant than econazole in cream form marketed as Pevaryl Cream.

While the drug is present in the tissue encapsulated in the lipid vesicle it may be not irritant, and it cannot be metabolized because it is protected by the lipid bilayers forming the vesicle. At the same time one cannot expect the encapsulated drug to produce any activity, as it has no access to its receptor to form the "drug–receptor complex" that is essential for biological activity. Consequently it is possible that the higher drug concentration measured in the liposome-treated animal will not have higher efficacy if the drug is still present in the encapsulated form. It is essential that the drug be released from the liposome if it is to produce its effect. Further studies were therefore directed to evaluate the efficacy of the liposomal products.

Results in human studies indicated enhanced local effect due to liposome encapsulation of local anesthetic agents [43]. In clinical investigations with econazole, hydrocortisone and betamethasone products contained lower concentrations of the active ingredient than the control produce, and yet a higher drug activity was found in the liposome-treated patients.

The liposomal form can also provide sustained-release delivery as documented in animal experiments [21,22] and in human experiments [43]. In clinical practice the recommended dosage regimen for Pevaryl cream is twice a day, and for Pevaryl Lipogel, only once a day.

That the liposomal form is cosmetically more acceptable than the ointment, cream, lotion, or gel was documented during clinical trials with the 0.5% liposomal hydrocortisone as compared with 1% hydrocortisone cream. Female patients treated with liposomal hydrocortisone for facial eczema requested more samples of the liposomal product even after the eczema cleared up, because it provided a "velvety" feeling at the site of application. It is not accidental that the first liposomal products (e.g., Capture) were cosmetic preparations.

X. MECHANISM OF LIPOSOMAL TOPICAL DRUG DELIVERY

To explain the mechanism by which liposomes achieve selective dermal drug delivery, we conducted ultrastructural electron microscopic evaluation of guinea pig skin treated with liposomes containing an electron-dense material, colloidal iron [44]. Intact liposomes and free colloidal iron were identified within the dermis, indicating that liposomes may penetrate the skin and serve as "drug carriers" even for those drugs that otherwise would not penetrate the barrier layers of the skin. While the drug is encapsulated in the lipid vesicles it is not available for absorption into the blood circulation, since the lipid vesicles do not penetrate into the blood vessels. Only the "free" drug molecules are able to diffuse into the capillary blood vessels. The liposomes, therefore, can serve as a depot, as a slow-release vehicle within the dermis, which is highly vascularized. By appropriate formulation one can regulate the in vivo drug release from liposomes and therefore control percutaneous absorption. Since liposomes can act as a depot for a slow-release vehicle, they can maintain a higher drug concentration in the skin than conventional vehicles.

Mezei [40] postulated the mechanism shown in Figure 7 for explaining the effect of liposome encapsulation on drug disposition. This figure illustrates the sequence of events related to a drug applied topically on the skin in the conventional dosage forms—ointment, cream, or lotion—free and in the liposome-encapsulated (LIP) form.

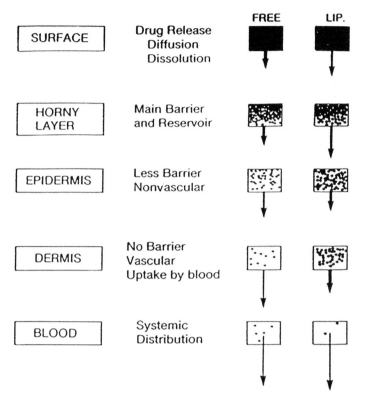

Figure 7 Schematic representation of the mechanism and rate of penetration of free and liposomal (LIP) drug. The density of spots indicates concentration; the relative length of arrow indicates the magnitude of the rate of diffusion.

In the conventional dosage form the "free" drug should be released, diffused to the surface of the skin, and dissolved (if it is not in solution form) before being absorbed into the horny layer. The drug in the liposomal form does not have to be released. Diffusion to the keratin layer is less of a problem, because the lipid vesicles are readily miscible with the skin surface lipid, which often serves as a barrier, especially to lipid-insoluble drugs.

At the second step, the drug should get through the horny layer, which is the main barrier. The vehicle may have an occlusive effect that enhances hydration of the keratin layer; this in turn increases the permeability of that layer. Many of the conventional dermatological vehicles have only a limited occlusive effect if any. The liposomal form has an excellent potential for hydrating the horny layer, for the lipid vesicles create a lipid film that supplements the skin surface lipids. Consequently the increase in the permeability of the main barrier layer is greater with the liposomal form than with some of the conventional forms (e.g., suspensions or emulsions of the oil/water type).

At the third step, when the drug reaches the epidermis, the diffusion rate of the "free" form is expected to be higher than that of the liposome-encapsulated form because of the difference in size. The "free" form is in the molecular state; the penetrating drug particles are smaller than the liposomes. The slower diffusion of the lipid vesicles provides a longer residency time for the encapsulated drug.

At the fourth step, because the dermis is highly vascularized, and because of a high concentration gradient, the "free" drug is quickly removed by the blood circulation. The larger liposomes, because of their size, are not able to penetrate the blood vessels; therefore the cutaneous clearance of liposomal drug is less than that of the "free" drug.

In our biodisposition studies comparing liposomal formulations with cream, ointment, or lotion preparations of triamcinolone, progesterone, econazole, minoxidil, retinoids, and local anesthetic agents, the liposomal drug concentration is 3–8 times that of the "free" form in the dermis, but most of the time the drug concentration in the blood is less than or the same as that resulting from use of the ointment, cream, or gel treatment.

One reason for the reduced epidermal/dermal clearance of the liposome-encapsulated drug may be the reduced drug metabolism; while the drug is encapsulated it is not available to the metabolic enzymes. A more likely reason, however, is that the liposomes probably do not penetrate the blood vessels— they are not removed from the site—and can therefore act as slow-release vehicles [21,22,54].

Liposomes may also penetrate via the lipid pathways. Several reports [8,12,15] claim that the lipid content of the stratum corneum exists as a lipid bilayer. This and the epidermal intercellular lipid bilayer could serve as pathways for the penetration of small and flexible lipid vesicles.

Keith and Snipes [57] emphasized in their work examining the permeability properties of the lipid-extracted epidermis and those of the lipid-extracted epidermis in which the phospholipids had been replaced that the diffusion of different molecules through the skin is determined by the physical properties of the molecular environment of the skin; consequently an easier diffusion of lipid-soluble molecules can be expected through the lipid channels. This may also imply that the diffusion of a number of liposomes via this route is possible.

Both autoradiographic and electron-dense marking techniques confirmed the presence of "free" and liposome-encapsulated drug within the skin [44]. This could be due to the release of drug from the liposomes at the skin surface and penetration of the "free" drug or the slow release of drug from the liposomes after their penetration into the skin. The simultaneous occurrence of these processes is also possible. "Liposome-like" material found between corneocytes points to a possible intercellular pathway as the penetration route. It is feasible to speculate that smaller liposomes, being flexible lipid vesicles, can penetrate through the "lipid channels," the lipidic material distributed in the intercellular spaces [58,59].

From the results of in vitro studies using hairless mouse skin in a diffusion cell, Ganesan et al. [60] and Ho et al. [61] concluded that liposome-encapsulated lipophilic drugs like progesterone and hydrocortisone seem to pass through the skin similarly to the free drug but that the more polar glucose entrapped in the aqueous compartment of liposomes is poorly available for transport. They suggest that the lipophilic drug is directly transferred from the liposome to the skin. The solubility of the lipophilic drug in liposomes allows greater payloads; thus more drug may be delivered through the skin via liposomes than by the simple aqueous solutions.

One can list a number of factors that influence drug diffusion in vitro differently than in vivo conditions. In addition to these factors, in the case of liposomes one should consider metabolic reactions that may lead to the destabilization of liposomal membranes and to the release of the entrapped drug. These might not be present in the dead skin tissues used in the in vitro experiments.

In addition, the distribution coefficient can greatly influence the fate of the lipid components. The receiver flask contained an aqueous buffer solution; consequently the lipoid ingredients preferred to stay in the skin tissue, which is more lipophilic than the aqueous solution.

These in vitro studies [60,61] measured only percutaneous (through the skin) and not cutaneous (into the skin) penetration. Since the skin samples were not analyzed for the presence of liposomes, the conclusion could be valid only for transdermal, rather than dermal, penetration.

One may argue that the lipid channels within the epidermis are too narrow for the penetration of liposomes 300–500 nm in diameter. But the diameters of lipid channels were measured after dehydration of the sample for EM examination, which does not necessarily represent the exact in vivo diameter. On the other hand, the liposomes are very flexible lipid vesicles. One can filter large liposomes, 5000–10,000 nm in diameter, through a polycarbonate filter with a pore size of 200–400 nm. Considering this and the dynamic nature of the lipid channels, it is possible that some liposomes can penetrate into the epidermis and dermis. The results of our electron microscopic studies prove this possibility [44].

It was also proposed [57] that the discontinuous phospholipid matrix of the extracted skin impedes the permeability of hydrophobic molecules. It is possible, therefore, that the major component of liposomes, the phospholipids, provide an aid to effectuate complete continuity of the epidermis, which maximally can

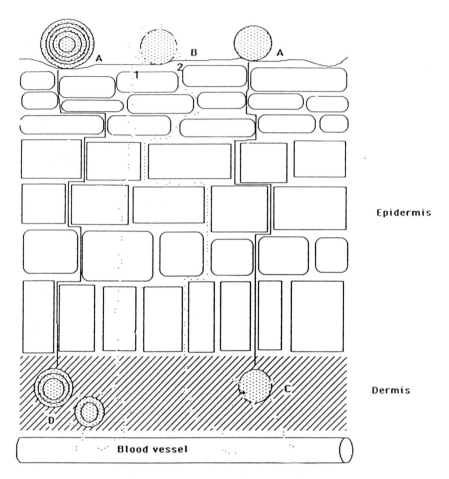

Figure 8 Proposed mechanism for the interaction of liposomes with the skin. A, Adsorption of liposomes to the skin surface; drug transfer from liposomes to skin. B, Rupture of vesicles, release of content, and penetration of free molecules into the skin via (1) intracellular or (2) intercellular route. C, Penetration of unilamellar vesicles via the liposome-rich channels to the dermis, where they slowly release their content due to disruption or degradation of liposomal membranes. D, Penetration of multilamellar vesicles via the lipid-rich channels. On the route of penetration, multilamellar vesicles can lose one or more outer lipid lamellae, which would lead to partial release of the encapsulated material.

facilitate the movement of the lipophilic drug molecules. This speculation is supported by findings that liposome-encapsulated lipophilic drugs are much more advantageous and successful for dermal delivery than liposome-encapsulated water-soluble drugs [40].

On the basis of autoradiographic and EM findings [44] coupled with previous in vivo experimental results and other literature data, we propose as possible pathways for liposome–skin interactions those illustrated in Figure 8. Multi- and unilamellar liposomes can be adsorbed onto the skin surface intact (Fig. 8A) before their penetration into the skin. Some liposomes can rupture on the surface of the skin (Fig. 8B). The penetration of smaller vesicles is more probable (Fig. 8C); however, it is possible that the intradermally localized uni- or oligolamellar vesicles are derived from multilamellar liposomes that lost their outer bilayers during penetration (Fig. 8D). The results of ongoing studies (to be published) with dual isotope labeling also confirm this conclusion; both the encapsulated drug ($[^3H]$minoxidil) and the liposomal membrane component ($[^{14}C]$phosphatidylcholine) are present within the skin and internal organs, although with a different isotope ($^3H/^{14}C$) ratio than that of the applied product.

XI. CONCLUSION

Both biodisposition and electron microscopic (in vivo) investigations indicate that liposomes can provide selective drug delivery: that liposomes penetrate the skin, carry their content into the skin, serve as a slow-release dosage form, and reduce or increase systemic absorption. Pharmacodynamic and clinical studies with hydrocortisone and local anesthetic agents have demonstrated higher efficacy of the liposomal products in comparison with the commercially available cream products. The first liposomal drug product, Pevaryl Lipogel, has been proved superior to Pevaryl Cream in clinical practice. Consequently, liposomes have a good potential to provide a safe and effective topical therapy.

These and other data presented herein clearly document that with proper liposomal formulation, targeting the drug can be achieved even within one tissue, i.e., the skin. In most cases the liposomal form provides higher drug concentration within the skin and lower or comparable drug concentration in the internal organs than the control formulas. The mechanism by which the liposomal encapsulation achieves selective drug delivery, localization of the drug at the target organ, is explained above. The principle is that liposomes enhance penetration of the drug into the skin and, more important, in the case of slow-release liposomes, decrease clearance of the drug by minimizing its absorption into the bloodstream. Experimental evidence indicates that intact liposomes penetrate the skin, and while the drug is encapsulated within the lipid vesicles it is not available for systemic absorption.

Although there are only limited data for liposomal transdermal drug delivery, it can be expected that liposomes can be useful for those drugs that do not penetrate the skin in the "free" molecular state. In these cases liposomes can be viewed as drug carriers. Since intact liposomes have been found in the dermis, they can carry their drug contents to the vascularized portion of the skin, where eventually the drug is released and can be absorbed into the bloodstream.

REFERENCES

1. H. J. Yardley, *Int. J. Cosmetic Sci. 9*, 13 (1987).
2. G. M. Gray, R. J. White, R. H. Williams, and H. J. Yardley, *Br. J. Dermatol. 106*, 59 (1982).
3. W. Curatolo, *Pharm. Res. 4*, 271 (1987).
4. V. A. Ziboh and R. S. Chapkin, *Prog. Lipid Res. 27*, 81 (1988).
5. R. M. Lavker, *J. Ultrastruct. Res. 55*, 79 (1976).
6. S. Grayson and P. M. Elias, *J. Invest. Dermatol. 78*, 128 (1982).
7. R. J. Scheuplein, *J. Invest. Dermatol. 45*, 334 (1965).
8. P. M. Elias, *J. Invest. Dermatol. 80*, 44 (1983).
9. R. C. Scott, R. H. Guy, and J. Hadgraft, Eds., *Prediction of Percutaneous Penetration*, IBC Technical Services, London, 1990.
10. P. A. Bowser and R. J. White, *Br. J. Dermatol. 112*, 1 (1985).
11. A.G. Matoltsy, *J. Invest. Dermatol. 67*, 20 (1976).
12. L. Landmann, *Anal. Embryol. 178*, 1 (1988).
13. W. Abraham and D. T. Downing, *J. Invest. Dermatol. 93*, 809 (1989).
14. G. Grubauer, K. R. Feingold, R. M. Harris, and P. M. Elias, *J. Lipid Res. 30*, 89 (1989).
15. S. E. Friberg, I. Kayali, L. D. Rhein, F. A. Simon, and R. H. Cogan, *Int. J. Cosmetic Sci. 12*, 5 (1990).
16. P. M. Elias, in *Models in Dermatology*, Vol. 1, H. I. Maibach and N. J. Lowe, Eds., Karger, Basel, 1985, p. 272.
17. J. Hadgraft, *Cosm. Toilet. 100*, 32 (1985).
18. B. Illel and H. Schaefer, *Acta Dermatovenerol. 68*, 427 (1988).
19. W. C. Fong, B. Harsanyi, and M. Mezei, *J. Biomed. Mater. Res. 23*, 1213 (1989).
20. G. Gregoriadis, Ed., *Liposomes as Drug Carriers*, Wiley, New York, 1988.
21. H. M. Patel, *Biochem. Soc. Trans. 13*, 513 (1985).
22. M. Mezei, in *Controlled Release Dosage Forms*, H. P. Tipnis, Ed., Bombay College of Pharmacy, Bombay, India, 1988, p. 37.
23. A. D. Bangham, M. M. Standish, and J. C. Watkins, *J. Mol. Biol. 13*, 238 (1965).
24. M. Mezei and F. J. Nugent, U. S. Patent 4,485,054 (1984).
25. D. Deamer and A. D. Bangham, *Biochim. Biophys. Acta 443*, 629 (1976).
26. S. Batzri and E. D. Korn, *Biochim. Biophys. Acta 298*, 1015 (1973).
27. H. G. Weder and O. Zumbuehl, in *Liposome Technology*, Vol. 1, G. Gregoriadis, Ed., CRC Press, Boca Raton, FL, 1984, p. 79.
28. Y. Barenholz, S. Amselem, and D. Lichtenberg, *FEBS Lett. 99*, 210 (1979).

29. X. X. Papahadjopoulos, U.S. Patent 4,234,871 (1980).
30. G. Gregoriadis, Ed., *Liposome Technology*, 2nd Edition, Vol. 1, CRC Press, Boca Raton, FL, 1993.
31. H. G. Weder et al., U.S. Patent 4,438,052 (1984).
32. T. Fredrikson, in *Percutaneous Absorption*, R.L. Bronaugh and H.I. Maibach, Eds., Marcel Dekker, New York, 1985, p. 513.
33. G. Herz, in *Topical Corticosteroid Therapy—A Novel Approach to Safer Drugs*, E. Christopher, A. M. Kligman, E. Schoph, and R. B. Stoughton, Eds., Raven Press, New York, 1988, p. 147.
34. M. Mezei and V. Gulasekharam, *Life Sci. 26*, 1473 (1980).
35. M. Mezei and V. Gulasekharam, *J. Pharm. Pharmacol. 34*, 473 (1982).
36. L. Krowczynski and T. Stozek, *Pharmazie 39*, 627 (1984).
37. W. Wohlrab and J. Lasch, *Dermatologica 174*, 18 (1987).
38. W. Wohlrab and J. Lasch, *Dermatol. Mon.-Schr. 175*, 344 (1989).
39. W. Wohlrab and J. Lasch, *Dermatol. Mon.-Schr. 175*, 348 (1989).
40. M. Mezei, in *Topics in Pharmaceutical Sciences 1985*, D. D. Breimer and P. Speiser, Eds., Elsevier, Amsterdam, 1985, p. 345.
41. M. Mezei, U.S. Patent 4,761,288 (1988).
42. H. Dalili and J. Adrian, *Clin. Pharmacol. Ther. 12*, 913 (1971).
43. A. Gesztes and M. Mezei, U.S. Patent 4,937,078 (1990).
44. M. Foldvari, A. Gesztes, and M. Mezei, *J. Microencap. 7*, 479 (1990).
45. W .C. Foong, B. B. Harsanyi, and M. Mezei, in *Phospholipids—Biochemical, Pharmaceutical and Analytical Considerations*, I. Hanin and G. Pepeu, Eds., Plenum, New York, 1992.
46. V. Masini, F. Bonte, A. Meybeck, and J. Wepierre, *Proc. Int. Symp. Controlled Release Bioact. Mater.*, Reno, NV, 1990, pp. 425–426.
47. N. Weiner, N. Williams, G. Birch, C. Ramaschandran, C. Shipman, Jr., and G. Flynn, *Antimicrob. Agents Chemother. 33*, 1217 (1989).
48. M. Foldvari, A. Moreland, R. B. Murray, and M. Mezei, *Int. Dermatol. Symp. Interferons Related Lymphokines*, Berlin, October 1989.
49. L. Leserman and P. Machy, in *Liposomes from Biophysics to Therapeutics*, M. J. Ostro, Ed., Marcel Dekker, New York, 1987, p. 157.
50. T. Ghose, M. Singh, G. Faulkner, A Goundalkar, and M. Mezei, in *Liposomes as Drug Carriers*, G. Gregorradis, Ed., Wiley, New York, 1988, p. 697.
51. M. Singh, T. Ghose, G. Faulkner, J. Kralovec, and M. Mezei, *Cancer Res. 49*, 3976 (1989).
52. G. Lopez-Berestein and R. L. Juliano, in *Liposomes from Biophysics to Therapeutics*, M. J. Ostro, Ed., Marcel Dekker, New York, 1987, p. 253.
53. N. C. Phillips and L. Chedid, in *Liposomes as Drug Carriers*, G. Gregoriadis, Ed., Wiley, New York, 1988, p. 243.
54. M. Mezei, in *Liposomes as Drug Carriers*, G. Gregoriadis, Ed., Wiley, New York, 1988, p. 663.
55. M. Schaefer-Korting, H. C. Korting, and O. Braun-Falco, *J. Am. Acad. Dermatol. 21*, 1271 (1989).
56. R. M. Handjani-Villa and J. Guesnet, *Ann. Dermatol. Venereol. 118*, 423 (1989).

57. A. D. Keith and W. Snipes, in *Principles of Cosmetics for Dermatologists*, P. Frost and S. Horowitz, Eds., C. V. Mosby, St. Louis, MO, 1982, p. 59.

58. P. Elias, *Int. J. Dermatol. 20*, 1 (1981).

59. P. Elias, in *Models in Dermatology*, H. I. Manibach and N. J. Lowe, Eds., Karger, Basel, 1985, p. 272.

60. M. G. Ganesan, N. D. Weiner, G. L. Flynn, and N. H. F. Ho, *Int. J. Pharm. 20*, 139 (1984).

61. N. H. F. Ho, M. G. Ganesan, N. D. Weiner, and G. L. Flynn, in *Advances in Drug Delivery Systems*, J. J. Anderson and S. W. Kim, Eds., Elsevier, New York, 1986, p. 61.

62. R. C. Wester and H. I. Maibach, in *Topics in Pharmaceutical Sciences, 1985*, D. D. Breimer and P. Speiser, Eds., Elsevier, New York, 1985, p. 359.

10

Barrier Properties of the Skin: Skin Development and Permeation

Tamie Kurihara-Bergstrom and William R. Good
CIBA-GEIGY Corporation, Summit, New Jersey

I. INTRODUCTION

Transdermal drug delivery can be defined as the delivery of a drug through the skin for systemic effect. The skin is, however, a very efficient barrier to the ingress of materials, allowing only small quantities of a drug to penetrate over a period of time. It is well accepted that the stratum corneum is the major rate-limiting barrier to molecular diffusion through mammalian epidermis [1–3]. This epidermal barrier limits the penetration of a wide variety of substances, the permeation of which most importantly depends upon their physicochemical properties as well as the normal and abnormal states of the skin. The ease with which most substances penetrate the skin after injury to [4,5] or removal of [6,7] the stratum corneum clearly indicates that this layer has a critical role in determining cutaneous permeability. Ultimately, success of the transdermal route of administration depends on the ability of the drug to permeate the skin in sufficient quantities to achieve its desired therapeutic effects.

The ability to enhance drug permeation to promote the absorption of drugs with low skin permeability is one of the important findings in the development of successful transdermal products. A deeper understanding of the barrier properties of the stratum corneum is needed not only to assess drug permeation enhancement but also to optimize transdermal dosage forms. In order to understand the form and function of the stratum corneum it is helpful to know the nature and origin of the barrier properties of skin in terms of physicochemical characteristics of the stratum corneum development. In this chapter we discuss the barrier characteristics of skin by studying fetal pig skin penetration, with emphasis on the influence of gestational age, and present a method of treating a premature neonatal infant using the incomplete skin barrier.

II. BARRIER PROPERTIES OF THE SKIN IN THE NEWBORN

Intact adult skin functions well as a barrier, but preterm infant skin is a less effective barrier. Differentiation of the epidermis to stratum corneum takes place in the third trimester of fetal life with the formation of completely keratinized cells, and by the time full-term gestation is reached the barrier property of the stratum corneum is essentially equivalent to that of adult skin [8]. Yet, not all babies are born full term, and therefore many new infants face the first few weeks of life with an incomplete skin barrier, which makes them particularly susceptible to excessive dehydration and absorption of potentially toxic substances.

The principal water barrier function of the epidermis resides almost entirely in the stratum corneum. A measurement of transepidermal water loss (TEWL) from the surface of anhidrotic skin provides a sensitive index of specific epidermal function, the barrier function. Comparison of TEWL in premature and term infants yields information about the maturity of the physical barrier in the newborn [9]. Premature infants of 29 weeks or earlier gestational age have significantly greater TEWL than older gestational age premature infants. On the other hand, older premature and term infants have similar TEWL. This also agrees with in vitro studies that premature infants of 26–30 weeks gestational age have significantly higher water skin permeability than that of full-term infants (37–40 weeks) [10].

The permeability of the preterm neonate skin to drugs was first noted by Nachman and Esterly [11] in their original description of the blanching response to topical application of phenylephrine. They demonstrated that blanching occurred in preterm infants but not in full-term infants and disappeared in preterm infants by 3 weeks of age. The blanching response shows the expected relationship to gestation and postnatal age, correlating closely with TEWL [9]. If preterm infants are susceptible to enhanced skin permeability, then they will also be more susceptible to systemic toxicity from a topically applied agent. Antiseptic agents used in neonatal care are absorbed through the preterm infant skin. Hexachlorophene, for example, is absorbed through immature or damaged skin to a significantly greater extent than through full-term infant skin, resulting in damage to the central nervous system [12–19]. It has been discovered that many other topical drugs are absorbed through preterm infant skin, causing systemic toxic effects [20–25]. The full-term newborn infant, on the other hand, has a well-developed skin that possesses excellent barrier properties. The permeabilities of most substances including water, gases [26,27], and drugs through mature newborn skin are similar to those of adult skin.

What is most interesting is that this incomplete skin barrier may provide a convenient route of administration for drugs intended for systemic therapy. In 1985, Evans et al. [28] exploited the enhanced permeability of preterm skin for the percutaneous delivery of theophylline from hydroxyethylmethylcellulose gels. These findings established that the premature infant has a greater permeability than the full-term infant, child, or adult. Further studies are necessary to link permeability phenomena directly with developing epidermal differentiation.

III. ANIMAL MODELS

Animal models of the newborn have been developed [29,30], and some have served as models for percutaneous absorption. In this context we have linked permeability phenomena directly with epidermal keratinization. Fetal pig skin has attracted interest because pig skin is often used as an experimental model for the study of the physiological and biochemical processes of human skin [2,31,32]. However, information on fetal pig skin is still sparse, although a few reports have been written regarding the histology of swine neonates [33]. A few transepidermal penetration studies with fetal pig skin have been undertaken specifically to correlate its permeation properties with epidermal keratinization and embryonic development [34]. We have examined the morphology of fetal epidermis to correlate, in vitro, skin penetration properties with differentiation of the epidermis. Fetal pigs, cross-bred of Landrace/Large White, at 55, 75, 84, and 96 days gestational age and full term (115 days) were used for light microscopic examination and skin transport studies.

A. Structure of Fetal Pig Skin

In the 55-day-old fetus (Fig. 1a), the epidermis has from 5 to 10 cell layers. It comprises an inner or basal layer (stratum germinativum), intermediate cells (stratum intermedium), and nonkeratinized transient outer layers, the periderm. Cords of cells of the developing hair follicles in the hair peg stage extend into the dermis, where they are surrounded by mesenchymal cells, the ancestor of most of the indigenous cells of adult connective tissues, of the developing hair bulb. Holbrook and Idkabd [35] reported the same observation in the developing human epidermis at 14–15 weeks gestational age (the beginning of the second trimester). The skin of the 55-day-old fetal pig resembles morphologically that of a human fetus during the early second trimester. In the 75-day-old fetus (Fig. 1b), the cells of the stratum intermedium appear to be enlarged and those of the

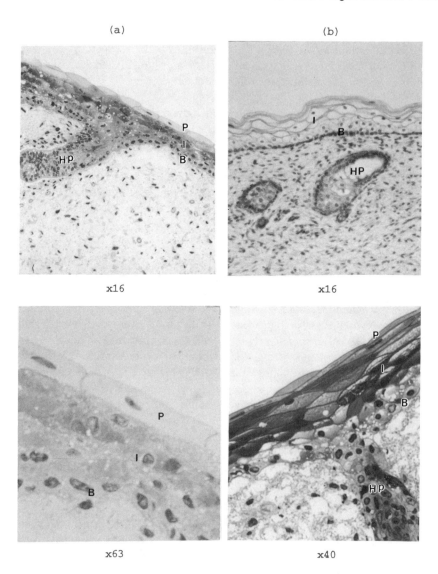

Figure 1 Microscopic cross-sectional views of fetal pig skin at varying stages of gestation. Skin taken at (a) 55, (b) 75, (c) 96, and (d) 115 (full-term) days of gestation. The paraffin section was stained by Gill's hematoxylin and eosin, and the plastic section was stained by 1% toluidine blue for microscopic observations. P, periderm; I, intermediate cells; B, basal layer; HP, hair peg; HF, hair follicle; SC, stratum corneum, SS, stratum spinosum. Upper panel: a–d, ×16. Lower panel: a, ×63; b, ×40; c, ×63; d, ×40.

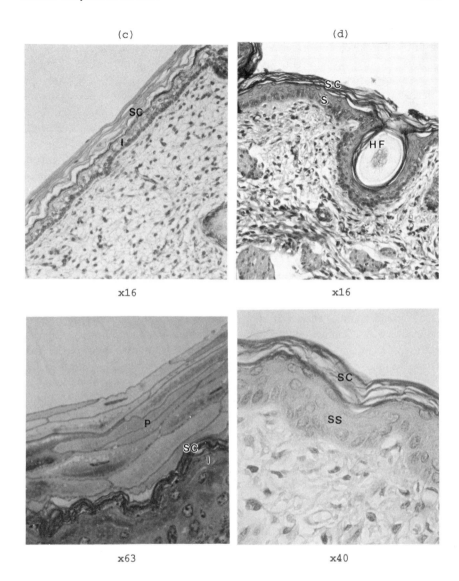

(c)

SC

I

x16

(d)

SC
S

HF

x16

P

SC
I

x63

SC

SS

x40

periderm somewhat flattened. The periderm is approximately one-third as thick as the epidermis. Hair follicles extend deep into the dermis. At this stage no evidence of keratinization appears in any part of the epidermis. Judging by these observations by light microscopy, the morphological characteristics of the 75-day-old fetal pig skin are qualitatively similar to those of the skin of a human fetus at the middle of the second trimester as described by Holbrook and Idkabd

[35]. Both 55- and 75-day-old fetal pig skins are morphologically similar to the stage of skin development during the second trimester in humans.

In the 96-day-old fetus (Fig. 1c), the morphology of epidermal cells appears to have progressed further toward flattened squamae. This stage of fetal skin is more accurately described as a stage of epidermal differentiation. The epidermis is partially keratinized, and the stratum corneum is just becoming visible, although its thickness is only about 9 μm, significantly less than that of the full-term pig. The beginning of the stratum corneum appears, correspondingly, in the human at the end of the second trimester. At first the stratum corneum consists of only a few cell layers, but it increases in thickness during the third trimester, and at full term it is approximately as thick as the adult stratum corneum [8]. It is also clear that fragments of degenerated periderm cells are all that remain above the keratinized cells of newly formed stratum corneum. In full-term pig skin (Fig. 1d), however, no remnants of the periderm remain in the entire epidermis. The granular cells also appear to be formed in the stratum intermedium of the 96-day-old fetus. In the human fetus, the granular layer is established at the sixth month, and the intermediate cells become known as spinous cells; thus, each layer of the epidermis assumes the adult nomenclature as the tissue assumes the adult characteristics [8]. These microscopic studies demonstrate that, in swine fetus, the periderm and stratum intermedium appear in the epidermis and then disappear when epidermal keratinization is completed. These findings with 96-day-old fetal pig skin are known to also occur in the third trimester of human fetal life. Collectively, these observations of fetal pig skin development show that it is morphologically comparable with developing human skin on a time scale roughly proportional with respect to the gestation periods for the two species.

B. In Vitro Skin Permeability

In vitro skin permeability studies can provide an understanding of the nature and origin of the barrier properties of skin in terms of physicochemical characteristics of stratum corneum development. In this section the barrier characteristics of skin will be examined by studying fetal pig skin penetration with emphasis on the influence of gestational age. All experiments performed in these studies involved use of full-thickness fetal pig dorsal skin. Arecoline and caffeine (Fig. 2) were chosen for the skin diffusion study. In studies of the effect of epidermal keratinization on transdermal penetration, they make a useful set of prototype compounds because of their varying physicochemical properties.

The permeation of arecoline and caffeine through fetal pig skin has been characterized as a function of gestational age. The permeability coefficients displayed in Figure 3 for arecoline and in Figure 4 for caffeine are clearly affected by the gestational age of fetal pig skin. In the profiles the patterns of behavior

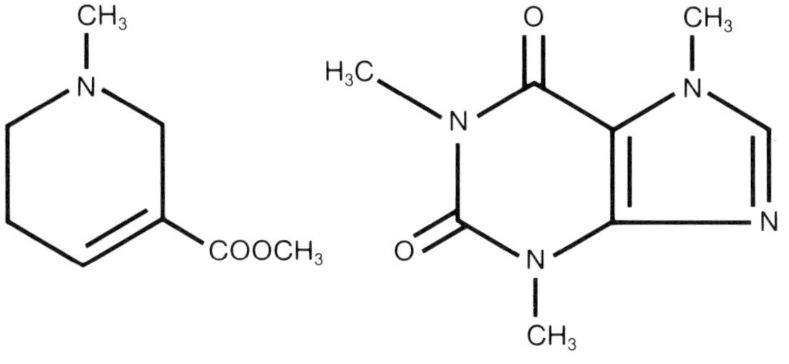

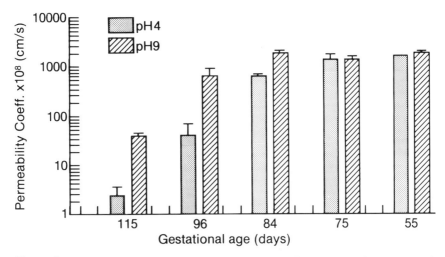

Figure 2 Chemical structure of (A) arecoline and (B) caffein.

for both compounds are similar. Fetal pig gestational age has been shown to markedly affect in vitro skin permeability of both charged and uncharged permeants. The stratum corneum, which represents the major barrier to drug absorption, appears to develop with increasing fetal pig gestational age. As it matures, fetal pig skin undergoes striking changes in its epidermal structure, especially the stratum corneum, which affect its properties as a barrier to drug

Figure 3 Permeability coefficients of arecoline through fetal pig skin from pH 4 and pH 9 aqueous solutions as a function of gestational age. The error bars represent $\pm\sigma$.

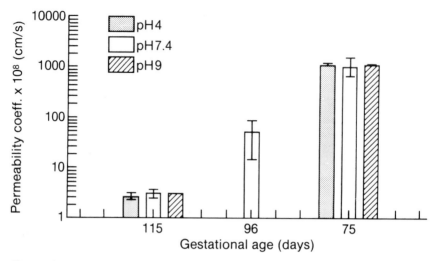

Figure 4 Permeability coefficients of caffeine through fetal pig skin from pH 4, 7.4, and 9 aqueous solutions as a function of gestational age. The error bars represent $\pm\sigma$.

diffusion. These functional changes of the epidermal barrier are also closely mirrored by histological changes.

Furthermore, a very significant finding is that permeation of fetal pig skin occurs not only for neutral species but also for charged species. The permeability of arecoline significantly increased as the pH of the aqueous solution increased from pH 4 to pH 9 in both full-term and 96-day-old fetal skin, but not in either 75- or 55-day-old fetal skin (Fig. 3). In contrast, the permeability of caffeine is independent of the solution pH in both full-term and preterm skin (Fig. 4). As has been known for adult human skin, the epidermal penetration is highly dependent upon the pH of the donor solution, which determines the activity of the transportable species, the uncharged form. Arecoline exists mostly in a protonated form at pH 4 and as a free base at pH 9, because its pK_a is 7.9. Caffeine, however, exists as an un-ionized form at all pH values. Indeed, in our experiment, the influence of skin development and gestational age on fetal skin properties is more clearly seen by examining the ratio of arecoline delivery rate at pH 9 and pH 4 (Fig. 5). This ratio is 15 for both full-term and 96-day-old fetuses. These findings implicate an aqueous pore pathway as the dominant route for transport of molecules across the fetal skin, particularly at early gestational age. These experimental results clearly demonstrate the significance of the lipid pathway in the stratum corneum as a function of epidermal keratinization.

Figure 6 depicts a general way to categorize the pathways for transport in pig skin as a function of gestational age. This schematic diagram provides par-

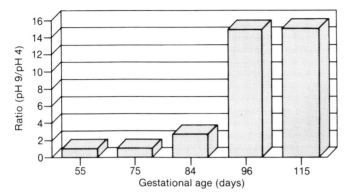

Figure 5 Ratio of arecoline permeability coefficient (P_{pH9}/P_{pH4}) through fetal pig skin as a function of gestational age.

allel lipoidal and aqueous pore pathways for the simple passive diffusion of drugs in the outer layer of the pig skin and is not intended to assign a pathway to a particular morphological structure. Fetal pig skin of early gestational period can be likened to a swollen hydrogen matrix. However, as the epidermis matures, keratinization increases. At 96 days gestational age, skin arecoline permeability coefficients of both ionized and un-ionized species increase although the permeability ratio (P_{pH9}/P_{pH4}) remains the same (Fig. 5). This indicates that the area fraction of both aqueous pore and lipid pathway remains the same as those of the full-term pig skin; however, the properties of both pathways appear to be altered. It is also observed histologically that an epidermal keratinization has been started by this gestational period. In 75-day-old or younger fetuses, there does not exist a parallel pathway in skin transport (Fig. 6). The skin offers little more than the resistance of a gelled aqueous phase to mass transfer. It resembles stripped skin when the stratum corneum is removed by stripping, as is suggested by Scheuplein [6]. Consequently, a critical gestational period of the fetal pig skin at which the stratum corneum starts developing appears to be between 75 and 96 days gestational age. The results presented here clearly demonstrate the significance of the lipid pathway in the stratum corneum as a function of epidermal keratinization.

IV. TRANSDERMAL DRUG DELIVERY TO THE PREMATURE INFANT

The conventional methods of administering systemically active therapeutic agents to preterm infants have distinct drawbacks. Oral administration of such agents generally leads to unpredictable absorption from the undeveloped gastro-

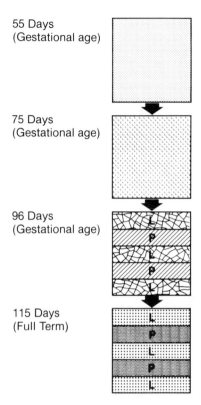

Figure 6 Idealized model of the fetal pig skin transport. L and P represent lipid and aqueous pore pathways for passive diffusion of drugs in the stratum corneum.

intestinal tract. Intravenous administration generally requires an access line that has a large dead volume compared with the generally small volume required by the patient. Moreover, the rather fragile and tiny vein size further introduces complications in attempts to administer drugs intravenously in such infants. Further, in preterm infants, inherent dangers are introduced due to the generally narrow therapeutic index of many neonatal therapeutic agents. Transdermal administration has thus been suggested as an alternative to traditional therapy to take advantage of the relatively high skin permeabilities of preterm infants resulting from their poorly developed stratum corneum.

A. Transdermal Delivery of Theophylline

Theophylline is an ideal candidate for transdermal administration to premature infants. It is widely used as a respiratory stimulant for the treatment or prevention of recurrent apnea of prematurity [36]. The therapy is usually started immediately after birth and continues for several weeks. The pharmacokinetics of theophylline in the preterm infant has been widely studied [37]. Data from studies of the premature infant are of interest because of their consistency in pattern: longer half-life, larger volume of distribution, and smaller body clearance compared with those of young children or adults. The effective serum levels, C_{ss}, of theophylline as treatment for recurrent apnea of premature infants are reported to be 4–12 μg/mL, and the plasma clearance, Cl_p of theophylline is 17.6 mL hr^{-1} kg^{-1} [37]. Then the steady-state flux, J_{ss}, for the required area, A, is given by

$$J_{ss} = C_{ss}\, Cl_p/A$$

Using this equation, the skin permeabilities of theophylline required to attain therapeutic plasma levels with a 2-cm^2 system are in the range of 35–105 μg cm^{-2} hr^{-1}.

B. Hydrogel Systems in the Transdermal Administration of Therapeutic Agents

Attempts have been made to deliver a systemically active agent, theophylline, to premature infants by the use of a hydroxymethylcellulose gel placed on the neonate abdominal skin under an occlusive patch [28]. However, in all cases removal of the patch was reported necessary owing to leakage of the gel after administration. Difficulties in handling and lack of uniformity in the administration were also reported. To overcome several drawbacks associated with a flowable gel it is necessary to provide a method of administering systemically active agents to the premature infant through intact skin.

The hydrogel provides a means of delivering water-soluble neonatal therapeutic agents through the intact skin of premature infants in a controlled continuous manner [38]. Hydrogel materials suitable for use as a drug reservoir include those cross-linked hydrophilic polymers that have been disclosed as compatible with human tissue, such as hydrogels described as useful in body implants or soft hydrophilic contact lens materials. In general, suitable cross-linked hydrogels include those prepared by copolymerization of a major amount of a hydrophilic monoolefinic monomer and a minor amount of a hydrophilic or hydrophobic cross-linking agent [39–41]. To increase the lipophilicity of the hydrogel, there may also be present, in addition to the hydrophilic monoolefin, a minor amount of a hydrophobic monoolefin. Alternatively, a hydrogel may be employed that is prepared by copolymerizing di- or polyvinylic macromer with a monoolefinic monomer, or mixture of monomers, having sufficient hydrophilicity that the resulting polymer is capable, upon equilibration, of absorbing between about 10 and 80 percent by weight water, based upon the total weight of the equilibrated polymer hydrogel.

C. Theophylline Hydrogel Disk

The hydrogel disk consists of a balanced hydrophilic/hydrophobic copolymer that is made by copolymerization cross-linking of poly-2-hydroxyethyl meth-acrylate monomer in the presence of a "macromer," polytetramethylene oxide [42]. The polymerized film is swollen in water, after which 2-cm² surface area disks are punched and vacuum-dried. Theophylline can be loaded into the hydrogel disks by solution sorption techniques. The disks are immersed in the saturated solutions for a minimum of 24 hr at 37°C in capped tubes. Drug loading is accomplished by both the drug solution uptake and drug partitioning into the hydrogel matrix. The drug-loaded "dissolved monolithic" hydrogel systems are then ready for transdermal application.

A plot of total cumulative drug release versus time for such theophylline systems is shown in Figure 7. Theophylline release from such systems can be described by

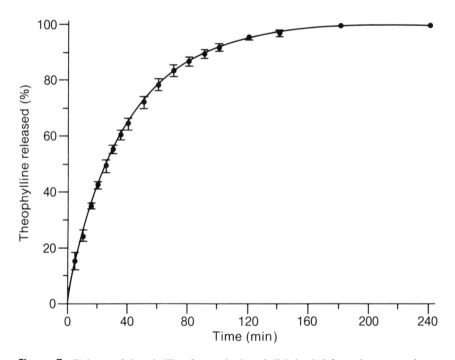

Figure 7 Release of theophylline from a hydrogel disk loaded from the saturated so-lution. The filled circles are the average of three experiments; error bars show standard deviation.

$$\frac{Q_t}{Q_\infty} = 1 - \sum_{n=0}^{\infty} \frac{8 \exp\left[-D(2n + 1)^2\pi^2 t/l^2\right]}{(2n + 1)^2\pi^2}$$

where Q_t is the total amount of drug released at time t, Q_∞ is the total drug loading, D is the drug diffusion coefficient, and l is the thickness of the disk. Theophylline diffusion coefficients can be calculated using an early time approximation of the above equation:

$$\frac{Q_t}{Q_\infty} = \frac{4(Dt)^{1/2}}{\pi l^2}$$

Square root time plots demonstrate excellent linearity out to approximately 50% total drug release as shown in Figure 8. The magnitude of the zero time Y-axis intercept is a measure of the "burst effect" due to surface-associated drug. All Y-axis intercept values are negligibly small and essentially equal to zero, demonstrating that systems are adequately rinsed of surface-associated drug from clinging loading solutions. Thus, the theophylline diffusion coefficient in the hydrogel system is determined to be 1.7×10^{-4} cm^2/hr.

Figure 9 presents representative transdermal theophylline delivery results for theophylline-loaded hydrogel disks using 96-day gestation and full-term (115-day) fetal pig skin. Nearly constant delivery rates are obtained out to 24 hr with both 96-day gestation and full-term skin. Significant delivery rate differences

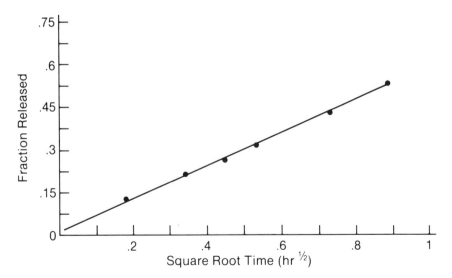

Figure 8 A typical time$^{1/2}$-dependent theophylline release curve from a hydrogel disk loaded from the saturated solution.

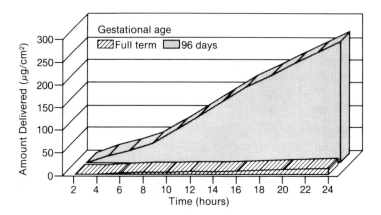

Figure 9 In vitro permeation of theophylline through 96- and 115-day gestational age fetal pig skin from theophylline hydrogel disks.

have also been observed between these skins. The decreased delivery rates observed with full-term skin relative to 96-day gestation skin is consistent with the previous transport studies using aqueous donor solutions and reflects reduced skin permeability with increased fetal maturation.

D. Clinical Evaluation of Theophylline Hydrogel Disk

The theophylline hydrogel disk loaded from aqueous solution saturated with choline theophylline was placed onto dry, untraumatized abdominal skin under occlusion [43–45]. Eleven premature infants were studied using the same formulation. Their gestation ranged from 25 to 30 weeks and postnatal age from 0.67 to 6 days. In six infants a single hydrogel was applied. In the other five infants, three or four hydrogel disks were applied consecutively. The first disk was placed on a site when the infants were between 26 and 76 hr of postnatal age. Subsequent disks were applied when the serum theophylline concentration obtained from the preceding disk started to decrease. No infant received theophylline prior to the study.

In all six infants treated with a single theophylline disk, therapeutic levels of 4–12 μg/mL were achieved after administration and maintained for 62–117 hr, on average. For example, Baby A, male, 25 weeks gestational age and postnatal age of 6 days, who had a birth weight of 0.83 kg and exhibited apneic syndrome, was treated by application of a disk prepared according to the above procedure. The therapeutic level was achieved within 3 hr and was maintained approximately for 100 hr (Fig. 10). Serum theophylline concentration shows generally

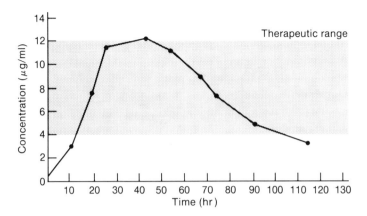

Figure 10 Typical serum theophylline levels in a premature infant after a single application of a theophylline hydrogel disk to the skin.

higher levels in infants of earlier gestations. This might be expected because these infants would tend to have more immature skin, lower birth weights, and lower clearance than those born at later gestations.

All five infants treated with multiple application of theophylline-loaded disks achieved serum concentrations within the therapeutic range. Theophylline serum concentrations were first attained between 8 and 25 hr after the initial application and were maintained within the therapeutic range for 6–15 days. A typical serum concentration profile is shown in Figure 11. Baby B, female, 26 weeks gestational age and postnatal age of 2 days, with a birth weight of 1.06 kg, was treated with three applications of a single disk. The therapeutic concentration was first attained 8 hr after the initial application, and C_{max} was 11.7 μg/mL. The second disk was applied on the 5th day, attaining C_{max} of 10.2 μg/mL, and the last disk on the 11th day, with C_{max} of 6.8 μg/mL. The amount of theophylline penetrating through the skin decreases with increasing number of subsequent disks, which indicates the maturation of skin with increased postnatal age. Babies in this study appeared to respond to theophylline in the same way as if the drug had been given orally or intravenously.

V. CONCLUSIONS

The results presented here clearly demonstrate the importance of the middle to end of the third trimester of pregnancy in the fetal pig to the development of an adequate skin barrier function in preparation for birth. There is much circumstantial evidence that the human fetus undergoes a similar sharp transition at the same relative gestational age and points out the importance of recognizing

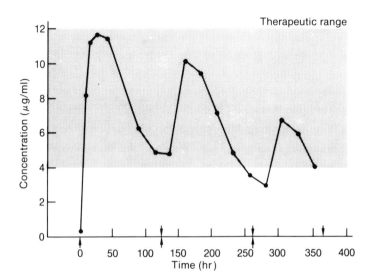

Figure 11   Serum theophylline levels in a premature infant after multiple applications of theophylline hydrogel disks to the skin. (↓) disk removal; (↑) disk application.

this in premature infants born in this period of gestation. Very significant is the finding that permeation of fetal pig skin as well as human premature infant skin occurs not only for neutral species but also for ionized species. The use of hydrogel systems in the transdermal administration of therapeutic agents to the premature neonate may be a viable method for delivering life-saving drugs intended for systemic treatment during the critical first weeks of life in the premature infant. The results of this investigation can apply not only to premature infant skin, but also to understanding the barrier properties of the stratum corneum with respect to drug transport in general.

REFERENCES

1. R. J. Scheuplein and J. H. Blank, *Physiol. Rev. 51*, 702 (1971).
2. T. Kurihara-Bergstrom, M. Woodworth, S. Feisullin, and P. Beall, *J. Lab. Animal Sci. 36*(4), 396 (1986).
3. M. Bartek, J. LaBudde, and H. Maibach, *J. Invest. Dermatol. 58*, 114 (1972).
4. R. K. Loeffler, J. W. Herron, and V. Thomas, *U.S. AEC Nucl. Sci. Abstr. 5*, 4959 (1951).
5. C. Behl, G. Flynn, T. Kurihara, W. Smith, O. Gatmaitan, W. Higuchi, N. Ho, and C. Pierson, *J. Invest. Dermatol. 75*(4), 340 (1980).
6. R. J. Scheuplein, *J. Invest. Dermatol. 45*, 334 (1965).

7. C. D. Yu, W. I. Higuchi, N. F. H. Ho, J. L. Fox, and G. L. Flynn, *J. Pharm. Sci.* *69*(7), 770 (1980).

8. K. A. Holbrook, in *Biochemistry and Physiology of the Skin*, L. A. Goldsmith, Ed., Oxford Univ. Press, Oxford, 1983, p. 64.

9. D. R. Wilson and H. I. Maibach, *Biol. Neonate 37*, 180 (1980).

10. L. Fisher, *J. Invest Dermatol. 64*(4), 291 (1975).

11. R. L. Nachman and N. B. Esterly, *J. Pediatr. 79*(4), 628 (1971).

12. A. Curley, R. E. Hawks, R. D. Kimbrough, C. Nathenson, and L. Finberg, *Lancet ii*, 296 (1971).

13. V. G. Alderm, D. Burman, B. D. Corner, and W. A. Gillespie, *Lancet ii*, 384 (1972).

14. A. E. Copelman, *J. Pediatr. 82*, 972 (1973).

15. E. E. Tyrala, L. S. Hillman, R. E. Hillman, and W. E. Dodson, *J. Pediatr. 91*, 481 (1977).

16. H. Powell, O. Swarmer, L. Gluck, and P. Lambert, *J. Pediatr. 82*, 976 (1973).

17. R. M. Shuman, R. W. Leech, and E. C. Akvird, *Pediatrics 54*, 689 (1974).

18. G. Martin-Bouter, R. Lebreton, M. Toga, P. D. Stolley, and J. Lockhart, *Lancet i*, 91 (1982).

19. S. J. Greaves, D. G. Ferry, E. G. McQueen, and P. M. Buckfield, *N. Zealand Med. J. 81*, 334 (1975).

20. S. P. Pyata, R. S. Ramanurthy, M. T. Krauss, and R. S. Pildes, *J. Pediatr. 91*, 825 (1977).

21. J. P. Chabrolle and A. Rossier, *Arch. Dis. Child. 53*, 495 (1978).

22. V. A. Harpin and N. Rutter, *Arch. Dis. Child. 57*, 477 (1982).

23. J. B. Schick and J. M. Milstein, *Pediatrics 68*, 587 (1981).

24. P. J. Aggett, L. V. Cooper, S. H. Ellis, and J. McAinsh, *Arch. Dis. Child. 56*, 878 (1981).

25. N. Rutter, *Clin. Perinatol. 14*, 911 (1987).

26. R. L. Cunico, H. U. Maibach, H. Kahn, and E. Bloom, *Biol. Neonate 32*, 177 (1977).

27. J. N. Evans and N. Rutter, *J. Pediatr. 108*, 282 (1986).

28. N. J. Evans, N. Rutter, J. Hadgraft, and G. Parr, *J. Pediatr. 107*, 307 (1985).

29. E. J. Singer, P. C. Wegmann, M. D. Christensen, and L. J. Vinson, *J. Soc. Cosmet. Chem. 22*, 119 (1971).

30. R. C. Webster, P. K. Noonan, and H. I. Maibach, *J. Soc. Cosmet. Chem. 30*, 297 (1979).

31. D. J. Bissett and J. F. McBride, *J. Soc. Cosmet. Chem. 34*, 317 (1983).

32. A. M. Kligman, *J. Soc. Cosmet. Chem. 34*, 317 (1983).

33. E. H. Fowler and M. Calhoun, *Am. J. Vet. Res. 25*, 156 (1964).

34. T. Kurihara-Bergstrom, C. Signor, M. Woodworth, and W. R. Good, *Pharm. Res. 7*(11), 1201 (1990).

35. K. A. Holbrook and G. F. Idkabd, *J. Invest. Dermatol. 65*, 16 (1975).

36. J. V. Aranda, D. Grondin, and B. I. Sasynuik, *Pediatr. Clin. N. Am. 28*(1), 113 (1981).

37. J. V. Aranda, D. S. Sitar, W. D. Parsons, P. M. Loughnan, and A. H. Neims, *N. Engl. J. Med. 295*, 413 (1976).

38. T. Kurihara-Bergstrom, W. R. Good, and C. D. Ebert, U.S. Patent 4,853,227 (Aug. 1, 1989).
39. O. Wichterle and D. Lim, U.S. Patent 27,401 (June 20, 1972).
40. T. H. Shepherd and F. E. Gould, U.S. Patent 3,520,949 (July 21, 1970).
41. K. F. Mueller and W. R. Good, U.S. Patent 4,177,056 (Dec. 4, 1979).
42. W. R. Good and K. F. Mueller, *AICE 77*(206), 42 (1981).
43. T. Kurihara-Bergstrom, N. Rutter, S. S. Davis, C. Ebert, and W. R. Good, Hydrogel systems in the transdermal administration of therapeutic agents to the premature neonate, *Proc. Int. Symp. Controlled Release Bioactive Mater. 15*, 219–220 (1988).
44. R. G. Cartwright, P. H. T. Cartlidge, N. Rutter, T. Kurihara-Bergstrom, C. D. Melia, and S. S. Davis, Percutaneous delivery of theophylline to neonates, *Proc. Int. Symp. Controlled Release Bioactive Mater. 15*, 396–397 (1988).
45. R. G. Cartwright, P. H. T. Cartlidge, N. Rutter, C. D. Melia, and S. S. Davis, *Br. J. Clin. Pharm. 29*, 533 (1990).

III

DRUG PERMEATION ENHANCEMENT VIA THE SKIN: PHYSICAL MEANS

11
Iontophoresis: Fundamentals

Ooi Wong
Cygnus Therapeutic Systems, Redwood City, California

I. INTRODUCTION

Delivery of drugs across membranes into the bloodstream requires energy. Various forms of energy have been employed to deliver drug molecules from a drug reservoir to the target area. Osmotic pressure has been applied successfully to an osmostic pump device [1]. Fick's diffusion laws have been applied to passive transdermal delivery systems [2]. An ion-pairing mechanism is used to explain facilitated transport, which is basically a chemical mechanism that lowers the activation energy of the passive transport barrier; many biological processes display facilitated transport [3]. Phonophoretic (ultrasonic) drug delivery systems [4] use wave energy, chemical potential energy is used in pH gradient delivery systems [5] to drive drug molecules through a membrane, and the prodrug approach of drug delivery [6] in many instances is another method of lowering activation energy.

Iontophoresis [7–17] has long been studied intensively as a means of delivering drugs through the skin or other membranes into the bloodstream with the assistance of a minute quantity of electric energy. Iontophoretic drug delivery is now a fast-growing field, as is evidenced by the large number of recent publications in this area and the iontophoretic institutions that are developing iontophoretic products [18]. Heat and light are other forms of energy that can also be used for drug delivery. In particular, it is well known that temperature can enhance the delivery rates of passive transdermal drug delivery.

Iontophoresis is defined as the introduction of therapeutic agents into the tissues of the body by means of electric current [19]. Historically, the idea of using electric current to drive medicine into the body was claimed by Pivati in 1747 [17]. Rossi tried to pass mercury through the skin electrically in 1802 [20]. Fabre-Palaprat claimed that he was able to introduce medication into the human body with direct current [21]. Wagner suggested the possibility of administering anesthesia by introducing cocaine electrically [22]. Le Duc was the first (in 1908) [23] to confirm that ions could be driven across the skin by means of an electric current. In 1911, Albrecht [24] studied the use of cocaine and epinephrine in iontophoresis for anesthesia to the external auditory meatus. Between then and 1921, numerous ophthalmological iontophoretic studies were carried out. Many difficulties were encountered, with some patients corneal scars, tissue burns, and electrical shocks.

Because of the major technical problems, iontophoresis was then virtually discarded until the early 1940s, when the successful iontophoretic delivery of penicillin and sulfadiazine into the infected eyes of animals renewed scientific interest in the technique [25]. Since then, interest in iontophoresis has shifted toward its use as a drug delivery system for a wide variety of medications. This is discussed in Section VI.

Iontophoresis has been found useful in the diagnosis of cystic fibrosis via the sweat test [36,154–163]. Iontophoresis of pilocarpine has been approved by the FDA for this purpose and is widely used by physicians. The device uses an extremely low level of electric current to assist the transport of pilocarpine into the skin to induce sufficient sweat for chloride assay. This method achieves better patient compliance than other methods. Currently, Medtronic, Inc. is marketing a CF Indicator device. Treatment of hyperhidrosis by iontophoresis of water is also widely used [26–29].

In this chapter, theories relative to iontophoresis given in the following sections include basic structures of electrochemical cells, electrochemistry of electrochemical cells, and principles of iontophoresis in terms of either Faraday's electrochemical law or electrodiffusion theory. Iontophoretic drug delivery rates can be easily related to Faraday's law. Techniques to obtain reliable iontophoretic delivery data are described in Section III. Selection of drug candidates are discussed on the basis of important physicochemical properties of drug candidates as they relate to drug delivery. Features of iontophoresis are described in Section V. Drugs that have been studied both in vitro and in vivo are discussed in Section VI.

II. THEORY

In principle, iontophoresis is very similar to electrophoresis, which is the migration of charged particles, especially colloidal particles, through a relatively

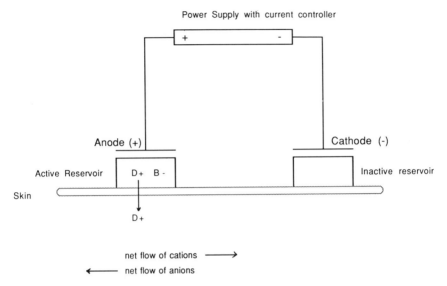

Figure 1 Schematic illustration of the basic features of an iontophoretic drug delivery system.

stationary liquid phase under the influence of an applied electric field provided, in general, by immersed electrodes [30]. Electrophoresis has been studied in great detail, and therefore its basic principles can be applied to iontophoresis. Both systems require electrodes and a power supply. In iontophoresis, the amount of electricity required to drive the molecules is small, and the skin acts as a drug transport barrier between the two electrodes. For electrophoresis, high voltage is required to drive the charged species, and the length of the medium through which the charged species travel under electrical influence is much greater than the thickness of the skin. In this way the charged species can be effectively separated in the medium. Both techniques resemble an electrochemical cell, and an understanding of what a cell is and how it functions is essential to understanding either technique. The migration rates of charged species through a medium during electrophoresis and iontophoresis depend on the magnitude of the applied electromotive force and the physical and chemical nature of the species and of the medium.

A basic design for an iontophoretic transdermal drug delivery device is shown in Figure 1, which will be used to explain iontophoretic drug delivery. An iontophoretic drug delivery system comprises a power supply; an anode connected to the active or drug-containing reservoir, which is in contact with the skin; and a cathode connected to the inactive reservoir, which contains buffers, ions, or other materials that can conduct electricity to complete the circuit. The inactive reservoir must also be in contact with the skin. The skin acts as an impedance barrier to drug transport. In the figure, a cationic drug is represented by D^+. When the battery is switched on, direct current flows from the positive pole of the battery toward the anode through the drug reservoir. The current flows through the skin and the tissues below the skin barrier to the inactive reservoir and back to the battery to complete the circuit. The cationic drug ions (D^+) are carried out of the reservoir and through the skin barrier, whereby they are absorbed into the bloodstream. Anionic drugs can be transdermally delivered in a similar fashion from the cathode.

A. Electrochemical Cells (31,32)

An electrochemical cell is generally composed of two conductors or electrodes immersed in the same electrolyte solution or in two different electrolyte solutions that are in electrical contact and separated by a porous diaphragm. Electrochemical cells can be classified into two types:

1. A galvanic cell in which electrochemical reactions occur spontaneously when the two electrodes are connected by a conductor, as shown in Figure 2, and
2. An electrolytic cell in which chemical reactions are caused to occur by the imposition of an external voltage greater than the reversible (galvanic) voltage of the cell.

Usually, a transdermal iontophoretic drug delivery device falls into the second class of electrochemical cells. Electrolytic cells are used to carry out chemical reactions at the expense of electric energy.

The galvanic cell can be illustrated by half-cell reactions using zinc and copper as examples. Oxidation occurs at the anode, where zinc is oxidized to zinc ions, and at the cathode, where copper ions in solution are reduced to copper metal. The charge on the ion is its oxidation state or oxidation number. Pulling electrons away from an atom is oxidation, and adding electrons to an atom is reduction.

Anode reaction (oxidation):

$$Zn \quad Zn^{2+} + 2e^- \quad E_{left}$$

Cathode reaction (reduction):

$$Cu^{2+} + 2e^- \quad Cu \quad E_{right}$$

Each half-cell reaction represents the change that occurs at a single electrode, and the two half-cell reactions can be added together to express the overall cell

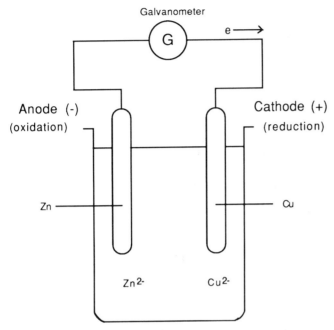

Figure 2 Schematic illustration of a galvanic cell. (Reproduced from Martin et al. [32].)

reaction:

$$Zn + Cu^{2+} = Zn^{2+} + Cu$$

$$E_{cell} = E_{left} + E_{right}$$

The individual electrode potentials (E_{left} and E_{right}) occur at the junction between each electrode and its surrounding solution. The sum of the two electrode potentials corresponds to E_{cell}, which is the *electromotive force* (emf) or *voltage* of the cell. The reactions occurring at the electrodes of the cell are always illustrated so that electrons are given up to the external circuit at the left electrode (anode) and accepted from the external circuit at the right electrode (cathode).

For an electrolytic cell, the electrode reactions and transport phenomena can be described in the following way. For an electric current to pass through the system, processes that facilitate its passage must occur at the electrodes. An immediate exchange of charged particles takes place between the electrode and the solution. Substances are reduced to a lower oxidation state at the cathode. Simultaneously, oxidation processes take place at the anode. The conditions during electrolysis can be characterized quantitatively by Faraday's law.

1. Faraday's Principles of Electrolysis

The electrochemical reactions at an electrode can be related to Faraday's electrochemical laws:

1. The mass of any substance that is oxidized or reduced at an electrode is proportional to the quantity of electricity that passes through the electrolyte.
2. The masses of different substances that are oxidized or reduced at an electrode by a given quantity of electricity are proportional to their equivalent weights and inversely proportional to their valence. One faraday (1F) is the quantity of electricity (96,500 coulombs) that will oxidize or reduce 1 equivalent weight of any substance.

These two laws can be combined into the equation

$$W = Itm/zF \tag{1}$$

where W is the number of grams oxidized or reduced, I the current in amperes, t the time in seconds, M the molecular weight, $F = 1$ faraday (96,500 coulombs/mole), and z is the valence charge of the reacting species.

2. Transport numbers

The fraction of the total current carried by a charged species is known as its transport number. For cations and anions, the transport numbers can be expressed as t_+ and t_-, respectively, where

$$t_+ = \frac{\text{current carried by cations}}{\text{total current}} \tag{2}$$

and

$$t_- = \frac{\text{current carried by anions}}{\text{total current}} \tag{3}$$

The sum of the two transport numbers is equal to unity:

$$t_+ + t_- = 1 \tag{4}$$

The transport number of an ion indicates two important characteristics of the ion:

1. Faster moving ions carry a greater fraction of the current.
2. The velocity of an ion depends on the degree of hydration of the ion and on its size and charge.

The velocity and transport numbers may be different for positive and negative ions. For example, the transport numbers of sodium and chloride ions in 0.01 M NaCl solution are $t_+(Na^+) = 0.385$ and $t^-(Cl^-) = 0.615$.

Transport numbers can be measured using a variation of the electromotive force method. The transport number of a drug ion is a very important parameter in iontophoretic drug delivery because it provides an indication of the speed of the drug ion moving through the skin. The higher the transport number, the higher the fraction of current that is carried by the drug ions. Therefore, an understanding of the factors influencing the ion transport number is helpful in optimizing ion permeation enhancement.

3. Ohm's law

Ohm's law states that

$$I = E / R \tag{5}$$

where I is the strength of an electric current in amperes, E is the applied potential or voltage in volts, and R is the resistance of the medium in ohms.

4. Conductance

The resistance R, in ohms, of any uniform material is directly proportional to its length L in centimeters and inversely proportional to its cross-sectional area A in square centimeters,

$$R = \rho L / A \tag{6}$$

where ρ is the resistance between opposite faces of a 1-cm cube of the conductor and is known as the specific resistance. The conductance C is the reciprocal of resistance.

$$C = \frac{1}{R} = \frac{1}{\rho} \left(\frac{A}{L} \right) \tag{7}$$

and hence can be considered a measure of the ease with which current can pass through the conductor. It is expressed in siemens units (S) or mhos.

B. Electric Energy for Drug Transport

The strength of an electric current is the flow rate of electricity (Q) in coulombs per unit time, or

$$I = Q / t \tag{8}$$

Electric power is equal to the product of the applied voltage and the electric current,

$$E \times Q = \text{voltage} \times \text{current} \tag{9}$$

The power required to overcome the stratum corneum penetration barrier can be expressed as

$$\text{Electric power} = EI = I^2 R \tag{10}$$

where E is the applied voltage, I the applied current, and R the resistance of the skin. When the resistance of the skin is reduced, less energy is required to overcome the barrier.

C. Drug Delivery Rates

Faraday's law can be applied to account for the drug delivery rate (D), which is defined as the amount of drug ions delivered across the skin barrier per unit time. Without a barrier between the electrodes, the drug delivery rate should perfectly follow Faraday's law. However, the skin barrier between the two electrodes influences the transport numbers of the ionic species.

$$D = W/t = MItt_D/zFt \tag{11}$$

$$D = MIt_D/zF \tag{12}$$

where W is the amount of drug ions (gm) delivered across the skin barrier, M the molecular weight of the drug, z the number of charges per drug ion, I current that passes through the skin barrier, t_D the transport number of the drug ion, t time, and F Faraday's constant (96,500 coulombs per equivalent).

The transport number of the drug ion through the skin must be considered in the delivery rate equation. Hence equation (12) accommodates practical drug delivery rates. Determination of t_D for a drug candidate is discussed in Section III.

D. Electrode Materials

Electrode materials used in iontophoresis include platinum, silver/silver chloride, brass, copper, zinc, gold-plated brass, conductive plastic, platinum-iridium, and steel [35–40].

E. Electrophoresis (41–51)

The rate of migration (mobility) of an ion in an electric field is the sum of two forces, the driving force and the resisting force.

The driving force depends on

1. The number of charges per molecule. Increasing the number of charges on the ion increases its rate of migration.
2. The sign of the charge on the ion. Cations will move from anode to cathode, while anions move in the opposite direction.
3. The degree of ionization of the species. The pK_a of the species affects the degree of ionization, which is a function of the pH of the medium [52].

4. The magnitude of the electric field potential. The rate of migration of an ionized species through a medium is directly proportional to the applied current.

5. The duration of exposure of the species to the field force. Longer exposure time will enhance the driving force, and this effect is also important to iontophoresis [53].

The factors relating the resistance to electrophoretic mobility are (1) the size and shape of the ion, (2) the viscosity of the medium, (3) the concentration of the ion, (4) the solubility of the ionizable species, and (5) the absorptive properties of the supporting medium.

Understanding the factors that control the migration of ions is very important. This allows one to design a more efficient system for iontophoresis in terms of (1) formulations in the drug and inactive reservoirs, (2) the type of materials to choose for building the system, (3) achieving high iontophoretic drug delivery efficiencies, (4) choosing a suitable drug candidate, and (5) the power supply.

The effect of a buffer on ion mobility [41] can be expressed as

$$\mu = \frac{4 \pi C e}{0.327 \times 10^8 \epsilon} \sqrt{I} \tag{13}$$

where e is the electric charge of an electron or proton, ϵ is the dielectric constant, I is the ionic strength, and C is a constant. This can be applied to the extraneous ions present in a drug reservoir competing with drug ions during iontophoresis. An ideal support medium should not adsorb the ion. In extreme cases, adsorption can prevent migration altogether. During iontophoresis, drug ions must be able to move through the drug reservoir medium and the skin. To enhance iontophoretic drug delivery, one can investigate the drug reservoir medium and mechanisms to reduce the resistance of the skin.

F. Iontophoresis

The drug delivery rate equations (11) and (12) can be used to describe the drug delivery rate due to the apparent electric energy. However, equations (11) and (12) do not account separately for electrodiffusion, passive diffusion, convective effects, or electro-osmotic effects. Applying kinetic electrodiffusion theory to the iontophoresis phenomenon is extremely complicated, even for a simple model system such as a charged particle diffusing through a simple homogeneous charge-free membrane [54]. Therefore, a complete understanding of the electrodiffusion phenomenon in the skin is expected to be extremely difficult. However, the phenomenon can be approximated for application and practical purposes.

The total flux of a component under the influence of a uniform electric field can be expressed as the sum of the flux due to passive diffusion, the flux due to electrodiffusion, and the flux due to convective effects:

$$J_{total} = J_p + J_{el} + J_{con} \tag{14}$$

This equation does not predict the effects of permselectivity or changes in transport numbers. When there are environmental changes such as changes in pH and/or transport numbers, the relative magnitudes of the electrical and convective terms for each charged species in the system will change in such a way that total current flow and the charge neutrality conditions are satisfied [13]. Burnette and Ongpipattanakul [55] demonstrated that the skin is a permselective membrane (isoelectric point, pH 3–4) and exists with an apparent net negative charge at the free solution pH of 7.4; during iontophoresis this permselectivity leads to current-induced volume flow. This induced volume flow will assist the permeation of neutral species, a phenomenon called electro-osmosis.

The equation most commonly used to describe electrically assisted transport is the Nernst-Planck equation for ideal solutions and for one-dimensional membrane transport of an ion under the influence of a uniform electric field. It is given as

$$J_i = D_i \frac{dC_i}{dx} + \frac{D_i z_i e E C_i}{kT} + V_i C_i \tag{15}$$

where J_i is the flux of the ion across the membrane, D_i the diffusion coefficient, C_i the concentration of the ion, e the electron charge of the ion, z_i the charge of the ion, E the electric field, k Boltzmann's constant, T the absolute temperature, and V_i the velocity of solvent flow (electro-osmotic flow).

The Nernst-Planck equation can thus be interpreted as implying that when a concentration gradient and an electric field both exist, the ionic flux is a linear sum of the fluxes that would arise from each effect alone.

G. Pathways of Permeation

Zankel and Durham [56] conducted a study in 1963 and concluded that transdermal absorption of ^{131}I could be reduced by prior application of heat, ultrasound, or histamine iontophoresis. Similarly, cooling could increase its absorption. Because heat enhances sweat secretion and cooling decreases the rate of sweat production, these findings point to the sweat glands as the most significant paths for conduction of charged ions into and through the skin. This conclusion was confirmed by Papa and Kligman [57].

III. PRACTICAL CONSIDERATIONS

Iontophoresis can be simplified to obtain meaningful experimental results. For in vitro experiments, a diffusion cell, a pair of electrodes, a membrane, and a power source are required.

An iontophoretic diffusion cell [37,38,131] is depicted schematically in Figure 3. Electrode materials used in iontophoresis are listed in Section II.D. Silver/silver chloride materials and platinum have been found to be excellent electrode materials for conducting current in an iontophoretic circuit [37].

A. Treatment of Electrically Assisted Transport Data (37)

Two approaches can be used for treatment of electrically assisted transport data. A simpler method is the thermodynamic approach of applying Faraday's electrochemical law. However, this approach does not account for the transport mechanism. The other is the more complicated kinetic approach of applying electrodiffusion theory to transport. The most commonly used equation for this approach is the Nernst-Planck equation, which includes passive and iontophoretic diffusion. For practical purposes, the use of Faraday's law seems to be simpler in terms of data manipulation. The drug delivery rate D, by applying Faraday's law, can be defined as the amount of drug delivered across the skin barrier per unit time:

$$D = W/t \tag{16}$$

where W is the amount of drug ions (mg) delivered across the skin barrier and t is time.

As given in equation (12),

$$D = MIt_D/zF$$

The transport number of the drug ion is defined as

$$t_D = \frac{\text{observed delivery rate}}{\text{maximum delivery rate}} \tag{17}$$

For a monovalent drug ion, $z = 1$, the maximum delivery rate of the drug ion (D_{max}) is defined as when $t_D = 1$,

$$D_{max} = MI/F \ (\text{mg sec}^{-1} \text{ mA}^{-1}) \tag{18}$$

The observed steady-state delivery rates, D (mg sec^{-1} mA^{-1}), can be obtained from the slopes of the permeation profiles, and they may, as a first approximation, be considered equal to the sum of the electrodiffusion delivery rate D_i, the passive delivery rate D_p, and the electro-osmotic delivery rate D_e,

$$D_{obs} = D_p + D_i + D_e \tag{19}$$

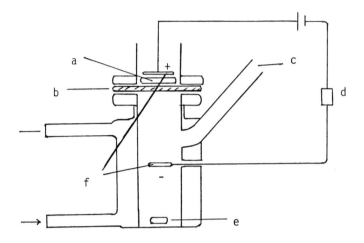

Figure 3 Schematic illustration of an iontophoretic diffusion cell assembly. (Reproduced from Bannon et al. [37].) a, drug reservoir or solution; b, skin or membrane; c, sampling port; d, ammeter; e, stir bar; f, electrode.

The iontophoretic rate can be expressed as the product of the current I and an iontophoretic constant, f_i,

$$D_i = f_i I \tag{20}$$

Combining equations (19) and (20) and assuming that $D_e \ll D_i$ gives

$$D_{obs} = D_p + f_i I \tag{21}$$

If the contribution from D_p is independent of the iontophoretic contribution, or at least affected only negligibly by this process, then equation (21) shows that D_{obs} should vary linearly with I to yield a line of slope equal to f_i. A series of steady-state fluxes or delivery rates D_{obs} can be obtained by performing a series of iontophoretic experiments using variable applied currents. A plot of the D_{obs} values versus the applied currents will yield an empirical linear line with the intercept corresponding to the passive flux where the applied current is zero. The slope of the line is f_i. A permeation experiment should also be done with zero current to obtain the experimental passive flux of the drug ion to confirm the extrapolated intercept value obtained from the plot of delivery rate versus applied current.

To calculate the transport number for the drug ion, the delivery rate obtained from an electrically assisted run is converted into units of milligrams per second per milliampere and then fitted into equation (17). This method of calculating the transport number does not exclude the passive flux of the drug ion. In cases where the passive fluxes are comparatively large, the variation of the transport number as a function of the applied current may become significantly large. Therefore, further treatment of the iontophoretic delivery data by the following equation may lead to a better refinement of the transport number.

$$t_D = \frac{\text{electrically assisted rate} - \text{passive rate}}{D_{max}} \tag{22}$$

This refined transport number would represent the efficiency of electrically assisted transport of the drug ion through the membrane in question.

Another way to calculate the transport numbers excluding the passive flux term is to convert the slope of the curve obtained from the plot of D_{obs} versus applied current into units of milligrams per second per milliampere. Subsequent division by the maximum delivery rate yields the desired transport number.

In actual devices, hydronium ions, extraneous ions, and chloride ions from the skin would be involved in conducting current. The total current passing through the skin will be the sum of the currents carried by each of these ions:

$$I_{total} = I_{M^+} + I_{D^+} + I_{Cl^-} + I_{H^+} + I_{OH^-} + I_{X^-} \tag{23}$$

where M^+ represents the positively charged ions present in the drug reservoir, X^- the negatively charged ions other than chloride ions, and D^+ the drug ions.

The current efficiency (CE) of the drug ion in question is

$$CE = (I_{D^+} / I_{total}) \times 100\% \tag{24}$$

To maximize the current efficiency of drug delivery, one can either design means to increase the fraction of current carried by the drug or decrease the fraction carried by the competing ions, particularly the protons, since proton transport has been implicated in the side effects of pain and burns [16].

Treatment of electrically assisted permeation data by electrodiffusion theory has been discussed by Kasting and Keister [8].

B. Enhancement Factor

The experimental enhancement factor (E.F.) can be calculated using the equation

$$\text{E.F.} = D_i/D_p \tag{25}$$

IV. FACTORS INFLUENCING IONTOPHORETIC DRUG DELIVERY

When selecting candidates for iontophoretic drug delivery, one must consider factors that may influence the iontophoretic drug delivery properties [9,14].

1. The charge of the drug ion. The drug molecules must be in an ionized state with either a positive or negative charge. The number of charges on the molecular ion has a direct proportional effect on the rate of its migration in an electric field, as evidenced by equations (12) and (15). Therefore a divalent molecular ion is expected to move faster than a monovalent ion through the same medium.

2. The applied current strength to be used. Drug ion transport is a function of the total current and the fluxes of other ions present. However, the rates of transport of the other species are also dependent upon the total current. The effect of current strength on the transport of benzoate ions has been studied [58]. The results suggest that there is a linear relationship between benzoate flux and the applied current. The steady-state flux of thyrotropin-releasing hormone is also directly proportional to applied current [59]. O'Malley and Oester [53], using iontophoresis of ^{32}P in rats and measuring its concentration in the urine, demonstrated that the amount of radioactive phosphorous distributed in the tissues was proportional to the current density, the duration of iontophoresis, and the concentration of the radioactive phosphorus.

3. The conductivity of the drug candidate. Conductivity of a drug in aqueous solution is a good parameter for selecting drug candidates [60]. However, the ultimate suitability of a given drug for iontophoretic application must be tested in vivo. The specific conductivities of drugs give an estimate of the ease of drug movement in solution when an electric current is applied. Suitable electrical conductivity is an important factor in the successful transdermal transport of drugs by iontophoresis. Gangarosa et al. [60] described the electrical characteristics of various drugs and the contribution to conductivity of buffers and nonspecific ions in the drug solution. They concluded that certain local anesthetics, vasoconstrictors, corticosteroids, anticancer drugs, and antiviral agents may be suitable for iontophoresis and that buffers or salt ions hinder iontophoretic transport due to competition between the extraneous ions and the drug ions for the current.

4. The pH of the vehicle used in the drug reservoirs. Most drug molecules are weak electrolytes and therefore poor passive percutaneous permeants. Under normal pH conditions, if the drug molecules can be kept in reasonably highly ionized form they can be administered transdermally using iontophoretic techniques. The effect of the pH of aqueous

vehicles on the rate and extent of lidocaine transport by iontophoresis through human stratum corneum was investigated by Siddiqui et al. [61]. Without iontophoresis, the rate of lidocaine penetration was highest at higher pH values where lidocaine existed mainly in the un-ionized form. With iontophoresis, lidocaine penetration was most effective at lower pH values where lidocaine existed mainly in the ionized form. An increase in the lidocaine flux of 8.5 and 4 times at pH 3.4 and 5.2, respectively, was observed for the iontophoretic flux over the flux of nonionic lidocaine.

5. The competition of extraneous ions in the drug reservoir [9]. The presence of buffer species or salt ions in the drug reservoir has a negative effect on the iontophoretic delivery of drug molecules owing to their competition with charged drug molecules for the applied electric current. However, the presence of any drug counterions carrying the opposite charge does not have any adverse effect on the iontophoretic delivery of charged drug molecules. Small, mobile ions of the same charge as the drug molecules should be avoided in the drug reservoir to minimize their competition for current. As long as there is sufficient ionized drug species in the reservoir, current can be conducted through the circuit. In the inactive reservoir, appropriate buffering should be maintained to complete the circuit. One should be aware of the fact that sodium ions and chloride ions in the body may act as competing ions. Therefore, the efficiency of the in vivo iontophoretic drug delivery will usually be less than the in vitro. The ionic strength is related to the concentration of various ions present in the solution. In solution each ion is surrounded by ions of opposite charge, and this may exert a retarding effect on the motion of the ion targeted for delivery into a tissue. When the ionic strength becomes greater, the concentration of extraneous ions will also become larger, resulting in higher competition for the electric current. An increase in ionic strength was reported to yield a reduction in the uptake of ^{32}P in tissues by iontophoresis [53].

6. The drug concentration in the reservoirs. In general, the effect of concentration can be predicted with the aid of the Nernst-Planck equation. An increased uptake of radioactive phosphorus by various tissues after iontophoresis was observed with an increase in the concentration of ^{32}P [53]. The flux of verapamil across excised hairless mouse skin was linearly dependent on the donor drug concentration in the range of 1–50 mg/mL [62].

7. The pK_a of the drug candidate [52]. Most iontophoretic experiments both in vitro and in vivo are carried out at a pH of about 5. The pH of the skin has been reported to be about 5. Therefore, it is wise to choose

a drug candidate that has a pK_a value that will maximize the amount of drug existing in ionized form.

8. The aqueous solubility of the drug candidate. The aqueous solubility of the drug candidate dictates the amount of the drug that can be dissolved into the reservoir. Most drug candidates are in salt form, so solubility is not usually a problem unless the drug candidate is highly lipophilic.

9. The molecular weight of the drug candidate. As predicted by Stokes's equation, the resisting force, F', on the migration of an ion is a function of ion size, ion shape, and the viscosity of the medium. The larger the molecule, the higher the resisting force and the slower the migration of the ion through the medium.

10. The lipophilicity of the drug candidate. This aspect of iontophoresis has been examined by Terzo et al. [63] on a homologous series of ionized and nonionized models.

11. The potential for skin irritation and sensitization.

12. The transport number of the drug candidate. The transport number of an ion has a direct effect on the mobility of the ion. The higher the number, the larger the fraction of total applied current it carries and the higher the rate of migration through the permeation medium.

13. The effect of temperature. The effect of temperature on the mobility of ions can be described by the equation

$$\log \mu = a\,\frac{1}{T} + b$$

Increasing the temperature will increase the mobility of the ions.

14. Electrochemical stability of the drug candidate. Drug candidates chosen for iontophoretic drug delivery systems should be electrochemically stable to avoid generation of any toxic degradant.

15. Electro-osmotic effects [32, p. 482]. Electro-osmotic flow is defined as the volume flux of a liquid through a membrane caused by an electric field imposed across the membrane. The imposed electric stimulus causes a net force on unpaired ions that exist in a very thin region near the liquid–solid interface within the structure of the membrane. This region is called the electrochemical double layer and results from the adsorption of ions to the surface of the solid. The counterions of these adsorbed ions are free to move in an electric field, and as they move they entrain bulk liquid, resulting in a net volume flux. Gangarosa et al. [64] showed that nonelectrolytes [^{3}H]9-β-D-arabinofuranosyladenine (Ara-A) and [^{3}H]thymidine (dThd) can be iontophoretically delivered to mouse tissues in aqueous NaCl solutions owing to the associated phenomenon of electro-osmosis. Attempts to deliver drugs by electro-osmosis have been reported. Iontophoresis of cortisone was unsuccess-

ful [65]. Iontophoresis of prednisolone was reported by James et al. [66]. Electro-osmotic and iontophoretic release of noradrenaline from micropipettes was reported by Bevan et al. [67].

V. FEATURES OF IONTOPHORESIS

1. Certain therapeutic compounds of larger molecular weight, including peptides and proteins, can be readily driven through the skin under the influence of an applied current whereas they can be delivered only with great difficulty, if at all, by the traditional passive route. Iontophoresis can therefore widen the spectrum of transdermal drug delivery.
2. Proteins and polypeptides can be delivered by iontophoresis through the skin route [55,68–73]. Oral delivery requires a larger dose because of heavy degradation of protein in the GI tract and first-pass effects. Nasal delivery of proteins and polypeptides may be discouraged by the active enzyme systems, irritation caused by the penetrants, and intersubject variability.
3. The area of drug administration on the skin can be considerably reduced compared to the transdermal passive systems.
4. Iontophoresis offers a high degree of control over the drug delivery rate.
5. Iontophoretic delivery provides a means of noninvasive administration of drugs to the body [74].
6. Iontophoresis delivery minimizes trauma, risk of infection, and damage to the wound.
7. For applications requiring local or topical delivery of drug, iontophoretic delivery has the advantage of high local drug concentration to reduce systemic side effects [10].
9. Delivery rates can be varied by alteration of the applied current at any time, and therefore iontophoresis can allow for different delivery rates at varying times.
10. Iontophoretic delivery allows for less interpatient variability.
11. Onset of action can be easily controlled by the applied current.
12. Iontophoretic administration can avoid first-pass hepatic circulation.

VI. APPLICATIONS OF IONTOPHORESIS

Table 1 shows numerous applications of iontophoresis to the delivery of medications for widely varying disorders such as melodinine for the treatment of vitiligo, glycopyrronium bromide for the treatment of palmer and plantar hyperhidrosis, and sodium salicylate for treatment of plantar warts. In muscle and

Table 1 Applications of Iontophoresis

	Drug	Target or condition	Ref.
Inorganic			
1.	Sodium fluoride	Dentin	75, 76
2.	Sodium fluoride	Tooth hypersensitivity	77
3.	Water	Hyperhidrosis	26–29
4.	Iodine	Scar tissue	78
5.	Iron and titanium oxides	Pigment for dermobraded tattoos	79
6.	Zinc	Ischemic skin ulcers	80
7.	Copper	Male contraceptor	81
8.	Copper	Fungi	82
9.	Copper	Allergic rhinitis	82
10.	Calcium	Hypo/hyperirritability	83
11.	Lithium chloride	Gouty tophi	84
12.	Sodium iodide	Electrolyte	85
Organic			
1.	Pilocarpine	Sweat induction for cystic fibrosis diagnosis	36
2.	Acetic acid	Calcific deposit	86
3.	Hydrocortisone, salicylate	Inflammation	87, 88 89
2.	Penicillin	Burns	90
3.	Histamine	Disease conditions of soft tissues, bursae, and tendons	91
4.	Sulfa drugs	Pyocyanic infection	92
5.	Dexamethasone, sodium phosphate, xylocaine	Musculoskeletal inflammatory conditions	93, 94
6.	Lidocaine HCl	Topical analgesia	75, 95–105
7.	Acetyl beta methylcholine chloride	Arthritis	106
8.	Idoxuridine	Herpes simplex keratitis	107
9.	Methylprednisolone succinate	Postherpetic neuralgia	108
10.	Sodium salicylate	Plantar warts	109
11.	Esterified glucocorticoids	Peyronie's disease	110
12.	Vasopressin	Lateral septal neuron activity	111
13.	Alkaloids	Chronic pain	112
14.	6-Hydroxydopamine	Ocular infection	113
15.	Metoprolol	Beta blocker (angina pectoris)	114

16.	Lidocaine HCl with epinephrine	Local anesthesia for painless cauterization of spider veins	115
17.	Triamcinolone	Aphthous stomatitis	116
18.	Methylprednisone	Aphthous stomatitis	117
19.	Meladine	Vitiligo	118
20.	Hyaluronidase	Scleroderma	119
21.	Hyaluronidase	Lymphedema	120
22.	Salbutamol	Bronchodilator	121
23.	Leuprolide acetate	Lutenizing hormone-releasing hormone agonist	122
24.	Poldine methyl sulfate	Hyperhidrosis	123
25.	Atropine sulfate	Hyperhidrosis	124
26.	Glycopyrronium bromide	Hyperhidrosis	125
27.	Vidarabine monophosphate (Ara-AMP)	Herpes simplex virus	126, 127

joint disorders, successful results were reported with acetic acid iontophoresis for the treatment of calcium deposits; α-chymotrypsin iontophoresis in patients with inflammatory reaction of joints and soft tissues decreased articular and periarticular edema. Iontophoresis of penicillin into burn eschars has been used to decrease severe infection in burn cases. Histamine iontophoresis has been used to induce local capillary dilatation to obtain accurate determinations of blood gases and was also suggested as an aid in the healing of chronic sclerotic ulcers. In dental work, iontophoresis of local anesthetic agents has been used for tooth extraction, treatment of infected root canals, and for deposition of fluoride into the dentin of teeth.

The interest in applying iontophoresis to transdermal drug delivery has increased dramatically in the past few decades [7–18,36–39,54,58,61,62,68–74,128–153]. It is anticipated that this interest will continue to increase.

VII. THE FUTURE OF IONTOPHORETIC DRUG DELIVERY

The future of iontophoretic drug delivery remains bright, as evidenced by research activity and the development of drug delivery devices in this field. However, there is still much research needed in various aspects of iontophoretic drug delivery, such as the development of drug formulations for these systems [13]. Iontophoresis can enhance the flux of drug ions through the skin, providing sufficient systemic concentrations for therapeutic effect [13]. Advantages of transdermal iontophoretic delivery of drugs include an enhanced transport rate, particularly important for large molecules such as protein and peptide drugs. In addition, the physician's or patient's ability to control the rate of drug delivery is also enhanced.

Disadvantages of iontophoresis   Although iontophoretic drug delivery has much to offer there are some disadvantages associated this technology. The delivery systems are much more complicated than the passive transdermal systems because power supply devices and circuitry, electrodes, and specific drug ion transfer are involved. In addition, electrochemical stability could be a serious problem for some drug candidates. Toxic effects are not clear when metal ions resulting from dissolution of the metallic electrodes get into the skin and tissues. The cost of developing and manufacturing iontophoretic drug delivery systems is much higher in comparison with that of passive transdermal systems.

Acknowledgements   I thank Dr. Ron Haak and Mr. B. Miller for their comments on the manuscript.

REFERENCES

1. F. Theeuwes and S. I. Yum, *Ann. Biomed. Eng. 4*, 343 (1976).
2. A. F. Kydonieus and B. Berner, Eds., *Transdermal Delivery of Drugs*, Vols. 1–3, CRC Press, Boca Raton, FL, 1987.
3. R. Neubert, Ion pair transport across membranes, *Pharm. Res. 6*, 743–747 (1989).
4. P. Tyle and P. Agrawala, Drug delivery by phonophoresis, *Pharm. Res. 6*, 355–361 (1989).
5. J. V. Bondi, A. E. Alic, and E. M. Cohen, pH mediated drug delivery system, U.S. Patent 720652, pending (1985).
6. T. Higuchi and V. Stella, Eds., *Pro-drugs as Novel Drug Delivery Systems*, American Chemical Society, Washington, DC, 1975.
7. R. Harris, Iontophoresis, in *Therapeutic Electricity and Ultraviolet Radiation*, 2nd ed., S. H. Licht, Ed., Yale Univ. Press, New Haven, 1967, Ch. 4, pp. 156–178.
8. G. B. Kasting and J. C. Keister, Application of electrodiffusion theory for a homogeneous membrane to iontophoretic transport through skin, *J. Controlled Release 8*, 195–210 (1989).
9. A. K. Banga and Y. W. Chien, Iontophoretic delivery of drugs: fundamentals, developments and biomedical applications, *J. Controlled Release 7*, 1–24 (1988).
10. J. B. Sloan and K. Soltani, Iontophoresis in dermatology, *J. Am. Acad. Dermatol. 15*, 671–684 (1986).
11. P. Tyle, Iontophoretic devices for drug delivery, *Pharm. Res. 3*, 318–326 (1986).
12. R. G. Hill, The use of microiontophoresis in the study of the descending control of noiceptive transmission, *Prog. Brain Res. 77*, 339–347 (1988).
13. J. Singh and M. S. Roberts, Transdermal delivery of drugs by iontophoresis: a review, *Drug Des. Delivery 4*, 1–12 (1989).
14. C. R. Behl, S. Kumar, A. W. Malick, S. Delterzo, W. I. Higuchi, and R. A. Nash, Iontophoretic drug delivery: effects of physicochemical factors on the skin uptake of nonpeptide drugs, *J. Pharm. Sci. 78*, 355–360 (1989).

15. Y. W. Chien and A. K. Banga, Iontophoretic (transdermal) delivery of drugs: overview of historical development, *J. Pharm. Sci. 78*, 353–354 (1989).
16. J. E. Sanderson, S. R. deReil, and R. Dixon, Iontophoretic delivery of nonpeptide drugs: formulation optimization for maximum skin permeability, *J. Pharm. Sci. 78*, 361–364 (1989).
17. A. L. Watkins, *A Manual of Electrotherapy*, 3rd ed., Lea and Febiger, Philadelphia, 1968.
18. S. Dueball, *Controlled Release Newslett. 7*(3), 4, 1989.
19. *Dorland's Illustrated Medical Dictionary*, 25th ed., W. B. Saunders, Philadelphia, 1974, p. 796.
20. L. Delherm and A. Laquerriere, *Electrologie*, Paris, 1921.
21. B. R. Fabre-Palaprat, *Arch. Gen. Med. 2*, 126 (1833).
22. M. A. Zimmern, L'ionization et se applications analgesiques, *Rev. Actinol. 5*, 11 (1929).
23. S. Le Duc, *Electric Ions and Their Use in Medicine*, Rebman Liverpool, 1908.
24. N. Albrecht, *Arch. Ohreheilkd. 85*, 198–215 (1911).
25. A. S. Rapperport, D. L. Larson, D. G. Henges, J. B. Lynch, T. G. Blocker, Jr., and R. S. Lewis, Iontophoresis: a method of antibiotic administration in the burn patient, *Plast. Reconstr. Surg. 36*, 547–552 (1965).
26. R. Tapper, *J. Clin. Eng. 8*, 253–259 (1983).
27. M. L. Elgart and G. Fuchs, Tapwater iontophoresis in the treatment of hyperhidrosis. Use of the Drionic device, *Int. J. Dermatol. 26*, 194–197 (1987).
28. F. Levit, Treatment of hyperhidrosis by tapwater iontophoresis, *Cutis 26*, 192–194 (1980).
29. K. Grice, Hyperhidrosis and its treatment by iontophoresis, *Physiotherapy 66*, 43–44 (1980).
30. *The American Heritage Dictionary*, 2nd ed., Houghton Mifflin, Boston, 1982.
31. J. E. O'Reilly, Potentiometry, in *Instrumental Analysis*, H. H. Bauer, G. D. Christian, and J. E. O'Reilly, Eds., 1978, Ch. 2, pp. 12–48.
32. A. Martin, J. Swarbrick, and A. Cammarata, *Physical Pharmacy: Physical Chemical Principles in the Pharmaceutical Sciences*, 3rd ed., Lea and Febiger, Philadelphia, 1983.
33. N. Lakshminarayanaiah, *Chem. Rev. 65*, 491–565 (1965).
34. M. J. Pikal and S. Shah, Transport mechanisms in iontophoresis. II. Electroosmotic flow and transference number measurements for hairless mouse skin, *Pharm. Res. 7*, 213–221 (1990).
35. G. B. Kasting and L. A. Bowman, DC electricity properties of frozen, excised human skin, *Pharm. Res. 7*, 134–143 (1990).
36. H. L. Webster, *CRC Crit. Rev. Clin. Lab. Sci. 18*, 313–338 (1983).
37. Y. B. Bannon, J. Corish, and O. I. Corrigan, Iontophoretic transport of model compounds from a gel matrix, *Drug Dev. Ind. Pharm. 13*, 2617–2630 (1987).
38. L. Wearley, J. C. Liu, and Y. W. Chien, Iontophoresis-facilitated transdermal delivery of verapamil, I. In vitro evaluation and mechanistic studies, *J. Controlled Release 8*, 237–250 (1989).

39. L. Wearley, J. C. Liu, and Y. W. Chien, Iontophoresis-facilitated transdermal delivery of verapami. II. Factors affecting the reversibility of skin permeability, *J. Controlled Release 9*, 231–242 (1989).

40. L. Wearley and Y. W. Chien, Enhancement of the in vitro skin permeability of azidothymidine (AZT) via iontophoresis and chemical enhancers, *Pharm. Res. 7*, 34–40 (1990).

41. G. Rendina, The electrophoretic separation of serum proteins, in *Experimental Methods in Modern Biochemistry*, W. B. Saunders, 1971, p. 79.

42. R. J. Block, E. L. Duyran, and G. Zweig, *A Manual of Paper Chromatography and Paper Electrophoresis*, Academic, New York, 1958.

43. L. Ornstein and B. J. Davis, *Disc Electrophoresis*, preprint by Distillation Industries, Eastman Kodak Co., Rochester, NY, 1962.

44. B. J. Davis, Disc electrophoresis: methods and applications to human serum proteins, *Ann. N.Y. Acad. Sci. 121*, 321 (1965).

45. D. E. Williams and R. A. Reisfeld, Disc electrophoresis in polyacrylamide gels: extension to new conditions of pH and buffer, *Ann. N.Y. Acad. Sci. 121*, 373 (1965).

46. L. Ornstein, Disc electrophoresis. I. Background and theory, *Ann. N.Y. Acad. Sci. 121*, 321–349 (1965).

47. J. T. Clarke, Simplified "disc" (polyacrylamide gel) electrophoresis, *Ann. N.Y. Acad. Sci. 121*, 428–436 (1965).

48. J. Broome, A rapid method of disc electrophoresis, *Nature 199*, 179 (1963).

49. H. Rilbe, Basic theory of electrophoresis: definitions, terminology and comparison of the basic techniques, in *Electrophoretic Techniques*, C. F. Simpson and M. Whitaker, Eds., Academic, New York, 1983, pp. 1–25.

50. J. Vacik, Theory of electromigration process, in *Electrophoresis: A Survey of Techniques and Applications*, Elsevier, New York, 1979, Ch. 1, p. 121.

51. L. Ornstein, Disc electrophoresis. 1. Background and theory, *Ann. N.Y. Acad. Sci. 121*, 321–349 (1965).

52. D. D. Perrin, B. Dempsey, and E. P. Serjeant, *pKa Prediction for Organic Acids and Bases*, Chapman and Hall, New York, 1981.

53. E. P. O'Malley and Y. T. Oester, Influence of some physical chemical factors on iontophoresis using radio-isotopes, *Arch. Phys. Med. Rehabil. 36*, 310–316 (1955).

54. R. A. Arndt and L. D. Poper, *Simple Membrane Electrodiffusion Theory*, Physical Biological Sciences, Misc., Blacksburg, VA, 1972.

55. R. R. Burnette and B. Ongpipattanakul, *J. Pharm. Sci. 76*, 765–773 (1987).

56. H. T. Zankel and N. C. Durham, Effect of physical modalities upon RA I[131] iontophoresis, *Arch. Phys. Med. Rehabil. 44*, 93–97 (1963).

57. C. M. Papa and A. M. Kligman, Mechanism of eccrine anhidrosis, *J. Invest. Dermatol. 47*, 1–9 (1966).

58. N. H. Bellatone, S. Ri, M. L. Francoeur, and B. Rasadi, Enhanced percutaneous absorption via iontophoresis. I. Evaluation of an in vitro system and transport of model compounds, *Int. J. Pharm. 30*, 63–72 (1986).

59. R. R. Burnette, and D. Marrero, Comparison between the iontophoretic and passive transport of thyrotropin releasing hormone across excised nude mouse skin, *J. Pharm. Sci. 75*, 738–743 (1986).

60. L. P. Gangarosa, N. H. Park, B. C. Fong, et al., Conductivity of drugs used for iontophoresis, *J. Pharm. Sci. 67*, 1439–1443 (1978).
61. O. Siddiqui, M. S. Roberts, and A. E. Polack, The effect of iontophoresis and vehicle pH on the in-vitro permeation of lignocaine through human stratum corneum, *J. Pharm. Pharmacol. 37*, 732–735 (1985).
62. L. Wearley, J. C. Liu, and Y. W. Chien, Iontophoresis-facilitated transdermal delivery of verapamil. I. In vitro evaluation and mechanistic studies, *J. Controlled Release 8*, 237–250 (1989).
63. S. D. Terzo, C. R. Behl, and R. A. Nash, Iontophoretic transport of a homologous series of ionized and nonionized model compounds: influence of hydrophobicity and mechanistic interpretation, *Pharm. Res. 6*, 85–90 (1989).
64. C. P. Gangarosa, N. H. Park, and J. M. Hill, Increased penetration of nonelectrolytes into mouse skin during iontophoretic water transport (iontohydrokinesis), *J. Pharm. Exp. Ther. 212*, 377–381 (1980).
65. A. Chantraine, J. P. Ludy and D. Berger, Is cortisone iontophoresis possible?, *Arch. Phys. Med. Rehabil. 67*, 38–40 (1986).
66. M. P. James, R. M. Graham and J. English, Percutaneous iontophoresis of prednisolone—a pharmacokinetic study, *Clin. Exp. Dermatol. 11*, 54–61 (1986).
67. P. Bevan, C. M. Bradshaw, R. Y. K. Dun, N. T. Slater and E. Szabadi, Electroosmotic and iontophoretic release of noradrenaline from micropipetters, *Experientia 37*, 296–297 (1981).
68. R. L. Stephen, T. J. Petelenz, and S. C. Jacobsen, Potential novel methods for insulin administration. I. Iontophoresis, *Biomed. Biochim. Acta 43*, 5, 553–558 (1984).
69. Y. W. Chien, O. Siddqui, W. M. Shi, P. Lelawongs, and J. C. Liu, Direct current iontophoretic transdermal delivery of peptide and protein drugs, *J. Pharm. Sci. 78*, 376–383 (1989).
70. P. Lelawongs, J. C. Liu, O. Siddiqui, and Y. W. Chien, Transdermal iontophoretic delivery of arginine-vasopressin I. Physicochemical consideration, *Int. J. Pharm. 56*, 13–22 (1989).
71. Y. W. Chien, O. Siddiqui, Y. Sum, W. M. Shi, and J. C. Liu, Transdermal iontophoresis delivery of therapeutic peptides/proteins. I. Insulin, *Ann. N.Y. Acad. Sci. 507*, 32–51 (1987).
72. B. Kari, Control of blood glucose levels in alloxan-diabetic rabbits by iontophoresis of insulin, *Diabetes 35*, 217–221 (1986).
73. R. L. Stephen, T. L. Petelenz, and S. C. Jacobsen, Potential novel methods for insulin administration. I. Iontophoresis, *Biomed. Chim. Acta 43*, 553–558 (1984).
74. R. L. Stephen, Answer to question on iontophoretic delivery of drugs, *J. Am. Med. Assoc. 256*, 769 (1986).
75. L. R. Gangarosa, Sr., *Iontophoresis in Dental Practice*, Quintessence, Chicago, 1983.
76. D. A. Kern, M. J. McQuade, M. J. Scheidt, B. Hanson, and T. E. Van Dyke, Effectiveness of sodium fluoride on tooth hypersensitivity with and without iontophoresis, *J. Periodontol. 60*, 386–389 (1989).

77. N. D. Lutins et al., Effectiveness of sodium fluoride on tooth hypersensitivity with and without iontophoresis, *J. Periodontol. 55*, 285–288 (1984).

78. M. Tannenbaum, Iodine iontophoresis in reducing scar tissue, *Phys. Ther. 60*, 792 (1980).

79. H. B. Batner, Cataphoresis in dermabrasion tattooing, *Plast. Reconstr. Surg. 27*, 613–617 (1961).

80. M. W. Cornwall, Zinc iontophoresis to treat ischemic skin ulcers, *Phys. Ther. 61*, 359–360 (1981).

81. S. S. Riar, R. C. Sawhney, J. Bardhan, P. Thomas, R. K. Jain, and A. K. Jain, Copper iontophoresis in male contraceptor, *Andrologia 14*, 481–491 (1982).

82. J. Kahn, Ed., *Clinical Electrotherapy*, 4th ed., Syoset, NY, 1985.

83. J. Kahn, Calcium iontophoresis in suspected myopathy, *Phys. Ther. 55*, 276–277 (1975).

84. J. Kahn, Lithium iontophoresis for gouty tophi, *JOSPT 4*, 113 (1982).

85. A. Strohl, J. Verne, J. C. Roucayrol, and P. F. Leccaldi, *C. R. Soc. Biol. 144*, 819–824 (1950).

86. J. Kahn, *Phys. Ther. 57*, 658–659 (1977).

87. L. E. Bertolucci, Introduction of anti-inflammatory drugs by iontophoresis, a double-blind study, *JOSPT 4*, 103 (1982).

88. J. Kahn, Iontophoresis with hydrocortisone for Peyronie's disease, *Phys. Ther. 62*, 995 (1982).

89. H. R. Harris, Iontophoresis—clinical research in musculoskeletal inflammatory conditions, *JOSPT 4*, 109 (1982).

90. A. S. Rapperport, D. L. Larson, D. F. Henges, J. B. Lynch, T. G. Blocker, and R. S. Lewis, *Plastic Reconstr. Surg. 36*, 547–552 (1965).

91. D. H. Kling and D. Sashin, *Arch. Phys. Ther. X-Ray Radium 18*, 333–338 (1937).

92. L. von Sallmann, *Am. J. Ophthalmol. 25*, 1292–1300 (1942).

93. P. R. Harris, *J. Orthopaed. Sports Phys. Ther. 4*, 109–112 (1982).

94. F. G. Delacerda, *J. Orthopaed. Sports Phys. Ther. 4*, 51–54 (1982).

95. M. Comeau and R. Brummett, *Laryngoscope 88*, 277–285 (1978).

96. J. Russo, Jr., A. G. Lipman, T. J. Cornstock, B. C. Page, and R. L. Stephen, *Am. J. Hosp. Pharm. 37*, 843–847 (1980).

97. D. F. Echols, C. H. Norris, and H. G. Tabb, *Arch. Otolaryngol. 101*, 418–421 (1975).

99. M. Comeau and J. Vernon, *Arch. Otolaryngol 98*, 114–120 (1973).

100. O. Siddiqui, M. S. Roberts, and A. Z. Polack, *J. Pharm. Pharmacol. 37*, 732–735 (1985).

101. T. Petelenz, I. Axenti, T. J. Petelenz, J. Iwinski, and S. Dubel, *J. Clin. Pharmacol. Ther. Toxicol. 22*, 152–155 (1984).

102. A. J. Schleuing, R. Brummett, and M. Comeau, *Trans. Am. Acad. Ophthalmol. Otolaryngol. 78*, 453–457 (1974).

103. L. P. Gangarosa, *Methods Find. Exp. Clin. Pharmacol. 3*, 83–94 (1981).

104. S. B. Arvidsson, R. H. Ekroth, A. M. C. Hansby, A. H. Lindholm, and G. William-Olsson, *Acta Anaethesiol. Scand 28*, 209–210 (1984).

105. J. B. Laffree, P. Vermeij, and J. H. Hulshof, The effect of iontophoresis of lig-nocaine in the treatment of tinnitus, *Clin. Otolaryngol. 14*, 401–404 (1989).
106. T. Cohn and S. Benson, *Arch. Phys. Ther. X-Ray Radium 18*, 583–587 (1937).
107. L. P. Gangarosa, N. H. Park, and J. M. Hill, *Proc. Soc. Exp. Biol. Med. 154*, 439–443 (1977).
108. L. P. Gangarosa, M. Haynes, S. Qureshi, M. M. Salim, A. Ozawa, K. Hayakawa, M. Ohkido, and P. E. Mahan, 3rd Int. Dental Congr. Modern Pain Control, 1982, *Abstr.* 1982, p. 221.
109. A. H. Gordon and M. V. Veinstein, *Phys. Ther. 49*, 869–870 (1969).
110. S. H. Rothfeld and W. Murray, *J. Urol. 97*, 874–875 (1967).
111. J. E. Marchand and N. Hagino, *Exp. Neurol. 78*, 790–795 (1982).
112. B. Csillik, E. Knyihar-Csillik, and A. Szucs, *Neurosci. Lett. 31*, 87–90 (1982).
113. J. W. Caudill, E. Romanowski, T. Araullo-Cruz, and Y. J. Gordon, *Curr. Eye Res. 5*, 41–45 (1986).
114. K. Okabe, H. Yamaguchi, and Y. Kawai, *J. Controlled Release 4*, 79–85 (1986).
115. J. L. Bezzant, R. L. Stephen, Y. J. Petelenz, and S. C. Jacobsen, Painless cauter-ization of spider vein with the use of iontophoretic local anesthesia, *J. Am. Acad. Dermatol. 19*, 869–875 (1988).
116. M. D. Lekas, Iontophoresis treatment, *Otolarnygol. Head Neck Surg. 87*, 292–298 (1977).
117. L. P. Gangarosa, Sr., *Iontophoresis in Dental Practice*, Quintessence, Chicago, 1983, pp. 40–52.
118. M. B. Moawad, Treatment of vitiligo with 1% solution of the sodium salt of meladine using the iontophoresis technique, *Dermatol. Monatsschr. 155*, 388–394 (1969).
119. R. J. Popkin, The use of hyaluronidase by iontophoresis in the treatment of gen-eralized scleroderma, *J. Invest. Dermatol. 16*, 97–102 (1951).
120. H. S. Schwartz, Use of hyaluronidase by iontophoresis in treatment of lymph-edema, *Arch. Intern. Med. 95*, 662–668 (1955).
121. Y. B. Bannon, J. Corish, O. I. Corrigan, and J. G. Masterson, Iontophoretically induced transdermal delivery of salbutamol, *Drug Dev. Ind. Pharm. 14*, 2151–2166 (1988).
122. B. R. Meyer, W. Kreis, J. Eschbach, V. O'Mara, S. Rosen, and D. Sibalis, Suc-cessful transdermal administration of therapeutic doses of a polypeptide to normal human volunteers, *Clin. Pharm. Ther. 44*, 607–612 (1988).
123. K. Grice, H. Satter, and H. Baker, Treatment of idiopathic hyperhidrosis with iontophoresis of tap water and poldine methosulfate, *Br. J. Dermatol. 86*, 72–78 (1972).
124. K. Gibinski, L. Giec, J. Zmudzinski, et al., Transcutaneous inhibition of sweat gland function by atropine, *J. Appl. Physiol. 34*, 850–852 (1973).
125. K. Morgan, The technic of treating hyperhidrosis by iontophoresis, *Physiotherapy 66*, 45 (1980).
126. J. M. Hill, L. P. Gangarosa, and N. H. Park, Iontophoretic application of antiviral chemotherapeutic agents, *Ann. N.Y. Acad. Sci. 284*, 604–612 (1977).

127. B. S. Kwon, L. P. Gangarosa, N. H. Park, D. S. Hull, E. Fineberg, C. Wiggins, and J. M. Hill, *Invest. Ophthalmol. Vis. Sci. 18*, 984–988 (1979).

128. J. C. Liu, Y. Sun, O. Siddiqui, Y. W. Chien, W. M. Shi, and J. Li, Blood glucose control in diabetic rats by transdermal iontophoretic delivery of insulin, *Int. J. Pharm. 44*, 197–204 (1988).

129. Y. Sun, O. Siddiqui, J. C. Liu, and Y. W. Chien, Transdermal modulated delivery of polypeptides: effect of DC pulse waveform on enhancement, *Proc. 13th Symp. Controlled Release Bioactive Mater. 13*, 175–176, 1986.

130. A. M. James, Electrophoresis of particles in suspension, in *Surface and Colloid Science* Vol. 11, *Experimental Methods*, R. J. Good and R. R. Stromberg, Eds., Plenum, New York, 1979, Ch. 4, pp. 121–185.

131. P. Glikfeld, C. Cullander, R. S. Hinz, and R. H. Guy, A new system for in vitro studies of iontophoresis, *Pharm. Res. 5*, 443–446 (1988).

132. P. Molyneux and H. P. Frank, *J. Am. Chem. Soc. 83*, 3169 (1961).

133. J. E. Sanderson and S. R. deReil, Method and appratus for iontophoretic drug delivery, U.S. Patent pending (Feb. 18, 1986).

134. J. E. Sanderson, R. W. Caldwell, J. Hsiao, R. Dixon, and R. R. Tuttle, Noninvasive delivery of a novel inotropic catecholamine. Iontophoretic versus intravenous infusion in dogs, *J. Pharm. Sci. 76*, 215–218 (1987).

135. E. Holzle and T. Ruzicka, Treatment of hyperhidrosis by a battery-operated iontophoretic device, *Dermatologica 172*, 41–47 (1986).

136. G. A. Leisten, Desensitization techniques [letter], *J. Am. Dent. Assoc. 112*, 160 (1986).

137. L. E. Linblad and L. Ekenvall, Electrode material in iontophoresis, *Pharm. Res. 4*, 438 (1987).

138. R. Kovacs, *Electrotherapy and Light Therapy*, 2nd ed., Lea and Febiger, Philadelphia, 1935.

139. Y. W. Chien and A. K. Banga, Iontophoretic (transdermal) delivery of drugs: overview of historical development, *J. Pharm. Sci. 78*, 353–354 (1989).

140. P. C. Kuo, J. S. Tien, J. C. Liu, S. F. Chang, and Y. W. Chien, Transdermal delivery of oxycodone hydrochloride. V. The role of stratum corneum under the influence of iontophoresis, *Chung-hua Yao Hsueh Tsa Chih 41*, 181–188 (1989).

141. P. C. Kuo, J. C. Liu, S. F. Chang, and Y. E. Chien, Transdermal delivery of oxycodone hydrochloride. IV. Enhancement of the percutaneous absorption of oxycodone-HCl by iontophoresis, *Chung-hua Yao Hsueh Tsa Chih 41*, 99–114, (1989).

142. O. Siddiqui, M. S. Roberts, and A. E. Polack, Iontophoretic transport of weak electrolytes through the excised human stratum corneum, *J. Pharm. Pharmacol. 41*, 430–432 (1989).

143. Y. B. Bannon, J. Corish, O. I. Corrigan, and J. G. Masterson, Iontophoretically induced transdermal delivery of salbutamol, *Drug Dev. Ind. Pharm. 14*, 15–17 (1988).

144. J. E. Sanderson, S. DeRiel, and R. Dixon, Iontophoretic delivery of nonpeptide drugs: formulation optimization for maximum skin permeability, *J. Pharm. Sci. 78*, 361–364 (1989).

145. C. R. Behl, S. Kumar, A. W. Malick, S. DelTerzo, W. I. Higuchi, and R. A. Nash, Iontophoretic drug delivery: effects of physicochemical factors on the skin uptake of nonpeptide drugs, *J. Pharm. Sci. 78*, 355–360 (1989).

146. J. C. Liu, Y. Sun, O. Siddiqui, Y. W. Chien, W. M. Shi, and J. Li, Blood glucose control in diabetic rats by transdermal iontophoretic delivery of insulin, *Int. J. Pharm. 44*, 197–204 (1988).

147. V. Miletic and H. Tan, Iontophoretic application of calcitonin gene- related peptide produces a slow and prolonged excitation of neurons in the cat lumbar dorsal horn, *Brain Res. 446*, 169–172 (1988).

148. L. C. Slough, M. J. Spinelli, and G. B. Kasting, Transdermal delivery of etidronate (EHDP) in the pig via iontophoresis, *J. Membrane Sci. 35*, 161–165 (1988).

149. G. B. Kasting, E. W. Merritt, and J. C. Keister, An in vitro method for studying the iontophoretic enhancement of drug transport through skin, *J. Membrane Sci. 35*, 137–159 (1988).

150. M. Levkut, V. Svidron, F. Lesnik, and R. Skarda, The effect of colchicine applied by iontophoresis on the growth of tumors induced by ASV in chickens, *Folia Vet. 31*, 135–140 (1987).

151. H. Pratzel, P. Dittrich, and W. Kukovetz, Spontaneous and forced cutaneous absorption of indomethacin in pigs and humans, *J. Rheumatol. 13*, 1122–1125 (1986).

151. L. E. Linblad, L. Ekenvall, K. Ancker, K. Rohman, and P. A. Oeberg, Laser Doppler flow-meter assessment of iontophoretically applied norepinephrine on human finger skin circulation, *J. Invest. Dermatol. 87*, 634–636 (1986).

152. K. Okabe, H. Yamaguchi, and Y. Kawai, New iontophoretic transdermal administration of the beta-blocker metoprolol, *J. Controlled Release 4*, 79–85 (1986).

153. J. M. Glass, R. L. Stephen, and S. C. Jacobson, The quantity and distribution of radiolabeled dexamethasone delivered to tissue by iontophoresis, *Int. J. Dermatol. 19*, 519–525 (1980).

154. A. J. Coury, E. J. Fogt, M. S. Norenberg, and D. F. Untereker, Development of a screening system for cystic fibrosis, *Clin. Chem. 29*, 1593–1597 (1983).

155. W. J. Warwick, N. N. Huang, W. W. Waring, A. G. Cherian, I. Brown, E. Stejskal-Larenz, G. Duhon, J. G. Hill, and D. Strominger, Evaluation of a cystic fibrosis screening system incorporating a miniature sweat stimulator and disposable chloride sensor. *Clin. Chem. 23*, 850–853 (1986).

156. W. H. Yeung, J. Palmer, D. Schidlow, M. R. Bye, and N. N. Huang, Evaluation of a paper-patch test for sweat chloride determination, *Clin. Pediatrics, 23*, 603–607 (1984).

157. L. E. Gibson and E. A. Cooke, A test for concentration of electrolytes in sweat in cystic fibrosis of the pancreas utilization of pilocarpine by iontophoresis, *Pediatrics, 23*, 545–549 (1959).

158. L. E. Gibson, P. A. diSant' Agnese, and H. Shwachman, *Procedure for Quantitative Iontophoretic Sweat Test for Cystic Fibrosis*, GAP Conference Reports; *Problems in Sweat Testing*, Cystic Fibrosis Foundation, Atlanta, 1975.

159. L. E. Gibson, Iontophoresis sweat test for cystic fibrosis, technical details, *Pediatrics, 39*, 465 (1967).

160. T. Berg and J. Wrance, Pilocarpine iontophoresis–practical aspects, *Acta Pediatric. Scand* [suppl], *177*, 94–95 (1967).

161. L. S. Prad, K. P. Sinha, and A. Rahman, Some observations on sweat test by pilocarpine iontophoresis, *Indian Pediatric*, *8*, 342–344 (1977).

162. B. C. Palombini and P. R. K. DeSonza, Cystic fibrosis–an improved diagnostic method using constant current iontophoresis, *Rev. Bras. Biol. 32*, 197–204 (1984).

163. C. J. Sawyer, A. V. Scott, and G. K. Summer, Cystic fibrosis of the pancreas: A study of sweat electrolyte levels in 36 families using pilocarpine iontophoresis, *South Med. J. 59*, 197–202 (1966).

12

Transdermal Delivery of Proteins and Peptides by Iontophoresis: Development, Challenges, and Opportunities

Jue-Chen Liu and Ying Sun
Topical Formulation and Drug Delivery Research Center, Johnson and Johnson, Skillman, New Jersey

I. BACKGROUND

A. Drugs of the Future

As a result of the recent advances in genetic engineering, more and more peptide and protein drugs are being developed for medical use. They are regarded as "the drugs of the future" for their extremely high potency and their endogenous origin, which minimizes the risk of unwanted side effects. Drugs of this type, however, are facing challenging delivery problems because of their poor oral efficacy and their short biological half-lives. These difficulties can be partially overcome through parenteral administration. Parenteral administration, however, often requires trained personnel and is painful and irreversible.

B. Noninvasive and Transdermal Delivery

Chronic complications associated with parenteral injections have always been a problem in peptide and protein therapy. Much effort has been dedicated to exploring novel delivery approaches via noninvasive routes such as nasal, rectal, and transdermal administration. The investigation of alternative routes for the delivery of proteins and peptides is desirable to achieve better patient compliance, to minimize the risk of contamination by pathogenic microorganisms associated with needle penetration, and to attain better pharmacological efficacy. Transdermal administration is one of the potential noninvasive routes to achieve these goals.

However, proteins and peptides, because of their hydrophilic nature and large molecular size, have limited permeabilities in the skin. Therefore, penetration enhancement is required to facilitate the migration of drug species across the skin and allow sufficient drug to be delivered to give the desired local or systemic effects. Iontophoresis could be an ideal method for the enhanced transdermal delivery of proteins and peptides.

C. Iontophoresis

The concept of using a low-intensity electric field to increase the tissue penetration of charged drugs or agents has been applied in dermatology for almost 100 years [1]. This technology, called iontophoresis, has been used to deliver anesthetics, anti-inflammatory drugs, and other therapeutic agents to treat skin disorders. It has been proved to be a clinically effective, safe, and painless noninvasive way to administer ionized drugs in dermatologic, physiotherapeutic, and diagnostic applications [1,2]. As a noninvasive therapy, iontophoresis is growing in popularity among anesthesiologists, pediatricians, general and orthopedic surgeons, burn specialists, and dental practitioners [3]. Many health professionals select iontophoresis as a cost-effective alternative to traditional therapy. In recent years, technological advancements in the fields of electrical chemistry, electronics, and polymer chemistry have revolutionized iontophoretic technology and brought it to the forefront of biomedical research. Many researchers are looking into the use of transdermal iontophoresis for systemic delivery of proteins and peptides because of its ability to enhance drug delivery. Table 1 lists some of the research work on the transdermal iontophoretic delivery of peptides, which will be discussed in detail in Section III. Iontophoresis technology is merging with biomedical technology in the development of programmable and closed-loop drug delivery systems for proteins and peptides. A pulsatile delivery pattern mimicking biological rhythms can be generated by programming the power source. In a closed-loop system, the delivery of a drug can be turned on and off in response to metabolic changes in the body. A transdermal iontophoretic delivery system can become a closed-loop self-regulating device with the addition of one or more biosensors, which would activate or deactivate the electric current, delivering the drug according to the need of the patient.

D. Need for Time-Based Delivery Systems

Most peptide and protein drugs require a dose regimen mimicking their physiological secretion patterns. For instance, the secretion of natural gonadotropin-releasing hormone (GnRH) follows a pulsatile pattern [4]. There is a pulsed

Table 1 Current Research on Transdermal Delivery of Macromolecules

Macromolecules	Molecular nature	Mol. wt.	Enhancement	Ref.
Thyrotropin-releasing hormone (TRH)	Peptide (1–3)	>350	Iontophoresis	14
Vasopressin	Peptide (1–9)	≈1,100	Iontophoresis	26, 29
Gonadotropin-releasing hormone (GnRH or LHRH)	Peptide (1–10)	≈1,200	Iontophoresis	30, 31
Desenkephalin-γ-endorphin	Peptide (6–17)	≈1,400	Chemical enhancer	32
Melanotropin-stimulating hormone (MSH)	Peptide (1–13)	≈1,600	none	33
Calcitonin	Peptide (1–32)	≈3,600	Iontophoresis	34
Growth hormone releasing factor (GRF)	Peptide (1–44)	≈5,300	Iontophoresis	35
Insulin	Peptide (1–51)	≈6,000	Iontophoresis	36–41
Grass pollen allergen	Glycoprotein	>10,000	Iontophoresis	42

secretion generated about every 90 min in men and women. Pulsatile delivery of GnRH is essential for the treatment of female infertility and hypogonadism, where the goal is to restore the natural fluctuation of GnRH levels. Constant infusion of GnRH has been reported to depress sexual function, resulting in an antagonistic effect. Currently, an external minipump (Lutrepulse®, Ortho) is used to infuse GnRH every 90 min, simulating the endogenous secretion patterns.

II. THEORY AND MECHANISMS

A. Transport Theories

Mathematically, steady-state iontophoretic transport can be expressed by the extended Nernst-Planck equation (in diluted solution form) [5],

$$J_i = \frac{-RT}{zF} \mu_i \left(\frac{dC_i}{dx_i} + C_i \frac{z_i F}{RT} \frac{dV}{dx} \right) + \beta C v_i \qquad (1)$$

the equation for flux contribution,

$$J_i = J_{ip} + J_{ie} + J_{ic} \qquad (2)$$

the continuity equation,

$$dJ_i/dx = 0,$$ (3)

the Poisson equation,

$$\frac{d^2V}{dx^2} = \frac{-F}{\epsilon} \sum_{i=1}^{n} z_i C_i$$ (4)

and the equation for electric current,

$$I_t = \sum_{i=1}^{n} z_i F_i J_i$$ (5)

where J_i is total fluxes of species i, J_{ip} the passive diffusion of species i, J_{ie} the electrical migration of species i, J_{ic} the convective flow of species i, n the number of ionic species, R the gas constant (8.314 J K^{-1} mole^{-1} or 8.314 V·coulomb K^{-1} mole^{-1}, T the absolute temperature (K), z ionic charge, F the Faraday constant (96,500 coulombs/mole), μ ionic mobility (cm^2 V^{-1} sec^{-1}, C concentration, V potential drop across the membrane, β a proportional constant, v volume flow of double-layer movement, ϵ the dielectric constant, and I_t the total current applied.

It can be seen from equations (1) and (2) that the total iontophoretic flux of a protein drug consists of three basic modes of mass transport: passive diffusion (J_{ip}), electrical migration (J_{ie}), and convection or electro-osmosis (J_{ic}). The driving forces responsible for iontophoretic transport are the chemical potential gradient (dC_i/dx) and the electrical potential gradient (dV/dx). Electrical migration, which is controlled by the electromotive forces, is the major component for the transport of charged species. On the other hand, convection, mainly resulting from electro-osmosis, is responsible for the transport of both ionic and nonionic drugs. The constant β is related to the physicochemical properties and molecular dimension of the permeating species. The volume flow (v) is a function of pH, ionic strength, and current intensity.

B. Intrinsic and External Factors Involved in Iontophoretic Enhancement

1. Properties of Drug and Formulation Conditions

As indicated in equation (1), the flux of a species i (such as a protein drug) is dependent upon its mobility μ, charge valence z, and concentration C. The diffusivity D can be expressed as

$$D = \frac{RT}{zF} \mu \qquad (6)$$

Since the mobility of a macromolecule is inversely proportional to the square root of its molecular weight ($M^{1/2}$) [6], it would be expected that macromolecules would possess much lower diffusivities than small electrolytes. Furthermore, protein molecules have a tendency to aggregate or polymerize, resulting in even lower mobilities. The passive diffusion of macromolecules across the skin is usually very small and is often negligible. The valence z of the charge of a protein drug can be optimized through the appropriate adjustment of pH. Gangarosa and coworkers [7] reported that a molecule with high conductivity would be a good candidate for iontophoretic enhancement. In general, the pH of the formulation should be adjusted to at least two units above or below the isoelectric point of a protein drug to achieve best iontophoretic enhancement. Siddiqui et al. [8] demonstrated that insulin could be delivered more efficiently when the formulation pH was above or below the isoelectric point.

In addition, higher drug concentrations are needed for greater iontophoretic enhancement. Since the total current is carried by both the drug and small ions, as indicated in equation (5), buffer ions and other charged excipients would compete for current, resulting in less iontophoretic enhancement for the drug itself, especially for large molecules such as proteins and peptides. In addition, when the ionic strength or concentration of buffer ions is high, the migration term becomes insignificant compared to the convective term. As a consequence, iontophoretic enhancement may result mainly from convection.

2. Electrical and biophysical properties of the skin and electrotransport

The skin is a heterogeneous membrane composed of 15–20% lipids, 40% proteins, and 40% water [9]. The skin is negatively charged at neutral pH because the isoelectric point of the horny layer is around pH 4.1 [10,11]. Burnette and Ongpipattanakul [12] demonstrated the permselective nature of the skin. Electroosmosis may become significant for iontophoretic enhancement when the formulation pH is above 4.1. Gangarosa and coworkers [13] observed increased transport of neutral species due to application of an electric field. Burnette and Marrero [14] also demonstrated the enhanced transport of neutral thyrotropin-releasing hormone when anodal iontophoresis was applied. Pikal and Shah [15–17] performed a series of studies investigating the electro-osmosis phenomena in ion-exchange membranes and hairless mouse skin. The skin manifests itself as a porous membrane with various pore size and charge distributions, i.e., neutral pores, positive pores, and negative pores. The effect of pH, ionic strength, and current intensity on the volume of electro-osmosis was investi-

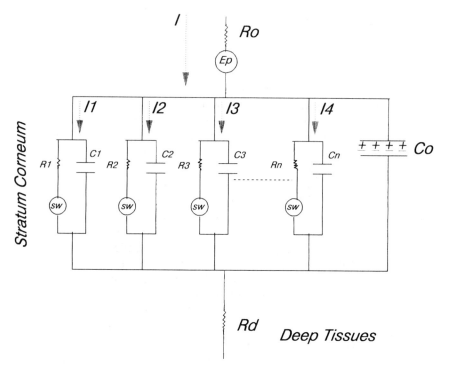

Figure 1   An equivalent circuit for the skin. R_0, intrinsic resistance of the stratum corneum (SC); C_0, capacitance of SC; I, applied current; I_i, current passed through channel i; R_i, resistance of channel i; C_i, capacitance of channel i; R_d, resistance of deep tissues.

gated. It was found that the magnitude of electro-osmosis decreased as the ionic strengths increased owing to a decrease in the double-layer thickness. The impact of electro-osmosis on the transport of high molecular weight solutes was also investigated. However, due to the heterogeneity and complexity of the pore system in the skin, theoretical predictions did not match the experimental observations [17].

It has been reported that the major impedance of the skin lies throughout the stratified layers of the stratum corneum [18,19]. Skin impedance changes in a very complex fashion. It can be resistive and capacitive [20–23]. A complex parallel RC circuit was used to show several conductive pathways (Fig. 1) [24]. The pathways or channels are both voltage- and time-dependent. Furthermore, the pathways are selective to ions of various molecular dimensions. The resistive components may be the protein domain or "pores" of the skin, whereas the capacitive components may be the lipid domain. It was reported that the impedance of the skin dropped initially after current application and reached a plateau value after about 30 min. The magnitude of the impedance drop is directly related to the intensity of the applied current [25]. The decrease of impedance in the skin was more pronounced when pulsed current was applied.

III. TRANSDERMAL IONTOPHORETIC DELIVERY OF PROTEINS AND PEPTIDES

Although there are no transdermal peptide dosage forms currently on the market, many research efforts have been dedicated toward this goal. Table 1 lists some of the published work on the transdermal delivery of proteins and peptides. Attempts were made to deliver proteins/peptides ranging from molecular weights of about 360 to >10,000 through the skin. Both chemical and physical (e.g., iontophoretic) methods were used to enhance the skin penetration of the drugs. A brief overview of the transdermal iontophoretic delivery of peptides is covered in the following subsections.

A. Thyrotropin-Releasing Hormone

Thyrotropin-releasing hormone, a tripeptide with a molecular weight of 362.42 and a pK_a value of 6.2 was shown to permeate through intact hairless mouse skin with the aid of iontophoresis [14]. The results showed that the permeation of uncharged peptide was enhanced more by iontophoresis than that of the charged species. In that study, however, the ionic strength used in the drug reservoir system was quite high (0.6 M), indicating that most of the current was carried by the smaller electrolytes present in the system. Therefore, the primary enhancement was due to convective flow or electromotive force–induced flow rather than electrical migration.

B. Vasopressin

The in vitro skin permeation of vasopressin, a nonapeptide with antidiuretic action, was enhanced up to 1000-fold by iontophoresis [26]. The enhancement was found to be highly dependent upon pH, ionic strength, and delivery pattern [26,27]. In in vivo studies in rabbits, the enhancement was observed to be further optimized by changing electrical parameters such as the on/off ratio and frequency [28].

A blanching test was used to determine the percutaneous permeation efficacy of ornipressin (a vasopressin derivative) enhanced by iontophoresis in men [29]. The degree of absorption was determined by the extent and duration of the blanching reaction in the skin. It was reported that iontophoretic delivery of ornipressin resulted in more intense blanches for longer durations, indicating the efficacy of iontophoretic enhancement.

C. Luteinizing Hormone-Releasing Hormone (LHRH) or GnRH

A GnRH analogue (a peptide with nine amino acids) was successfully delivered through the skin of nine men in a clinical study conducted at North Shore University at Manhasset, New York [30]. Serum luteinizing hormone (LH) was found to be significantly elevated after the application of an iontophoretically active patch. No change in serum LH levels was observed when a passive patch was applied. The iontophoretic patches were well tolerated without having significant cutaneous toxicity. Miller et al. [31] reported that both GnRH and its analogues can be delivered through the skin in vitro with the assistance of iontophoresis. One unique point in their experimental design was the arrangement of the electrodes. A pair of salt bridges were used to prevent the direct contact of the electrodes with the peptide solutions to minimize the electrical degradation of peptides. It was also reported that GnRH would metabolize in the skin, causing a dramatic decrease in GnRH concentrations in the receptor solutions [31].

D. Desenkephalin-gamma-Endorphin and Melanotropic Stimulating Hormone

Chemical enhancers were used to enhance the delivery of neuropeptides such as desenkephalin-gamma-endorphin [32], which has been implicated in schizophrenic psychoses. Melanotropic stimulating hormone (a peptide with 13 amino acid residues) was delivered through the skin without enhancement [33]. Iontophoretic technology could also be a viable enhancement method for these peptides.

E. Calcitonin

Calcitonin, a peptide with about 32 amino acid residues, indicated for the treatment of osteoporosis, was demonstrated to penetrate through the skin with the assistance of iontophoresis [34].

F. Growth Hormone Releasing Factor

An endogenous hypothalamic peptide with a 44-amino-acid sequence (GRF 1-44) was delivered through the skin of hairless guinea pigs with the assistance of iontophoresis. A steady-state plasma concentration of about 0.25 ng/mL was achieved after a lag time of 2 hr. Negligible amounts of GRF were detected in the plasma after the application of passive patches [35].

G. Insulin

Transdermal delivery of insulin of iontophoresis was first reported by Stephen et al. [36]. They reported that a highly ionized monomeric form of insulin (51 amino acid residues) was delivered through pig skin by iontophoresis to achieve systemic effects. However, their attempts using human subjects failed. This was attributed to the fact that the regular soluble insulin used in human studies was weakly charged and much of it was present in a polymeric form under their experimental conditions. Kari [37] also reported that reductions of blood glucose levels of diabetic rabbits could be achieved by insulin delivered transdermally with a direct-current iontophoretic device. In his experiment, however, the stratum corneum was disrupted by a surgical scalpel. Using streptozocin-induced diabetic hairless rats as an animal model, Sun et al. [38] found that iontophoresis with a pulsed dc waveform delivered insulin more effectively across intact skin than the commonly used dc to achieve normoglycemia. Liu et al. [39] attributed the high effectiveness of this technique to the depolarization of skin associated with the pulsed dc waveform, which significantly decreased the skin impedance.

Meyer et al. [40] achieved transdermal delivery of insulin by iontophoresis to control the blood glucose levels of alloxan-induced diabetic rabbits. They concluded that low levels of electric current might induce changes in stratum corneum permeability that are sufficient to induce transdermal absorption of physiologic doses of protein drugs such as insulin. It was speculated that the process involved in the transport was electro-osmosis. Whether the skin permeability was altered in the process of electro-osmosis remains to be investigated.

Sun and coworkers [41] demonstrated the reduction of blood glucose levels in diabetic hairless rats by transdermal iontophoretic delivery of insulin (TIDI) using a skin pretreatment technique. The skin was pretreated with freshly prepared calamine lotion (U.S.P.), followed by iontophoretic delivery of insulin for 30 min [41]. It was found that the hyperglycemic blood glucose levels of diabetic rats were not improved and the insulin levels in the plasma remained low when passive insulin patches were applied on the pretreated skin (Fig. 2). This indicated that the pretreatment process did not significantly damage the skin barrier function. On the other hand, the blood glucose levels were significantly reduced when insulin was delivered iontophoretically across the pretreated skin (Fig. 3).

The same paper introduced a unique technique called alternating reverse electrical polarity (AREP), which uses both the anode and cathode as active driving electrodes (Fig. 4). It was found that insulin can be delivered more efficiently to control hyperglycemia through AREP than using the unipolar iontophoretic device. The pharmacokinetics of insulin as indicated by the reduction of blood glucose levels and elevated insulin concentrations in the plasma was observed

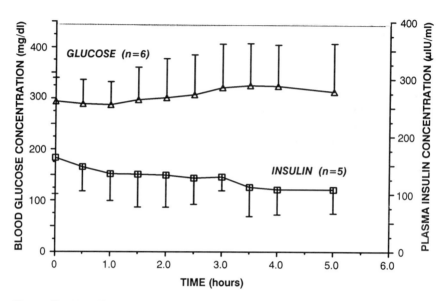

Figure 2 The effect of skin pretreatment on blood glucose levels and plasma insulin concentrations after the passive diffusion of insulin. Skin was pretreated with calamine lotion for 30 min.

(Fig. 5). The concept of AREP is discussed more in Section V.B. There was a slight pH shift (~0.5 unit) in the insulin reservoirs after 30 min of current application. In contrast, dramatic pH changes were found when current was applied with a fixed polarity. The insulin retrieved from the reservoirs after iontophoresis was found to remain active, as determined from its hypoglycemic effect on rats.

The feasibility of using this design for multidose administration was also demonstrated [42]. Blood glucose levels were controlled to simulate biological patterns through the temporal delivery of insulin using the AREP device (Fig. 6). It can be seen that normoglycemia was achieved with multiple doses of insulin delivered in a pulsatile fashion. A glucose challenge test was performed to examine whether a 30-min duration of iontophoretic delivery of insulin was sufficient for blood glucose control. It was found that the blood glucose levels of diabetic rats rose immediately after ingestion of 2 g of glucose delivered via a stomach tube (glucose challenge test) after the termination of 30-min transdermal delivery of insulin (TIDI). The experimental results suggested that longer duration of TIDI might be needed for the control of diabetes. A recovery to normoglycemia conditions was observed after the glucose challenge test when the duration of transdermal iontophoretic delivery of insulin (TIDI) was ex-

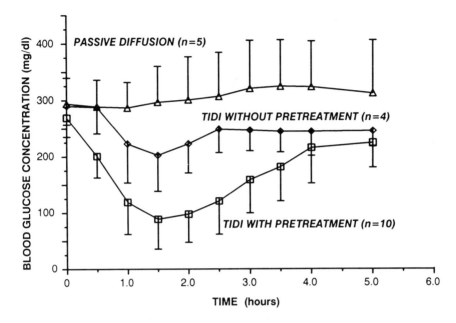

Figure 3 The effect of skin pretreatment on blood glucose levels of diabetic rats after passive delivery of insulin (△), transdermal iontophoretic delivery of insulin (TIDI) without pretreatment (◇), and TIDI with pretreatment (□). Iontophoretic treatment: 2 mA pulse dc with AREP for 30 min.

tended to 60 min. This demonstrated that the duration of application was important because it could control the amount of insulin delivered.

H. Grass Pollen Allergen Extracts

The percutaneous absorption of grass pollen allergen extracts (peptides and glycoproteins) under the influence of iontophoresis was tested using the IgE-mediated skin reaction (wheal) [43]. Pollen extracts with molecular weights greater than 10,000 were delivered through the skin by iontophoresis at a current density of 0.05 mA/cm^2 for 10 min. All 10 volunteers (with grass pollen allergies) tested showed allergic reactions. It was believed that iontophoresis enhanced the penetration of the allergen extracts.

IV. CHALLENGES TO OVERCOME

Although transdermal iontophoretic delivery is capable of providing precise and convenient drug administration of proteins and peptides, several technical prob-

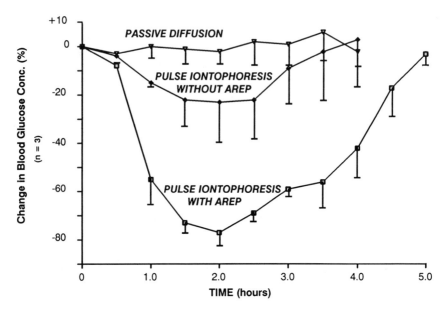

Figure 4 The effect of AREP on blood glucose levels of diabetic rats after passive delivery of insulin (▽) and transdermal iontophoretic delivery of insulin without AREP (◇) and with AREP (□).

lems must be solved before this approach can be efficiently utilized. These challenges include physicochemical compatibility, aggregation and adsorption, stability under an electric field, electrical relative mobility, skin irritation, bioactivity, and bioavailability.

A. Physicochemical Compatibility

First, protein molecules such as insulin are generally surface-active and have a high propensity to adsorb to the surfaces of containers [44,45], resulting in a reduction of available free protein molecules for iontophoretic delivery. It was reported that insulin molecules have a higher tendency to adsorb onto hydrophobic polymers (e.g., Teflon and silicone rubber) than onto hydrophilic materials (e.g., polyacrylamide). Insulin was also observed to adsorb onto metal surfaces. The adsorption of insulin on a platinum surface was found to be irreversible [46]. In addition, the conformation of the protein, which could be directly related to the bioactivity, may be altered through the adsorption process. Therefore, the selection of materials for the device's drug reservoir plays a significant role in the design of an iontophoretic delivery system.

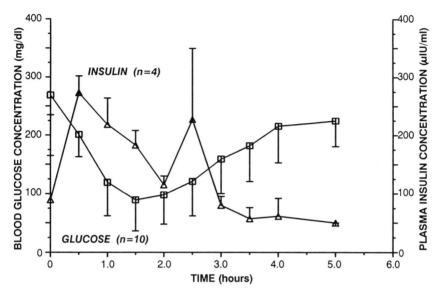

Figure 5 Blood glucose levels and plasma insulin concentration of diabetic rats after TIDI with AREP.

Some pharmaceutical excipients, such as human serum albumin, glycine, glycerin, urea, and surfactants, can be added into the formulation to stabilize the protein providing that the excipients do not create too much competition for current. The tendency of proteins to aggregate in the medium will increase the molecular dimension of the drug, leading to lower electrical mobility under an electric field.

In most cases, hydrophilic polymeric gels are used as a matrix base for the drug reservoir in iontophoretic devices [47]. Nonionic hydrophilic gels such HPMC and polyacrylamide are recommended for the delivery of proteins and peptides because of their unreactive nature. Anionic or cationic polymers may react with proteins, causing undesirable precipitation. For instance, Carbopol, an anionic polymer at neutral pH, may interact with positively charged proteins, resulting in a decrease in the concentration of free protein molecules for iontophoretic enhancement.

B. Chemical and Electrical Stability

Proteins are labile and are more subject to degradation and denaturation than most chemical compounds. Appropriate pH's should be chosen to attain maximum stability. The additional energy generated from the iontophoretic process may further accelerate degradation. One possible reason for the instability of

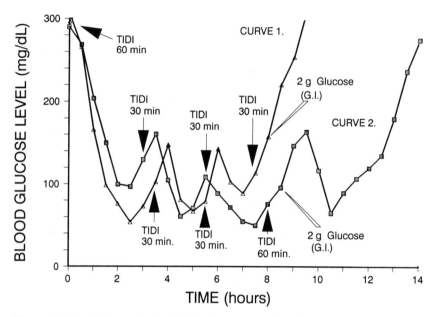

Figure 6 Blood glucose levels of diabetic rats controlled by pulsatile delivery of insulin (TIDI + AREP) challenged with 2 g of glucose.

drug under iontophoresis is the electrochemical degradation on the electrode surfaces and pH shift from water electrolysis when platinum electrodes are used in iontophoresis.

The electrochemical reaction occurring at the cathode ($-$) is

$$2e^- + 2H_2O \rightarrow 2OH^- + H_2 \tag{7}$$

The simultaneous reaction at the anode ($+$) is

$$H_2O \rightarrow 2H^+ + (1/2)O_2 + 2e^- \tag{8}$$

During anodal iontophoresis, the increase in oxygen content at the anode may facilitate the oxidation of a drug, especially for proteins and peptides that contain tryptophan, methionine, and cysteine, which are susceptible to oxidation [48]. Therefore, the first task in iontophoretic development is to develop a stable formulation and/or design a reservoir device that separates the proteins from direct contact with the electrodes.

In addition, the above reaction indicates that 1 mole of hydronium ions [H^+] at the anode will be generated with the passage of 1 mole of electrons.

For example, vasopressin formulated at pH 7 (without buffers) was delivered transdermally by anodal ($+$) iontophoresis at a current density of 0.05 mA/cm^2

for 10 min, 20 min, 40 min, and 1 hr with a reservoir capacity of 1 mL and effective contact area of 10 cm². The final pH can be estimated using the equation

$$pH = -\log [H^+] = -\log [(60\ IAt)/(FV)] \tag{9}$$

where I is the current density (mA/cm² or 10^{-3} coulomb sec^{-1} cm^{-2}), A the effective contact area (cm²), t the application time (min), F the Faraday constant (96,500 coulombs/mole), and V the volume of the drug reservoir or donor electrode (mL).

The final pH in the drug reservoir (anode) after iontophoresis was calculated to be 2.51, 2.20, 1.90, and 1.30 after 10 min, 20 min, 40 min, and 1 hr, respectively, of current application. This demonstrates the significance of pH shift after iontophoresis. The change of pH at the cathode can be estimated using a similar equation:

$$pH = 14 + \log [OH^-] = 14 + \log [(60\ IAt)/(FV)] \tag{10}$$

The excess hydrogen and hydroxyl ions produced on the anode and cathode that shift pH to a lower or higher value will lead to undesirable stability problems. The large number of hydronium ions or hydroxide ions produced through electrochemical reaction, which are highly mobile, will also compete for current, resulting in less iontophoretic enhancement.

C. Addition of Buffer Ions and Relative Electrical Mobility

Since an appropriate pH is required to make a protein or peptide highly charged for iontophoretic enhancement as well as to ensure chemical stability, the addition of buffer species is a common practice to maintain constant pH. However, highly mobile buffer ions will compete with the high molecular weight protein drug for the current, leading to a slowdown in the movement of the protein molecules. The fraction of current carried by a charged molecule (transfer number t) or the ability of the molecule to compete for iontophoretic transport is a function of its concentration C, valence z, and mobility μ; that is,

$$t_i \propto C_i z_i \mu_i \tag{11}$$

The transfer number of large molecules (t_A) in the presence of a buffer (B) can be simplified as follows:

$$t_A = C_A Z_A \mu_A / [C_A Z_A \mu_A + C_B Z_B \mu_B) \tag{12}$$

Therefore, the addition of buffer ions such as citrate or phosphate ions to proteins and peptides may cause a significant decrease in iontophoretic enhancement. It has been shown that iontophoresis efficiency is inversely influenced by the ionic strength because the ion transfer number of the drug (defined as the fraction of the total electric charge carried by the drug species) decreases as the concentration of buffer electrolytes increases. This indicates that a minimal buffer concentration is a necessity in the development of an effective iontophoretic delivery system.

D. Electrode Compatibility

Two recent studies reported that there was extensive insulin loss from the donor solution during iontophoresis [49,50]. The use of Ag/AgCl electrodes in direct contact with protein and peptide solutions could cause a drug loss due to the precipitation of proteins and peptides by Ag^+ ions.

E. Skin Irritation

One of the concerns in transdermal iontophoretic delivery is the possible skin irritation caused by electric current. It is generally accepted that skin irritation can be minimized when the current density is controlled below 0.2–0.5 mA/cm^2 [51]. Good contact between the patch surface and the skin is important to avoid uneven distribution of the applied electric current. It was reported that the use of pulsed current could reduce the irritation potential of iontophoresis [52,53].

F. Bioavailability

As the costs of protein and peptide drugs are very high, the percent of the drug available in the drug reservoir for therapeutic responses is crucial in the development of a transdermal iontophoretic device. The bioavailability of proteins and peptides delivered by transdermal iontophoresis could be improved through better permeation enhancement and stabilization of formulations for multiple application.

V. APPROACHES TO IMPROVE THE BIOAVAILABILITY OF TRANSDERMAL DELIVERY SYSTEMS FOR PROTEIN/PEPTIDES

A. Current Mode

Theoretically, when simple direct current is used to facilitate the transport of charged molecules through the skin, the polarization impedance developed in the skin due to charge accumulation operates against the applied electric field, resulting in a decrease in the effective current for the transport of charged molecules. In the case of pulsed current (Fig. 7), the applied electric field is switched alternately on and off depending upon the frequency used. Therefore, the skin will have an opportunity to dissipate the charge buildup or depolarize completely in each on/off cycle. In addition, skin impedance decreases with increases in

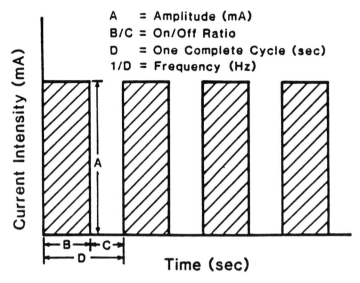

Figure 7 A diagram of pulsed dc profiles. A, amplitude (mA); B/C, on/off ratio; D, one complete cycle (sec); $1/D$ = frequency (Hz).

pulse frequency. Maximum iontophoretic enhancement could be achieved at an optimal frequency and on/off ratio. Liu et al. [24] proposed an equivalent circuit model to describe this phenomenon. The optimal on/off ratio depends not only on frequency but also on current intensity (Fig. 8). Liu et al. [39] demonstrated that pulsed direct current is better than simple direct current in the delivery of insulin for the control of diabetes. They found that a higher frequency and a lower on/off ratio led to better iontophoretic enhancement.

B. Electrode Design

Several iontophoretic devices have been described that have improved electrode designs. The improved electrodes may be designed to prevent the system pH from shifting, to avoid direct contact between the drug solution and the electrodes, and to eliminate the need for unwanted competing buffer ions.

Sanderson and coworkers [54] described an iontophoretic delivery device to minimize the change in subcutaneous pH produced by the iontophoretic treatment (which might cause burns) and to prevent the competition of buffer species. Its working electrode device consisted of two chambers molded from polyvinyl chloride. The upper chamber contained buffer solution gelled with karaya gum and glycerin. The lower chamber contained only drug solution and was enclosed by a microporous polypropylene membrane. These chambers were separated by

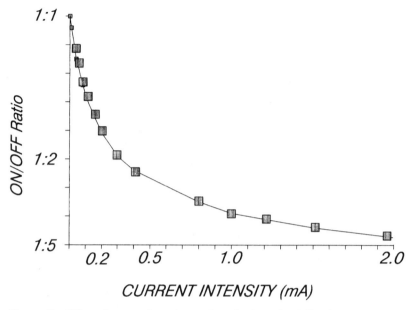

Figure 8 Effect of current intensity on the selection of on/off ratio.

an ion-exchange membrane to inhibit the flow of ionic electrolysis products into the drug solution compartment and then into the skin. This ion-exchange membrane also served to keep the drug away from direct contact with the metal electrode to minimize any possible electrode reaction of the drug.

Sun et al. [41] took a different approach, using the electrochemical reaction that occurs on the electrodes during iontophoresis to maintain the system pH. Figure 9 shows a typical in vivo conventional iontophoresis device that is currently being used. A drug solution is placed in the drug reservoir of the working electrode. The working electrode may be either the anode or the cathode depending on whether the drug is cationic or anionic. The dispersive (or receiving) electrode is usually made of electrically conducting gel to complete the circuit.

The design of Sun's device is shown in Figure 10. Unlike the conventional iontophoresis device with only one working electrode, both electrodes are working electrodes in this system. The metal electrode is located in a chamber separated from the drug reservoir by a porous polymer partition membrane of controlled pore size. The diameter of the pores is smaller than that of the protein molecules. The function of the porous partition membrane is to prevent the electrochemical degradation of the drug on the electrode. Another distinct feature of this system compared to conventional transdermal iontophoresis is the use of an alternating

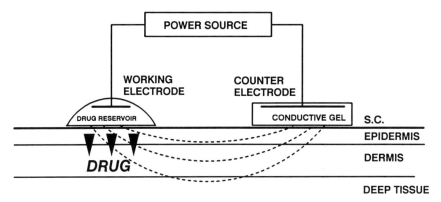

Figure 9 A schematic diagram of a conventional iontophoretic device.

reverse electrode polarity (AREP) of dc or pulsed dc waveform. The following examples and Figure 11 can be used to illustrate how this system works.

Design 1

An insulin solution of pH 8 (negatively charged, insulin's pH_{iso} = 5.3) is placed into the drug reservoirs of both working electrodes. When the power is switched on, the cathode (electrode I) acts as the working electrode to drive insulin molecules into the skin. Meanwhile, hydroxyl ions (OH^-) are produced on the cathode [see equation (7)]. The excess hydroxyl ions produced shift the pH towards a higher value. The simultaneous reaction on the anode (electrode II) leads to the production of hydrogen ions (H^+), resulting in a pH change to a lower value. The porous partition membrane allows only the small ions to pass through to complete the electric circuit while preventing the negatively charged insulin from

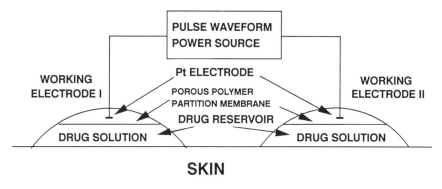

Figure 10 A schematic diagram of AREP design using pulsed direct current.

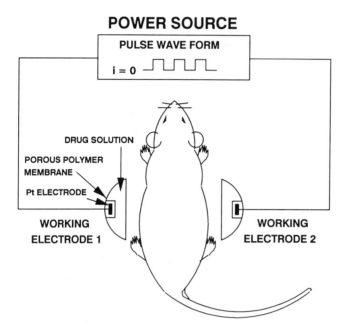

Figure 11 An experimental layout of in vivo transdermal iontophoretic delivery using AREP technique.

reacting on the electrode to cause degradation. After a short time period, the polarity of the electric circuit is reversed: electrode I is now the anode and electrode II the cathode. Insulin will be driven into the skin by electrode II, and the electrochemical reactions on the two electrodes are completely reversed so that the pH is restored to the original condition. After insulin molecules have been delivered into the skin, reversing the electric polarity will not pull them back, because the abundance of small ions in the epidermal tissues (i.e., Na^+ and Cl^-) will take over the task of transporting electrons and therefore leave the much larger insulin molecules in the skin for further absorption.

Design 2

The same insulin solution as in design 1 (pH 8, negatively charged) is placed in the reservoir of electrode I. A second insulin solution of pH 3 (positively charged) is placed in the electrode II reservoir. When the power is on, both electrodes drive insulin into the skin. When the polarity is reversed, the pH in both electrodes is restored to the original condition.

The advantages of these systems are that (1) they eliminate the requirement for buffers, therefore minimizing the amount of competing ions present;

(2) they prevent the electrochemical degradation of drugs; (3) they increase the electrodes' functioning area without actually increasing the size of the skin contact area. These three advantages address the major problems faced by all iontophoretic systems currently in existence—the limited drug delivery efficiency due to poor absorption, the influence of competing buffer ions, and drug instability due to electrochemical degradation.

The third advantage is of practical importance, because it is directly related to skin irritation. It has been known that the skin's tolerance to applied electricity is measured by the current density (mA/cm^2). Since there is a practical limitation on the size of the skin contact area, this delivery system may clear some of the major technical obstacles for commercialization of transdermal iontophoretic drug delivery systems, especially for peptide/protein drugs. The optimal AREP for iontophoretic enhancement is under investigation.

C. Formulation Optimization

The selection of pH, buffer species and concentration, and other excipients in the formulation plays a significant role in determining the degree of enhancement. As discussed in the previous section, a minute change in pH in the drug reservoir can cause a drastic decrease in transfer efficiency (transfer number). Since the efficiency of enhancement in transdermal iontophoretic delivery is highly dependent upon the charge on the drug ions, the pH of the formulation should be maintained in an appropriate range to create highly charged species.

D. Delivery Pattern

The rate of current input and duration of application also play an important role in determining the degree of iontophoretic enhancement. Lelawongs et al. [27] found that the cumulative amount of vasopressin permeated was higher with higher current density despite the fact that the same amount of total electric energy was applied. In that study [27], pulsed current was applied at current densities of 0.078, 0.31, and 0.47 mA/cm^2 for 240, 60, and 40 min, respectively; i.e., the total energy applied was about 1.12 coulombs/cm^2. The combination of 0.47 mA/cm^2 for 40 min yielded the highest permeation. Lelawongs [28] also illustrated the effect of the mode of applied current, continuous or periodic, on enhancement efficacy. In that experiment, current was applied continuously for 120 min or for 10 min on and 30 min off for 12 cycles. The results indicated that the continuous mode achieved higher flux [28].

E. Additional Chemical and/or Physical Enhancement

Many researchers recommend the combination of chemical enhancers and iontophoresis for maximum enhancement with minimum irritation. Table 2 lists the

Table 2 Chemical Enhancers Used in Combination
with Iontophoresis

Chemical	Enhancement effect
Absolute alcohol	+
L-Ascorbic acid	+
Calamine lotion	+
DMSO	−
Decyl MSO	−
75% Alcohol/N.S.	−
Sodium bisulfite	+
Sodium taurocholate	−
Sodium lauryl sulfate	−
Thioglycolate	+

chemical enhancers used in combination with iontophoresis. Depending upon their mechanisms of action, the results were found to be synergistic or nonadditive. Srinivasan et al. [55] observed a synergistic effect of iontophoresis and a chemical enhancer for the delivery of a polypeptide. It was shown that a 2-hr pretreatment with absolute ethanol followed by iontophoresis dramatically increased the permeability coefficient of insulin through human skin. In contrast, Lelawongs [28] demonstrated an unfavorable nonadditive effect when decylmethyl sulfoxide (DeMSO) and iontophoresis were applied together. The mode of action for DeMSO has been shown to be related to its interaction with the protein [56]. As a surfactant, it changes the conformation of protein and then opens up aqueous channels [57]. The alkyl part of DeMSO (C_{10}) could also insert between the structured lipids, resulting in increased lipid fluidity. It was speculated that DeMSO may reduce the potential gradient across the skin, resulting in less enhancement from iontophoresis because the major driving force for transdermal iontophoresis is the potential drop across the skin.

Therefore, the selection of a chemical enhancer and its concentration plays a critical role in achieving the desired permeation enhancement. The chemical enhancers used in combination with iontophoresis should not perturb the resistive components (such as the protein domain) of the skin to achieve a synergistic effect.

Sun et al. [41] reported a pretreatment process to further improve iontophoretic insulin delivery. The skin of hairless rats was pretreated with various pharmaceutical excipients. During the pretreatment, the test solution was placed in the electrode reservoirs with iontophoresis at 2 mA for 4 min. The choice of test substances was based on the fact that the drug transport route for transdermal iontophoresis is different from that for a passive diffusion process. The experimental results indicated that 75% ethanol in normal saline, 1% sodium tauro-cholate, and 1% sodium lauryl sulfate did not increase the iontophoretic insulin delivery, but L-ascorbic acid, sodium bisulfite, and thioglycolic acid improved the iontophoretic insulin delivery. Skin pretreatment with 0.05% calcium thioglycolate significantly improved the efficiency of iontophoretic delivery.

The use of ultrasound energy (phonophoresis) to further facilitate the penetration of macromolecules has also been proposed [58]. It was believed that iontophoresis and phonophoresis should work synergistically, with the former providing a driving force and the latter accelerating the absorption process, to enhance the transdermal delivery of macromolecules for systemic medication.

F. Miscellaneous

The possible metabolism of peptides and proteins in the skin can be minimized by the addition of an enzyme inhibitor or by molecular modification (analogues). For instance, GnRH was found to be more subject than its analogues to biodegradation in the skin [31].

VI. PROGRESS IN THE DESIGN OF TRANSDERMAL IONTOPHORETIC DELIVERY SYSTEMS

Many companies and research institutes are actively designing iontophoretic delivery systems independently or through collaborative efforts. The following are some of the development activities.

Panoderm. A patented watch-size transdermal drug transport system developed through the joint efforts of Elan Pharmaceuticals and Swiss Corporation for Microelectronics and Watchmaking Industries (manufacturer of Swatch watches) [59]. Elan formulated the products and Swatch manufactured the electronics, sensors, and case of the device. The future of the system lies in the biofeedback control for individualized patient therapy.

Bioelectro Systems. Alza and Medtronics are under a "collaborative arrangement" to develop electrotransport technology [60]. They currently are evaluating electrotransport for the delivery of proteins and peptides developed by the biotech industry. Medtronic has one electrotransport product on the market: a cystic fibrosis indicator for pediatric use. It has been approved by the FDA for this purpose and is widely used by pediatricians. The battery-powered device delivers pilocarpine with a low-level electric current to excite the sweat glands. The clinician then removes the device and applies a patch, which analyzes the chemical content of the sweat and indicates the likelihood of cystic fibrosis via a color change.

Powerpatch. This patented system, developed by Drug Delivery Systems, is capable of inducing transport of compounds across the skin based on the use of electrically induced phenomena in human skin [30,40]. The Powerpatch applicator is a bandagelike device that contains an intrinsic power source, electronic conditioning components, and usually two drug reservoirs. The patch is thin, flexible, self-adhering, and easily applied by the patient. Patch components are assembled on an inert film substrate coated with an adhesive. The power source is a coin-size sealed battery with appropriate electronics to control the current. A drug reservoir is located in each electrode, and the electric circuit is completed when the Powerpatch is applied to the skin surface.

Phoresor. This is an iontophoretic therapeutic drug delivery device marketed by IOMED. It is indicated for the administration of dexamethasone sodium phosphate to treat acute or subacute inflammations. Phoresor is also indicated for the administration of lidocaine hydrochloride as an alternative to hypodermic injection to produce local anesthesia.

VII. FUTURE PERSPECTIVES

The use of iontophoresis in the pharmaceutical and cosmetic industries is steadily increasing. It has been accepted by the FDA for diagnostic purposes and for the treatment of localized diseases and may offer new horizons for the delivery of proteins and peptides. Based on the report from the Technology Management Group Conference on worldwide activities and market opportunities in delivery of proteins [34], there are at least 26 companies and institutions involved in enhanced transdermal technology. Bioavailability and long-term safety are the major challenges to overcome. Continued success in the development of transdermal iontophoretic drug delivery systems will depend upon a better understanding of the physicochemical and biophysical characteristics of a drug and the skin under an electric field and the enhancement mechanisms.

Acknowledgements We thank Drs. Michael Corbo, Diane Calvosa Corbo and Hong Xue for their kind assistance in the preparation of this chapter.

REFERENCES

1. J. Sloan and K. Soltani, *J. Am. Acad. Dermatol. 15*, 671 (1986).
2. J. E. Griffin and T. C. Karselis, *Physical Agents for Physical Therapists*, Charles C. Thomas Publisher, Springfield, 1988, Ch. 3.
3. M. F. Fay, *Today's OR Nurse 11*, 10 (1989).
4. B. H. Vickery, J. J. Newtor, and E. S. E. Hafez, Eds., *LHRH and Its Analogs*, MTP, Boston, MA, 1984.
5. F. Helfferich, *Ion-Exchanger Membranes*, McGraw-Hill, New York, 1962, p. 344.

6. N. Lakshminarayanaiah, *Equations of Membrane Biophysics*, Academic, New York, 1984, p. 52.
7. L. Gangarosa, N. H. Park, B. C. Fong, D. F. Scott, and J. M. Hill, *J. Pharm. Sci.* 67, 1439 (1978).
8. O. Siddiqui, Y. Sun, J. C. Liu, and Y. W. Chien, *J. Pharm. Sci.* 76, 341 (1987).
9. P. Tyle, *Pharm. Res. 13*, 318 (1986).
10. H. Schade and A. Marchionini, *Munchen. Med. Wochnschr. 74*, 1435 (1927).
11. P. Keller, *Arch. Dermatol. Syph. 160*, 136 (1930).
12. R. R. Burnette and B. Ongpipattanakul, *J. Pharm. Sci. 76*, 765 (1987).
13. L. Gangarosa, N.-E. Park, C. A. Wiggins, and J. M. Hill, *Pharmacol. Exp. Ther. 212*, 377 (1980).
14. R. R. Burnette and D. Marrero, *J. Pharm. Sci. 75*, 738 (1986).
15. M. J. Pikal, *Pharm. Res. 7*, 118 (1990).
16. M. J. Pikal and S. Shah, *Pharm. Res. 7*, 222 (1990).
17. M. J. Pikal and S. Shah, *Pharm. Res. 7*, 230 (1990).
18. C. Lawler, M. J. Davis, and E. C. Griffin, *J. Invest. Dermatol. 34*, 301 (1960).
19. R. T. Tregear, in *Physical Function of Skin*, R. T. Tregear, Ed., Academic, New York, 1966, p. 64.
20. A. Barnett, *J. Physiol. 93*, 349 (1938).
21. W. Geets and J. Colle, *Compt. Rend. Soc. Biol. 140*, 701 (1946).
22. H. Gerstner, *Arch. Ges. Physiol. 250*, 125 (1948).
23. T. Yamamoto and Y. Yamamoto, *Med. Biol. Eng. Comput. 15*, 219 (1977).
24. J. C. Liu, W. M. Shi, and Y. Sun, *Pharmacol. Exp. Ther. Suppl.* A27 (1988).
25. P. Lelawongs, J. C. Liu, and Y. W. Chien, *Pharmacol. Exp. Ther. Suppl.* A27 (1988).
26. P. Lelawongs, J. C. Liu, O. Siddiqui, and Y. W. Chien, *Int. J. Pharm. 56*, 13 (1989).
27. P. Lelawongs, J. C. Liu, and Y. W. Chien, *Int. J. Pharm.* (1990).
28. P. Lelawongs, Transdermal Iontophoretic Delivery of Arginine Vasopressin, Ph.D. Thesis, Rutgers Univ., 1990.
29. W. Remy, M. Demmler, and O. Mielcke, *Allergologie 12*, 224 (1989).
30. B. R. Meyer, W. Kries, J. Eschbach, V. O'Mara, et al., *Clin. Pharmacol. Therap. 44*, 607 (1988).
31. L. L. Miller, C. J. Kolaskie, G. A. Smith, and J. Rivier, *J. Pharm. Sci. 79*, 490 (1990).
32. H. E. Bodde, J. C. Verhoef, and M. Ponec, *Biochem. Soc. Trans. 17*, 943 (1989).
33. B. Dawson, M. E. Hadley, N. Levine, K. L. Kreutzfeld, et al., *J. Invest. Dermatol. 94*, 432 (1990).
34. J. Devane, Drug delivery of proteins, Proc. Technology Management Group Conf., Boston, 1989.
35. S. Kumar, H. Char, S. Patel, D. Piemontese, et al., In-vivo transdermal iontophoretic delivery of GRF (1-44) in hairless guinea pigs, *Proc. Int. Symp. Controlled Release Bioact. Mater. 17*, 435–436 (1990).
36. R. L. Stephen, T. J. Petelenz, and S. C. Jacobsen, *Biomed. Biochim. Acta 43*, 557 (1984).

37. B. Kari, *Diabetes 35*, 217 (1986).
38. Y. Sun, O. Siddiqui, J. C. Liu, and Y. W. Chien, Important parameters affecting iontophoretic transdermal delivery of insulin, *Proc. Int. Symp. Controlled Release Bioact. Mater. 13*, 175–176 (1986).
39. J. C. Liu, Y. Sun, O. Siddiqui, Y. W. Chien, et al., *Int. J. Pharm. 44*, 197 (1988).
40. B. R. Meyer, H. L. Katzeff, J. C. Eschbach, and J. Trimmer, *Am. J. Med. Sci. 297*, 321 (1989).
41. Y. Sun, J. C. Liu, and H. Xue, Important parameters affecting iontophoretic transdermal delivery of insulin, *Proc. Int. Symp. Controlled Release Bioact. Mater. 17*, 202–203 (1990).
42. Y. Sun and H. Xue, in *Temporal Control of Drug Delivery*, W. J. M. Hrushesky, R. Langer and F. Theeuwes, Ed., Annals of the New York Academy of Sciences, Vol. 618, 1991, p. 596.
43. J. Gauger, W. Remy, and H. U. Voigt, *Allergologie 12*, 227 (1989).
44. M. V. Sefton and G. M. Antonacci, *Diabetes 33*, 674 (1984).
45. T. Arnebrant and T. Nylander, *J. Colloid Interface Sci. 122*, 557 (1988).
46. V. Razumas, J. Kulys, T. Arnebrant, T. Nylander, et al., *Sov. Electrochem. 24*, 424 (1988).
47. H. Pfefferova, J. Marek, and H. Bockova, Czech. Patent CS 238517 B1 (1987).
48. Y. J. Wang and M. A. Hanson, *J. Parenter. Sci. Technol. 42*, S3 (1988).
49. A. K. Banga and Y. W. Chien, *Pharm. Res. 6*, S109 (1989).
50. K. H. Valia and M. J. Pikal, *Pharm. Res. 6*, S146 (1989).
51. R. Harris, in *Therapeutic Electricity and Ultraviolet Radiation*, S. Licht, Ed., Wiley, New York, 1967, p. 168.
52. K. Okabe, H. Yamaguchi, and Y. Kawai, *J. Controlled Release 4*, 79 (1986).
53. C. R. Behl, S. Kumar, A. W. Malick, S. D. Terzo, et al., *J. Pharm. Sci. 78*, 355 (1989).
54. J. E. Sanderson, R. W. Caldwell, R. W. Hsiao, J. Dixon, et al., *J. Pharm. Sci. 76*, 738 (1986).
55. V. Srinivasan, W. I. Higuchi, S. M. Sims, A. H. Ghanem, and C. R. Behl, *J. Pharm. Sci. 78*, 370 (1989).
56. B. W. Barry, *J. Controlled Release 6*, 85 (1987).
57. P. S. Banerjee and W. A. Ritschel, *Int. J. Pharm. 49*, 199 (1989).
58. J. Singh and M. S. Roberts, *Drug Des. Delivery 4*, 1 (1989).
59. T. J. Roseman, Ed., *Controlled Release Newslett. 8*, 8 (1990).
60. *FDC Reports 6*, Feb. 12, 1990.

13

In Vivo Experience with Electrically Mediated Transdermal Drug Delivery

B. Robert Meyer
Albert Einstein College of Medicine, Bronx, New York

I. INTRODUCTION

The transdermal route of drug administration has several potential advantages over other routes of administration. For selected drugs in which oral administration is prohibited by the extent of enteric degradation and first-pass metabolism, the transdermal route offers an alternative pathway that avoids gastrointestinal and first-pass liver effects. The transdermal route also has the potential for the continuous infusion of medication instead of intermittent bolus administration. This is an advantage for drugs in which peak concentrations are a significant cause of additional toxicity or where trough concentrations are a potentially serious cause of treatment failure. The use of a single application for sustained therapy (from 1 day to as much as 7 days) also suggests the possibility of improved patient compliance with therapy.

The permeability characteristics of the human skin have significantly limited the development and exploitation of the theoretical advantages of the transdermal route for drug delivery. The stratum corneum is an effective barrier to the passive penetration (by diffusion along a concentration gradient) of a wide variety of chemical compounds. As a result, the number of products available as transdermal preparations has remained small. If the advantages of transdermal drug delivery are to be realized, then new techniques for the enhancement and control of transdermal drug absorption need to be developed.

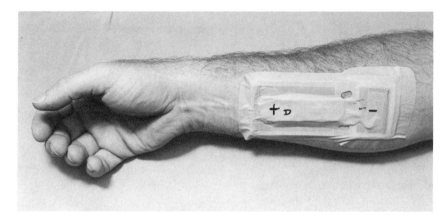

Figure 1 View of patch as applied to the forearm of a volunteer for leuprolide study. For the duration of the study, the arm was wrapped in an ace bandage to ensure adherence of the patch to the skin. Positive and negative electrodes are identified.

II. EXPERIMENTAL DATA WITH ELECTRICALLY MEDIATED TRANSDERMAL DELIVERY

We have investigated the possibility of using an electric current to alter stratum corneum permeability and enhance the absorption of a variety of chemical entities. The theoretical basis for such a technique is discussed elsewhere in this book. In theory, this technique has all of the potential advantages of transdermal delivery outlined in the opening paragraph of this chapter. In addition, as transdermal absorption in such a system would be controlled by the applied electric field, it would also offer the possibility of turning delivery ''on'' or ''off'' by the application or removal of current or by the reversal of current direction. This could permit the development of programmed drug delivery over the course of a day or patient-initiated ''prn'' delivery by activation of the electric current.

A critical step in the development of such an electrically powered transdermal delivery system is the development of a small, self-contained, relatively inexpensive, and easily applied patch. The powerpatch drug delivery system developed by Drug Delivery Systems Inc. (New York, NY) is a small (10 cm × 7 cm) patch that can be easily be applied to the forearm, trunk, or abdomen (Figs. 1 and 2). In the studies discussed here, the power source for the patch consisted of three 3-V disk batteries identical to those found in watches. This 9-V power source is connected to an integrated circuit with variable resistance that controls current at a constant value. The patches used in these studies delivered direct current at levels between 0.2 and 0.4 mA. The electrodes are graphite. There are drug reservoirs at the positive and negative electrodes that can range in

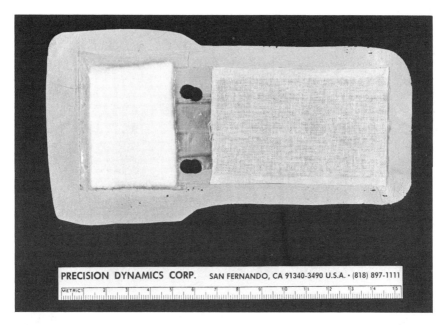

PRECISION DYNAMICS CORP. SAN FERNANDO, CA 91340-3490 U.S.A. · (818) 897-1111

Figure 2 View of the surface of the patch that is applied to the skin. The smaller surface on the left is the drug reservoir at the negative electrode, and the larger surface on the right is the positive reservoir. The reservoir volume for the leuprolide studies is either 1 mL or 0.4 mL for the positive reservoir and 3 mL for the negative reservoir.

volume from less than 0.5 mL to greater than 3 mL. More recent developments allow for a thin, flexible solid-state lithium battery and for drug reservoirs composed of various hydrogels.

We have used the powerpatch system to investigate the practical feasibility of using electric current to enhance the transdermal absorption of drugs. This chapter summarizes some of that work.

A. Transdermal Administration of Peptides

An increasing number of peptide drugs are being developed for clinical use. The next decade will see a vast increase in the number of such drugs and their potential indications. These compounds are potent, frequently are relatively short acting, and are not absorbed in therapeutically relevant amounts from the gastrointestinal tract. Therefore they usually must be administered by intermittent subcutaneous or intravenous injection. An alternative technique for administration would be a major advantage in the development of these compounds.

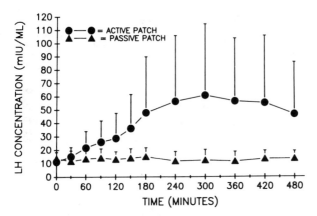

Figure 3 Serum LH response to the administration of leuprolide by electrically powered patches to 13 normal human male volunteers. The active patches with 0.2 mA of current differ significantly from the passive patches without current. Error bars represent standard deviations. (Reproduced with permission from Meyer et al. [2].)

Leuprolide is a nine-amino-acid polypeptide with a molecular weight of 1209. It is a useful model polypeptide for the study of electrically mediated transdermal absorption. Because of its safety with short-term dose administration, it is relatively easy to conduct human studies with it. We conducted a series of experiments documenting the transdermal absorption of leuprolide in normal human volunteers.

Our initial study consisted of a double-blind, randomized, crossover study of the luteinizing hormone (LH) response to the administration of leuprolide by the patch system. The patches for this study contained 5 mg of commercially available leuprolide (TAP Pharmaceuticals, North Chicago, IL) added to the positive reservoir of the patch, 5 mg/mL. The patches delivered an electric current of 0.22 mA. The negative reservoir of the patch was loaded with 3 mL of a sodium phosphate buffering solution. The "control" patches for this study were identical patches loaded with identical solutions but without any electric current. Patches were applied to the volar forearm of study subjects. The skin was not prepared in any way prior to patch application. Eleven normal male volunteers had serum LH concentrations obtained at baseline and serially over a 10-hr study period. Volunteers received either control or active patches on the first study day. They were then asked to return 1 week later, at which time they received the alternate arm of the study. An LH response was seen with the electrically powered patches but was not seen with the "control" patches (Fig. 3). This LH response peaked approximately 2 hr after the application of the patch and persisted for the duration of the study period [1].

Table 1 Mean Serum Leuprolide Concentrations in Normal Human Volunteers (10 mg/mL Leuprolide)

	0.05 M Na acetate (ng/mL ± SD)	0.5 M Na acetate (ng/mL ± SD)
0 min	0.00 ± 0.00	0.07 ± 0.10
30 min	0.77 ± 0.29	0.52 ± 0.30
60 min	0.59 ± 0.25	0.36 ± 0.17
90 min	0.65 ± 0.39	0.36 ± 0.31
120 min	0.94 ± 0.31	0.30 ± 0.11
150 min	0.81 ± 0.38	0.83 ± 0.90
180 min	1.28 ± 0.90	0.41 ± 0.16
240 min	0.73 ± 0.38	0.65 ± 0.60
300 min	0.93 ± 0.95	0.48 ± 0.19
360 min	0.75 ± 0.52	0.69 ± 0.58
420 min	0.77 ± 0.23	0.55 ± 0.51
480 min	0.69 ± 0.36	0.45 ± 0.32
600 min	0.84 ± 0.59	0.54 ± 0.23

SD = Standard deviation.

Subsequent studies in volunteers have compared the LH response seen after the application of leuprolide by patch to that seen after subcutaneous injection. The response after patch administration is slower to develop but is similar in overall magnitude and duration to that obtained after the administration of comparable subcutaneous doses of the drug [2,3].

Measurements of serum leuprolide concentrations using a radioimmunoassay have shown that serum leuprolide concentrations in the range of 0.5–1 ng/mL can be achieved and maintained with this technique over a study period of up to 12 hr (Table 1) [4]. These concentrations are in the range that is usually needed for most therapeutic applications of this drug.

The patches have been well tolerated by the volunteers in all studies thus far. The adverse effects seen during human use are summarized in Table 2. All reactions were transitory. Most resolved between 1/2 and 3 hr after patch removal. In no case was it necessary to prematurely discontinue the study.

The current density in these studies is well below the threshold for pain sensation. Some volunteers reported a tingling sensation beneath the patch. Since this was reported equally in both active and control patches, it does not seem reasonable to attribute this sensation to the electric current. Many of the adverse effects noted have been seen at the negative electrode, where sufficient buffering capacity must be present to control for changes in hydrogen ion concentration associated with the electric current. Further studies will also be needed to op-

Table 2 Adverse Cutaneous Effects Seen with
Transdermal Leuprolide in 54 Studies in
Normal Human Volunteers

1. Marked erythema at site of application
   (1.5%)
2. Transient mild erythema at site of patch
   application (40%) (resolving within 15–120
   min after patch removal)
3. Pruritus at site of patch application (1.5%)
4. Mild localized rash or scaling (4.7%)

timize the adhesive for the system. This was a source of irritation and contributed to the observed reactions.

Analysis by HPLC of leuprolide extracted from patches after sustained periods of application showed no evidence of biochemical alteration by the electrochemical environment of the patch (Fig. 4).

These data demonstrate that in short-term dosing studies a polypeptide such as leuprolide can be safely administered in therapeutic quantities to normal human volunteers.

B. Transdermal Administration of Proteins

All of the potential advantages associated with transdermal administration techniques for peptides are equally applicable to the administration of proteins. Ad-

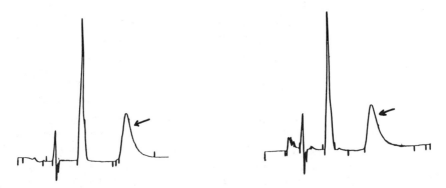

Figure 4 HPLC tracings of drug solution before application to a patch (left panel) and after application to patch, 8 hr of use, and back-extraction from the drug reservoir (right panel). Leuprolide peak is identified with an arrow.

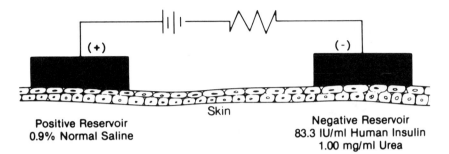

Positive Reservoir
0.9% Normal Saline

Skin

Negative Reservoir
83.3 IU/ml Human Insulin
1.00 mg/ml Urea

Figure 5 Patch design and loading for transdermal insulin administration to albino rabbits with alloxan-induced diabetes. (Reproduced with permission from Meyer et al. [5].)

ministration of proteins will of necessity be more problematic than that of peptides, given their larger size.

We have conducted studies on the transdermal administration of human insulin to albino rabbits [5]. For the purposes of these studies, a diabetic state was induced in the rabbits by the short-term intravenous administration of 125 mg/kg of alloxan. Prior studies had shown that streptozocin was ineffective for this purpose in rabbits. After 48 hr the diabetic state was confirmed by a random blood glucose determination, and animals were then treated with patches containing human insulin and delivering an electric current of 0.4 mA (Fig. 5). As in our human studies, a control arm was provided. Animals in the control arm received patches with identical amounts of drug but without an electric current. Patches were applied to the backs of the animals. In contrast to other studies reported in the literature [6], care was taken not to mechanically disrupt skin integrity at the site of application. Blood glucose concentrations and serum insulin levels were determined over the course of a 12-hr study period.

Blood glucose levels declined steadily during the study period for those with active patches (Fig. 6). Levels were in the normal range by the 10-hr mark and were maintained in that range for the duration of the study. Serum insulin levels rose appropriately and were maintained between 20 and 30 mIU/mL for the duration of patch application. The animals appeared to tolerate the patch well. No evidence for cutaneous injury was seen at the time of patch removal. HPLC data confirmed that the insulin was stable in the patch for the duration of the study period.

These data document the ability of an electric current to alter cutaneous permeability in such a way as to induce the transdermal transport of therapeutically relevant amounts of insulin. Other investigators have also reported upon the use of this technique for the transdermal administration of insulin [6,7]. Chien and coworkers [7] reported on the successful administration of insulin

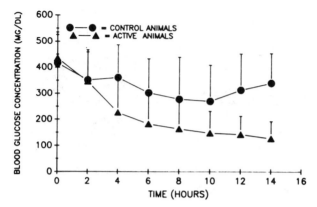

Figure 6 Blood glucose concentrations from rabbits treated with active patches delivering 0.4 mA of current or passive patches with no current. All blood glucose levels greater than 500 mg/dL were calculated as 500 mg/dL. Error bars represent standard deviations.

across hairless mice with streptozocin-induced diabetes mellitus. The animals were treated with 0.4 mA of pulsed direct current at various frequencies. The hypoglycemic effect of the insulin was accentuated by the use of pulsed (as opposed to constant) direct current.

Extensive further work on the transdermal delivery of human insulin will obviously be required before the clinical utility of the technique can be evaluated. There are considerable dangers associated with the administration of this drug, and a delivery technique must be predictable and precise before it can be used in the clinic. A variety of techniques should be used to optimize the formulation of insulin and to produce more consistent insulin response. These studies are ongoing.

C. Transdermal Administration of "Traditional" Drugs

A variety of traditional pharmacologic drugs have bioavailability problems similar to that of peptides and proteins, or have specific therapeutic situations where parenteral administration is indicated. One such compound is hydromorphone. Animal studies with this compound have been performed in a fashion identical to that used with insulin. The patches used a current of 0.2 mA, and hydromorphone was added to the positive reservoir of the patch. Serum hydromorphone levels were determined using an HPLC assay technique with electrochemical detection. Mean hydromorphone concentrations in the animals receiving active patches and control patches are shown in Table 3. The levels

Table 3 Mean Serum Hydromorphone
Concentrations in Albino Rabbits

Time (min)	Concentration (ng/mL ± SD)
0	0
60	24 ± 10
120	28 ± 11
180	34 ± 12
240	32 ± 12
300	25 ± 15
360	24 ± 18
420	25 ± 28

achieved with the active patches are in the range necessary for analgesic effects. The control patches showed no significant concentrations of hydromorphone.

D. Summary

The theoretical basis for electrically mediated transdermal drug delivery is not the subject of this chapter. This chapter provides a demonstration of the practical feasibility of the technique when applied to animals and humans. The data cited support four distinct conclusions.

1. Electrically mediated transdermal drug delivery is able to deliver therapeutically significant doses of a polypeptide drug to normal human beings. The drug is stable in the patch for the duration of these short-term dosing studies.
2. Electrically mediated transdermal drug delivery is able to deliver therapeutically significant doses of a protein such as insulin in an animal model. The drug is stable in the patch for the duration of the short-term dosing study.
3. An electrically mediated transdermal drug delivery system is able to administer traditional drugs not otherwise administered by passive transdermal systems. Once again, the stability of the drug is not affected by the patch system over the course of short-term dosing studies.
4. Electrically mediated transdermal drug administration is well tolerated by animals and by humans in short-term dosing studies.

III. FUTURE DIRECTIONS

There are four fundamental issues that will have to be more fully evaluated before this technique can become a clinical reality. These four issues involve the clarification of the mechanism of action for this technique, its reproducibility, its toxicity, and its efficiency.

A. Mechanism of Action

The data presented in this chapter represent the first steps in the development and optimization of this technique. Considerable effort still needs to be undertaken. The most basic need is for more investigation of the mechanism of transdermal transport in this system. Although the term "iontophoretic delivery" is frequently used to describe this type of system, it is unlikely that the transport observed can be fully explained as being due to routine iontophoretic transport. It is more likely that most of the observed transport occurs by means of electroosmosis or by some other process [9–13]. It is essential that a better understanding of these processes be developed and that we develop an ability to predict the effects of various aspects of the patch "formulation" on drug absorption. An essential aspect of this work will involve the calculation of transdermal flux of the drugs of interest and the relation of this flux to the variables in the "electrochemical environment" of the patch.

B. Reproducibility

A common criticism of this technique has to do with the rather large interindividual variability noted in all published studies. A review of all the data presented in this chapter will show that the standard deviations noted in the transdermal data are fairly large. It should be granted at the outset that the reproducibility of this technique will never be that of intravenous or subcutaneous dosing. It is more appropriate to expect the transdermal route to have the variability in absorption that is seen with oral rather than with traditional parenteral dosing. In this regard, the problem of interindividual variation may be dealt with in the same way it has been dealt with in the case of oral medications: by the use of different dosage strengths. It should be possible to develop different patches with different potencies for delivery. Individualization of dose would then proceed with patches in the same fashion as for oral therapy.

There is very little information available at this time about the occurrence of intraindividual variation. Our own observation in individuals who have participated in multiple studies is that there is substantial reproducibility over time in the bioavailability of the drug. More formal studies will be needed to document this fact, to determine the effect of application on different parts of the body and the effect of environmental changes on cutaneous response to the patch. At the present time it does not appear that the issue of intraindividual variation will be a significant problem in the development of an electric patch.

C. Toxicity

The dosing studies reported here were all short-term studies. Although no acute cutaneous injury was seen, the issue of toxicity associated with repeated dosing has not been addressed. Long-term dosing in the range of 60–90 days together with the analysis of appropriate biopsy material will be necessary before the safety of long-term administration can be ensured. Peptides and proteins are antigenic, and traditional techniques for induction of antibody reactions in animals involve the intradermal injection of these agents. Whether this system will lead to a similar response in our patients needs to be investigated.

D. Efficiency

The ultimate utility of this technique will depend in part on the bioavailability that can be achieved. From a scientific point of view the absolute bioavailability is not critical to the success of this technique. The critical issue from a pharmacologic point of view is the reproducibility of the delivery. A low bioavailability can be compensated for by loading a larger amount of drug onto the patch, by increasing the size of the patch, or by otherwise adjusting the electrochemical environment of the patch. Efficiency of delivery (bioavailability) is an issue when the practical reality of cost is concerned. Since peptides and proteins can be very expensive to produce, an inefficient (although effective) system could become prohibitively expensive for some compounds.

IV. CONCLUSION

This work shows that electrically mediated transdermal delivery is a promising new technique that can afford the opportunity for an effective alternative route of administration for peptides, proteins, and other drugs. Further work is needed to define the mechanisms of action and the ultimate utility of this technique.

REFERENCES

1. B. R. Meyer, *Clin. Pharm. Ther. 44*, 607–612 (1988).
2. B. R. Meyer, W. Kreis, V. O'Mara, J. Eschbach, S. Rosen, and D. Sibalis, *Clin. Pharm. Ther. 45*, 129 (1989).
3. B. R. Meyer, W. Kreis, J. Eschbach, V. O'Mara, S. Rosen, and D. Sibalis, *Clin. Pharm. Ther. 48*, 340 (1990).
4. B. R. Meyer, V. O'Mara, J. Eschbach, P. M. Conn, S. Rosen, and D. Sibalis, *Skin Pharm. 2*, 120 (1989).
5. B. R. Meyer, H. Katzeff, J. Eschbach, S. Rosen, and D. Sibalis, *Am. J. Med. Sci. 297*, 321–325 (1989).
6. B. Kari, *Diabetes 35*, 217–221 (1986).

7. Y. W. Chien, O. Siddiqui, Y. Sun, W. M. Shi, and J. C. Liu, *Ann. N.Y. Acad. Sci.* *507*, 32–51 (1987).

8. J. Eschbach, B. R. Meyer, A. Manzell, S. Rosen, and D. Sibalis, *Clin. Res. 37*, 337A (1989).

9. R. R. Burnette, in *Transdermal Drug Delivery: Developmental Issues and Research Initiatives*, J. Gadgraft and R. H. Guy, Eds., Marcel Dekker, New York, 1989, pp. 247–291.

10. Y. W. Chien, O. Siddiqui, W. M. Shi, P. Lelawongs, and J. C. Liu, *J. Pharm. Sci.* *78*(5), (1989).

11. M. J. Pikal, *Pharm. Res. 7*(200), (1990).

12. M. J. Pikal and S. Shah, *Pharm. Res. 7*, 213 (1990).

13. M. J. Pikal and S. Shah, *Pharm. Res. 7*, 222 (1990).

14

In Vivo and In Vitro Characteristics of Electro-Transdermal Drug Delivery

Mary Martin
Elan Corporation , Monksland, Athlone, County Westmeath Ireland

John Devane
Elan Pharmaceutical Research Corporation, Gainesville, Georgia

I. INTRODUCTION

For centuries dermatological agents have been applied to the skin for the purpose of beautification or to achieve localized effects. Of late, however, there is increasing recognition that the skin can also serve as a port of administration for systemically active drugs. The increasing number of passively delivered transdermal agents reaching the market is proof of the efficiency, safety, convenience, and popularity of this route of administration [1–3].

Limited by the fact that few drugs readily permeate the lipids of the stratum corneum and thereafter enter the systemic circulation, attention is now being focused on ways of enhancing transdermal drug transfer by either chemical or energy-assisted means including the use of electric current. The study of the migration of ions through the skin following application of an electric current should not, however, be considered just a science of the past decade. Although great interest has recently been channeled into the development of effective iontophoretic drug systems, the transdermal delivery of chemical agents was first demonstrated in the early 1900s [4,5]. By 1936, Ichihashi [6] had established a therapeutic use for iontophoresis and showed that hyperhidrosis could be induced by ionic transfer of certain solutions. Gibson and Cooke [7] found in 1959 that iontophoretic delivery of pilocarpine could induce sweating, and this is now an FDA-approved method used by pediatricians in the diagnosis of cystic fibrosis.

Table 1   A Model R&D Program

Stage 1: Preformulation
Stage 2: In vitro flux studies
Stage 3: In vivo animal studies
Stage 4: In vivo human studies

Although a number of alternative theoretical models have been developed to examine the transfer of drugs across the skin under the influence of an electric field, the primary goal of electro-transdermal drug absorption is to achieve the efficient and effective systemic delivery of an agent in a well-tolerated and ultimately economical manner. To do so necessitates following a systematic research and development program encompassing all relevant considerations and appropriate disciplines and ultimately concluding in the demonstration of clinical effectiveness in humans. We have coined the acronym ETDAS to describe an integrated electro-transport drug administration system designed to achieve drug transfer across the skin under the influence of an electric current. The in vitro and in vivo characteristics at issue in a practical ETDAS development program are outlined in the following sections.

II. A MODEL DEVELOPMENT PROGRAM

Although each specific drug substance and therapeutic indication will have its own requirements, a general development program for this system is outlined in Table 1. Commencing with extensive preformulation investigation and progressing through in vitro study, the program is focused toward early in vivo testing, i.e., human and/or animal study.

A. Preformulation Considerations

The increasing number of drugs successfully delivered electrically across the skin has led to a better understanding of the factors that determine the rate and extent of electrically controlled delivery. As the complexities of electro-transdermal delivery become more clearly defined, the primary factors that must be considered in the development of an electro-transdermal delivery system become more apparent. All these factors should be considered at the preformulation stage of a development program (Table 2).

1. Drug-Related Considerations

Although the size of the drug molecules to be delivered may be a rate-limiting feature in electro-transdermal delivery, the upper limit with regard to molecular weight for effective transfer across the skin has not been established. With the

Table 2 Preformulation Considerations

Drug
- Solubility/concentration considerations
- Stability
- Partition coefficient
- Molecular weight/size
- Ionization/pK_a or pI
- Ionic charge
- Mobility

Device
- Current/current density
- Voltage requirements
- Electrodes—materials, size, configuration, incompatibilities
- ETDAS formulation vehicle, formulation/stability
- Extraneous ions

Biological
- Skin resistance/impedance
- Skin tolerability
- Skin metabolism/degradation
- Binding in skin

successful delivery of macromolecules up to a molecular weight of 6000 clearly established [8,9], the potential for delivery of higher molecular weight drugs, including larger peptides and proteins, remains to be characterized.

Electric conductivity is an important factor in the successful transport of drugs by electro-transdermal means. Gangarosa et al. [10] measured the conductivity of a range of drugs suitable for iontophoretic delivery and highlighted the fact that buffers and salt ions hinder iontophoretic transfer owing to competition between the extraneous ions and the drug ions for current. Work we have been associated with has shown that the choice of drug salt can influence the rate of drug transport (Fig. 1). In this case the highest transport rate was associated with the salt that had the highest conductivity. Interestingly, the solubility of the salt was not connected with the transport rate [11].

2. Device-Related Considerations

Siddiqui and coworkers examined the relationship between the degree of ionization of a drug and its electrically enhanced transport. Initially using lignocaine as a model [12] and subsequently a range of drugs including salicylic acid, acetylsalicylic acid, methotrexate, ephedrine hydrochloride, chlorpromazine hy-

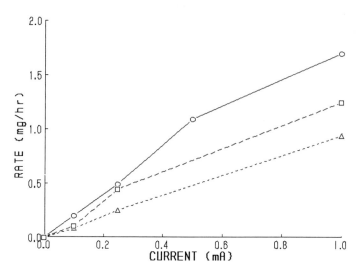

Figure 1   The relationship between the rate of morphine transport for the hydrochloride (solid), acetate (long dashes), and sulfate salt (short dashes) and current.

drochloride, and chlorpheniramine maleate [13], their studies showed that the rate of transfer of drugs through the stratum corneum is greatest when the drug exists in a highly ionized form. By formulating the drug-containing vehicle at a pH appropriate to the pK_a (or pI) of the drug, the molecule may be induced to carry charge and thus be delivered across the skin. Maintenance of a stable pH can therefore influence the ionization of the drug. Alterations in pH may also be relevant with regard to skin tolerability [13].

The data presented in Figure 2 show the pH of vehicles containing the sympathomimetic agent salbutamol sulfate measured before and after a 2-hr in vitro period of electro-transdermal drug transfer. A large drop in pH was apparent in vehicles where the electrodes were composed of an inert material. This pH drop was absent in systems in which the electrodes were composed of silver or silver chloride. It is interesting, however, to note that the observed change in pH in Figure 2 may promote the electrically induced transfer of a positively charged molecule.

3.   Biological System–Related Considerations

As the results in Figure 1 demonstrate, the delivery of a drug is usually directly related to the applied current, and these observations are supported by those of Bannon et al. [14] and Del Terzo et al. [15]. The selected current must be high enough to provide the desired delivery rate but should not produce any harmful

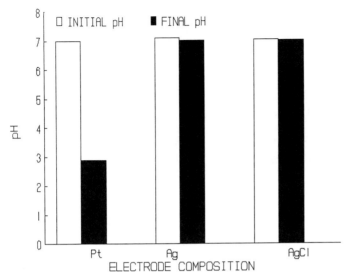

Figure 2 Measurements of pH before and after a 2-hr electro-transdermal experiment using salbutamol sulfate. The pH of the gel containing the active agent was measured using a surface electrode.

effects on the skin. However, transfer of a drug through the skin may be limited by skin polarization, which occurs with time during application of a continuous direct current [16]. It has been suggested that this may be prevented or minimized by using a pulsed current that allows the skin to repolarize during the "off" period. The waveform, current density, on/off ratio, and frequency of periodic current may be altered to provide the optimal delivery parameters for each individual agent [17].

Monitoring of skin impedance, and in particular skin resistance, is an essential feature of electro-transdermal research. Because of its lower water content of 20% compared with the normal physiological level of 70%, the stratum corneum is a layer of high electrical resistance. In addition, the skin has a capacitance element. Over the last few years, attention has been focused on the relationship between impedance and hydration, temperature, pH, solvents, and iontophoresis [18–20].

Impedance studies we have collaborated in reveal that a marked decrease in skin impedance occurs during electro-transdermal drug delivery (Fig. 3) [21]. Separation of impedance into its resistance and capacitance components shows an initial drop in resistance but not capacitance with application of an electric current. Upon removal of the current the resistance is seen to return toward its

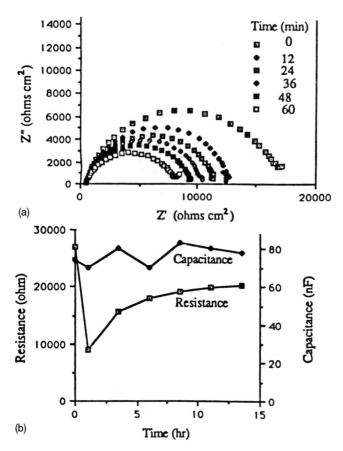

Figure 3 The decrease in impedance with time during delivery of a constant dc potential (2 V). (a) The data are presented as a Nyquist plot, (b) and show the recovery in skin resistance after the cessation of current delivery.

original level with time (Fig. 3). Further application of this technique will enable a better understanding of the events that occur during electrical transport of drugs across the skin.

Biological factors such as binding, metabolism, and degradation in the skin warrant attention in the preformulation stage of a development program. Siddiqui and coworkers [22] propose that insulin, delivered electrically across the skin, may form an initial reservoir in the skin, an observation supported by Kari [23]. Metabolism of a salicylate diester has been shown both in vitro and in vivo following electro-transdermal delivery by Gusek et al. [24].

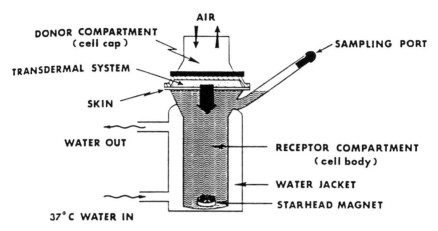

AIR

DONOR COMPARTMENT
(cell cap)

SAMPLING PORT

TRANSDERMAL SYSTEM

SKIN

WATER OUT

RECEPTOR COMPARTMENT
(cell body)

WATER JACKET

STARHEAD MAGNET

37°C WATER IN

Figure 4 Diagrammatic illustration of a Franz cell. (From Crown Glass Co., Inc., Somerville, NJ.)

B. In Vitro Studies

1. Experimental Setup

With all the relevant considerations having been evaluated in a preformulation phase, the parameters for a particular drug must be established in vitro. The influence of drug loading, surface area, current density, electrode configuration, vehicle formulation, drug flux, current waveform, and rate of transport must be established using a relevant in vitro model. The apparatus most commonly used by researchers in the transdermal field to measure in vitro flux is the Franz diffusion cell [25]. The Franz diffusion cell (Fig. 4) allows the use of liquid or solid dosage forms placed directly in contact with the membrane, thereby mimicking the in vivo situation. The skin is in contact with buffer in the receptor compartment, and samples can be taken periodically to assess drug transfer.

The arrangement of the electrodes with regard to the membrane varies between research groups. In their 1989 review article, Singh and Roberts [26] describe the two most popular arrangements, one in which the active and counter electrodes are placed on either side of the membrane and one in which both electrodes are placed on the same side of the membrane. The latter arrangement facilitates the use of a simple experimental design and most closely represents the ultimate in vivo situation.

The choice of membranes used in in vitro studies is determined by the requirements of the particular phase of study. Preliminary in vitro transdermal studies are routinely performed using well-defined synthetic membranes. Because the physiochemical properties of such membranes are established, variability associated with the use of skin may be eliminated for initial development work [27]. Although human cadaver skin is widely used and considered by many next in line to in vivo human skin, the model does possess difficulties in controlling the integrity and conditions of skin samples. For this reason, a number of animal skin models are studied, including hairless and nude mice, hairless and nude rats, guinea pigs, and mini-pigs [28].

The mouse SKH/MF1 strain is widely used in transdermal research [29]. The results presented in Figure 5 were generated using abdominal skin taken from female SKH/MF1 mice that were killed at 45–47 days of age. This study is an example of how to establish a total mass balance for drugs during electro-transdermal drug delivery. Skin strips were collected. The removal of the layers of stratum corneum was carried out by the method described by Tregear [30] and Yamamoto and Yamamoto [18], and skin biopsy was performed on the remaining skin at the active site and on the skin under the counter electrode. Analysis of the transferred drug, the drug in the stratum corneum and underlying skin, and any untransferred drug and drug in the counter gel showed 99.4% accountability.

2. *Establishment of Key Parameters*

Using salbutamol sulfate as a model, characterization of the relationship between current and the rate of transfer of the drug across the skin was established (Fig. 6). The rate of transfer of the drug was shown to be related to the current and the loading of drug in the vehicle. The duration of the period of current application (Fig. 7) is also a factor to be considered. Establishment of these parameters is essential at an early point in the development program to appropriately design the in vitro studies for extrapolation of findings to in vivo situations. Performance of ''on/off'' experiments at this stage in a development program allows examination of any possible permanent changes in skin permeation under conditions where the current has been stopped but the drug-containing vehicle may be left in contact with the skin. Establishment of such a characteristic is important in situations where intermittent drug therapy is required, possibly for short periods of time throughout the course of a day.

In a separate series of experiments and using visking membrane as a model, almost the entire drug loading of a nine-amino-acid peptide was successfully transferred during application of a current of 0.4 mA/cm^2 (Fig. 8a). With the same ETDAS system and using human stratum corneum as a model, over 50% of the drug was delivered in an 8-hr period (Fig. 8b).

C. In Vivo Animal Studies

As is the case for other routes of drug delivery, the use of in vivo animal models may be optional as part of a development program. Inclusion of in vivo animal studies is dependent on the drug involved and the extent to which its safety has

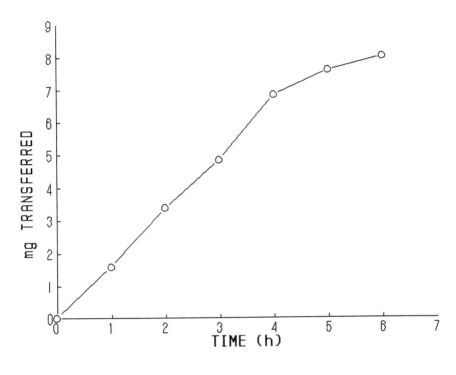

LOCATION	mg salbutamol present mean ± sd
Skin strip 1	0.023 ± 0.014
Skin strip 2	0.013 ± 0.0057
Skin strip 3	0
Skin strip 4	0
Skin strip 5	0
Active skin site	0.033 ± 0.014
Counter skin site	0.04 ± 0.027
Active gel	0.79 ± 0.0848
Counter gel	0.027 ± 0.0141

Figure 5   Transfer of salbutamol sulfate across hairless mouse skin over a 6-hr period. The values represent the mean ± SD of three individual experiments on separate skins. The quantity of drug present in the first five skin layers (skin strips 1–5), the skin under the active and counter electrodes, and the drug remaining in the active gel and detected in the counter gel are shown.

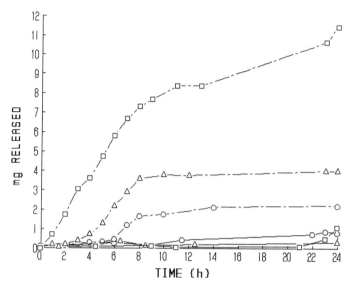

Figure 6 Transdermal delivery of 2 mg (○), 4 mg (△), and 11 mg (□) of salbutamol under passive (continuous line) and active (discontinuous line) conditions. Delivery was performed over a 24-hr period. Under active conditions a constant direct current was applied.

been previously established. However, the use of in vivo animal models does have a role in the study of many of the drugs currently under review for delivery by the electro-transdermal route.

The choice of animal depends on the drug in question, the required response, blood sample volume requirements, and the design of the electro-transdermal device itself. Hairless and normal rats have been successfully employed in in vivo electro-transdermal studies. Siddiqui and coworkers [22] demonstrated a reduction in blood glucose following electro-transdermal delivery of insulin in rats made diabetic by streptozocin injection. However, because of the size of the animals it was not possible to withdraw sufficient quantities of blood to measure plasma insulin concentrations at less than 10-min intervals. Despite these limitations, because of the large amount of in vitro work performed using hairless and nude mice, these animals are a popular choice for in vivo work where an in vitro/in vivo comparison can be made.

The passive transdermal delivery of nicotine has been widely studied [2,3], and a passive transdermal patch has been developed and commercialized. Nicotine was therefore an obvious choice of drug to use in studying the enhancement of transdermal delivery under electrical conditions. We have been involved in studies using hairless mice as a model in which the transdermal delivery of nicotine was

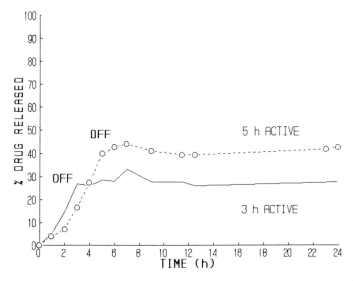

Figure 7 The delivery of salbutamol from a gel containing 8 mg of drug. A current of 0.4 mA was applied for a 3- or 5-hr period and subsequently removed. The gel was left in contact with the skin, and sampling continued to 24 hr.

evaluated over a 2-hr period under passive and active (0.1 and 0.2 mA) conditions (Fig. 9). Both the rate and extent of transdermal delivery were greatly enhanced under active conditions and were shown to be controlled by current.

D. In Vivo Human Studies

In terms of the technical development of an electro-transdermal drug absorption system, the final stage in a development program is the testing of its efficiency and effectiveness in humans. The 1986 study performed by Okabe et al. [31] and the 1988 study associated with Bannon et al. [32] demonstrated the in vivo electro-transdermal delivery of metoprolol and salbutamol, respectively. In the latter study, salbutamol sulfate was delivered from a 4-mg patch using currents of 0.1 and 0.2 mA. Plasma drug levels were seen to vary with applied current (Fig. 10) and reached therapeutically relevant concentrations. The in vivo delivery of leuprolide has also been demonstrated in human volunteers [33].

III. IN VIVO TOLERABILITY

Tolerability to both the drug and the electro-transdermal device must be clearly established. Knowledge of tolerability issues learned from the passive transdermal products currently available on the market will be of considerable aid in

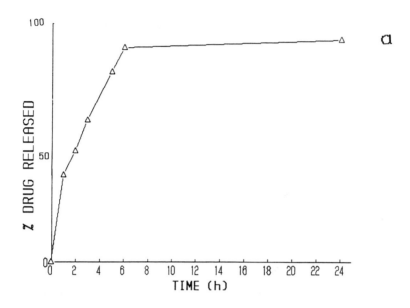

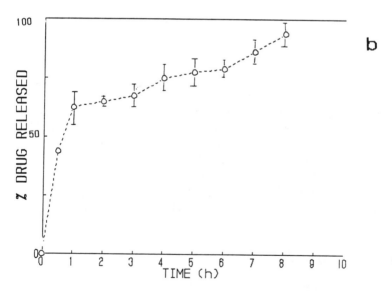

Figure 8   Delivery of desmopressin across (a) visking membrane and (b) human stratum corneum.

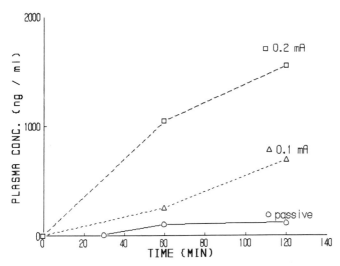

Figure 9 In vivo delivery of nicotine in hairless mice under passive and active (0.1 and 0.2 mA) conditions. The transdermal device, containing 2 mg of nicotine, was applied to the surface of the skin, and the experiment was performed over a 2-hr period. Samples were withdrawn by tail venipuncture, and plasma was assayed for nicotine content using an HPLC technique. Each data point represents the mean of three observations.

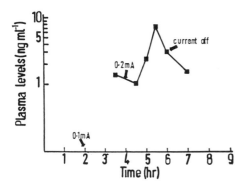

Figure 10 Semilog plot of salbutamol plasma levels versus time for electro-transdermal delivery from a gel containing 4 mg of salbutamol sulfate using currents of 0.1 and 0.2 mA in a human volunteer.

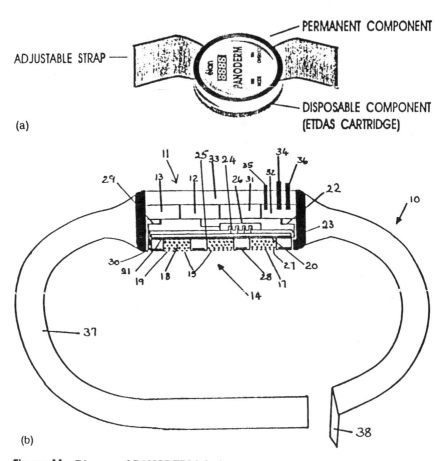

Figure 11   Diagram of PANODERM device.

Table 3   PANODERM Key Features

- Finely controlled pulsatile and/or continuous current
- Clock/timer, with automatic up/down counting facility for programming dosing periods in advance
- Visual display of time, dosage interval, dosing time remaining, current and voltage
- An alarm system to signal failure
- An override system for incremental therapy
- A replacement electrode system, which when interlocked with the PANODERM device sets the correct delivery for the specific drug

anticipating future drug-related tolerability issues. Gordon and coworkers [34] pointed out a high rate (10%) of contact dermatitis in response to transdermal hyoscine in naval crew members using this product to prevent motion sickness. On a more positive note, however, delayed hypersensitivity to transdermal glyceryltrinitrate is rare [35].

Electro-transdermal devices raise the additional issue of tolerability to the device itself, the electric current used, and, in particular, the electrochemical reaction. The issues, investigated at the preformulation stage, regarding the choice and configuration of electrodes become relevant in determining potential in vivo safety issues. In an in vivo skin tolerability study performed to assess the suitability of a variety of electrode configurations, erythema was visible on the skin surface for two of the configurations studied at current densities of 0.04 mA/cm^2. In addition, 24 hr after removal of the electrode, erythema was still clearly visible. However, the ETDAS system used with a current density of 0.15 mA/cm^2 was well tolerated, with no local skin effects evident.

IV. PANODERM DESIGN FEATURES

Developing an optimized drug absorption device means selecting a system that will provide the required delivery of therapeutic quantities of the drug using materials and currents that are well tolerated and meet specific requirements. It also involves design of a device that is economical to produce and convenient to use as a system for a long-term drug dosing regimen. Although some systems have been successfully applied in iontophoretic transdermal delivery [22], their large size does not facilitate convenient long-term use. With the continuing developments in microelectronics and microcircuitry, a novel miniaturized electro-transdermal drug absorption device, PANODERM, has been developed.

The PANODERM device (Figure 11) consists of three main components: a power source, control circuitry, and the electro-transdermal drug absorption system (ETDAS) incorporated into a cartridge containing drug reservoirs and electrodes. The essential features, outlined in Table 3, allow the accurate and safe delivery of a drug from the device, which can be programmed to meet the delivery requirements of each therapeutic agent. The cartridge composition and configuration as well as the selected currents have been designed to reduce skin resistance, making the device efficient with regard to power and convenient and safe with regard to use. Miniaturized to a wrist watch size, the PANODERM device is not only efficient and safe to use but also comfortable and convenient to wear.

V. PRESENT APPLICATIONS AND FUTURE CHALLENGES

As the extent of knowledge regarding electro-transdermal drug absorption has widened over the past decade, so too has an awareness of the potential of the transdermal route for systemic delivery. The basis of any development in this area is a well-designed feasibility and development program that considers electrical, microelectronic, pharmaceutical, and biological aspects in an integrated manner. The format and methods presented in this chapter provide the basis for a rational development program.

Acknowledgements We would like to acknowledge the contributions of members of the Departments of Chemistry and Pharmaceutical Sciences, Trinity College, Dublin, Ireland, in particular Professor John Corish, Dr. Owen I. Corrigan, and Dr. Desmond Foley (present address: Elan Corporation, Monksland, Athlone, Ireland).

REFERENCES

1. J. W. Fara, *Pharm. Technol. 7*, 33 (1984).
2. Y. B. Bannon, J. Corish, O. I. Corrigan, J. G. Devane, M. Kavanagh, and S. Mulligan, *Eur. J. Clin. Pharmacol. 37*, 285 (1989).
3. S. C. Mulligan, J. G. Masterson, J. G. Devane, and J. G. Kelly, *Clin. Pharmacol. Ther. 47*(3), 331 (1990).
4. S. Leduc, *Ann. Electrobiol. 3*, 545 (1900).
5. S. Leduc, *Electric Ions and Their Uses in Medicine*, Rebmorm, London, 1908.
6. T. Ichihashi, *J. Orient. Med. 25*, 101 (1936).
7. L. E Gibson and R. E. Cooke, *Pediatrics 23*, 545 (1959).
8. R. Burnette and D. Marrero, *J. Pharm. Sci. 75*, 738 (1986).
9. J.-C. Liu, Y. Sun, O. Siddiqui, Y. W. Chien, W. M. Shi, and J. Liu, *Int. J. Pharm. 44*, 197 (1987).
10. L. P. Gangarosa, N. H. Park, B. C. Fong, D. F. Scott, and J. M. Hill, *J. Pharm. Sci. 67*, 1439 (1978).
11. J. Corish, O. I. Corrigan, and D. Foley, in *Prediction of Percutaneous Penetration, Methods, Measurements and Modelling*, R. C. Scott, R. H. Guy, and J. Hadgraft, Eds., IBC Technical Services, p. 302.
12. O. Siddiqui, M. S. Roberts, and A. E. Polack, *J. Pharm. Pharmacol. 37*, 732 (1985).
13. O. Siddiqui, M. S. Roberts, and A. E. Polack, *J. Pharm. Pharmacol. 41*, 430 (1989).
14. Y. B. Bannon, J. Corish, and O. I. Corrigan, *Proc. 7th Pharm. Technol. Conf., 11*, 400 (1988).
15. S. Del Terzo, C. R. Behl, and R. A. Nash, *Pharm. Res. 6*, 85 (1989).
16. J. C. Lawler, M. J. Davies, and E. Griffith, *J. Invest. Dermatol. 34*, 301 (1960).
17. Y. W. Chien, O. Siddiqui, W.-M. Shi, P. Lelawongs, and J.-C. Liu, *J. Pharm. Sci. 78*(5), 376 (1989).
18. T. Yamamoto and Y. Yamamoto, *Med. Biol. Eng. 14*, 151 (1976).
19. A. C. Allenby, J. Fletcher, C. Schock, and T. F. S. Tees, *Br. J. Dermatol. 81*, 31–39 (1969).
20. R. R. Burnette and B. Ongpipattanakul, *J. Pharm. Sci. 77*, 132–137 (1988).
21. D. Foley, J. Corish, and O. I. Corrigan, *Proc. Int. Symp. Controlled Release Bioact. Mater. 17*, 427 (1990).
22. O. Siddiqui, Y. Sun, J.-C. Liu, and Y. W. Chien, *J. Pharm. Sci. 76*(4), 341 (1987).

23. B. Kari, *Diabetes 33*, 181A (1984).

24. D. B. Guzek, A. H. Kennedy, S. C. McNeill, E. Wakshull, and R. O. Potts, *Pharm. Res. 6*(1), (1989).

25. J. J. Franz, *J. Invest. Dermatol. 64*, 190 (1978).

26. J. Singh and M. S. Roberts, *Drug Des. Delivery 4*, 1 (1989).

27. Y.-H. Tu and L. Y. Allen, *J. Pharm. Sci. 78*(3), 211 (1989).

28. C. R. Behl, S. Kumore, A. W. Malick, S. Del Terzo, W. I. Higuchi, and R. A. Nash, *J. Pharm. Sci. 78*(5), 355 (1989).

29. V. Srinivasan, W. I. Higuchi, and M.-H. Su, *J. Controlled Release 10*, 157 (1989).

30. R. T. Tregear, *Physiological Functions of the Skin*, Academic, New York, 1966.

31. Y. Okabe, H. Yamaguchi, and Y. Kawai, *J. Controlled Release 4*, 79 (1986).

32. Y. B. Bannon, J. Corish, O. I. Corrigan, and J. G. Masterson, *Drug Dev. Ind. Pharm. 14*(15–17), 2151 (1988).

33. R. Meyer, W. Kreis, V. O'Mara, J. Eschbach, S. Rosen, and D. Sibalis, *Clin. Pharmacol. Ther.*, PDF-2 (1989).

34. C. R. Gordon, A. Shupak, I. Doweck, and O. Spitzer, *BMJ, 298*, 1220 (1989).

35. R. Weickel and P. J. Frasch, *Hautarzt 37*, 511 (1986).

15

Transdermal Drug Delivery by Phonophoresis: Basics, Mechanisms, and Techniques of Application

Ying Sun and Jue-Chen Liu
Topical Formulation and Drug Delivery Research Center,
Johnson and Johnson, Skillman, New Jersey

I. INTRODUCTION

A. Definition

Phonophoresis is defined as the movement of drugs through intact skin and underlying soft tissues under the influence of an ultrasonic perturbation [1].

B. Advantages and Potentials

Phonophoresis has been established as a safe and effective therapeutic technique since its first successful application in treating polyarthritis of the digital joints with hydrocortisone in 1954 [2]. Since then, numerous studies have been conducted with various drugs [3–10]. Because of its transdermal characteristics and noninvasive nature, phonophoresis shares most of the advantages of conventional (passive diffusion type) transdermal delivery systems and other noninvasive techniques (e.g., iontophoresis) and in addition has some of its own distinct advantages.

The advantages of phonophoresis can be summarized as follows:

1. Bypasses the gastrointestinal degradation and hepatic first-pass metabolism.
2. Improves patient compliance because it is noninvasive.
3. May eliminate the need to use chemical skin enhancers.

4. Can provide temporal drug delivery, i.e., pulsatile delivery.
5. Can be used to deliver drugs in either ionic or nonionic form.
6. Works well with either aqueous or oily vehicles.
7. Can deliver drug into deep subcutaneous tissues.
8. Can be used synergetically with other transdermal drug delivery systems (e.g., with transdermal patches of the passive diffusion type) to enhance the delivery rate, to reduce the lag time, and to provide a pulsatile delivery mode in addition to a basal delivery from passive diffusion.

The first two advantages in this list are shared by all the transdermal drug delivery techniques. The third and fourth are also exhibited by another skin permeation enhancement technique: iontophoresis. The last four advantages, however, are possessed only by phonophoresis. It is this unique broad applicability that offers phonophoresis a bright future as an enhancement technique in transdermal drug delivery. Many formulation difficulties that are often encountered in conventional transdermal drug delivery and iontophoresis may not present a problem in phonophoresis. Because ultrasound has extraordinary penetration capability, especially through solid materials, it is quite feasible that phonophoresis may be used as an ''add-on'' technique in conjunction with other transdermal delivery systems to give them an additional technological ''edge,'' such as reduced onset time, or pulsatile delivery (superimposed on the basal drug delivery by passive diffusion) for drugs requiring temporal administration.

Clinical evidence has clearly confirmed that phonophoresis is a safe technique for enhancing drug administration and is effective in clinical applications when used with a proper frequency and power level for an appropriate duration. The exact mechanism of phonophoresis is, however, still not well understood. This chapter provides the reader with some basic information about ultrasound, its effect on biological systems, and possible mechanisms for enhanced drug penetration by phonophoresis. Literature surveys of studies using phonophoresis with various drugs are summarized in excellent review papers by Skauen and Zentner [1] and Tyle and Agrawala [3] and therefore will not be duplicated here except for some pertinent examples of work published since these reviews.

II. BASICS OF ULTRASOUND: GENERATION AND PROPAGATION

A. Piezoelectric Effect and Ultrasonic Transducer

Ultrasound is a form of acoustic vibration propagated in the form of longitudinal compression waves at frequencies beyond the human auditory range (i.e., frequencies above 20 kHz). This form of energy is used extensively in medical diagnosis as well as in therapeutic applications such as physiotherapy and sports

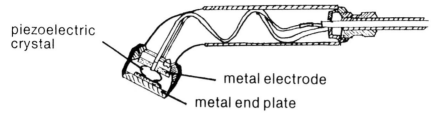

piezoelectric
crystal

metal electrode
metal end plate

Figure 1   A schematic diagram showing the structure of an ultrasonic transducer used
for phonophoresis (From Wadsworth and Chanmugan [12].)

medicine. An ultrasonic therapeutic system consists of a generator that produces
a high-frequency alternating voltage. The high-frequency electric voltage is then
converted by a transducer into mechanical (i.e., acoustic) vibrations. The transducer is made of a piezoelectric crystal inserted between two electrodes.

The conversion of the high-frequency alternating voltage into mechanical
vibration is accomplished by reversal of the piezoelectric effect [11]. The piezoelectric effect is a phenomenon whereby positive and negative charges appear
on opposite crystal faces when pressure is applied to a crystal of asymmetric
structure, such as the barium titanate and lead zirconate crystals used in clinical
ultrasonic generators. If this process is reversed—when an electric potential is
applied to the crystal—its dimension changes. If the imposed electric potential
alternates at a frequency higher than 20 kHz, the crystal expands and contracts
with the same frequency to produce ultrasound. A schematic diagram of an
ultrasound transducer is shown in Figure 1.

Like audible sound, ultrasound is propagated through small fluctuations in
the pressure of the medium surrounding the vibrating object. The speed at which
fluctuations of pressure spread out from their source is a constant for the medium
in which they are traveling, with only small variations due to the differences in
temperature and pressure. The speed of the pressure waves equals wavelength
(i.e., the distance between successive pressure crests) times frequency. Whereas
gases are very poor conductors of sound, acoustic energy is transmitted well
through degassed liquid and travels best through high-density solids.

B.   Ultrasonic Frequency

The frequency of ultrasound is the number of complete waves of the longitudinal
wave motion passing through a reference point per second. For instance, 1 million compressional waves pass a reference point in a medium when 1-MHz
ultrasound is applied to it. The shorter the wavelength, the higher the frequency.
Most medical applications use ultrasonic frequencies between 0.75 and 15 MHz;
for example, physiotherapy, 1–3 MHz; diagnostic, 1–10 MHz; general ultra-

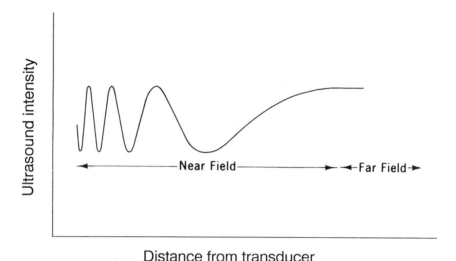

Distance from transducer

Figure 2   Ultrasound intensity distribution along the central axis of the ultrasonic beam.

sonic, 4–8 MHz [12]. Because every crystal has a resonance frequency at which resonance occurs when the electric frequency matches the natural vibrational frequency of the crystal, leading to a maximal efficiency in electrical–mechanical energy conversion, different transducers are often used for different ultrasonic frequencies if maximum conversion efficiency is desired.

C.   Ultrasonic Energy: Intensity

The acoustic energy transferred from a transducer into tissues is carried by compressional waves in the form of pressure fluctuations. The amplitude of the pressure fluctuations increases as the acoustic energy level increases. The total acoustic energy emitted in an ultrasonic beam is measured in watts (W). Intensity is a quantity used to establish exposure level to the ultrasound beam. It is measured in watts per square centimeter of effective radiating surface. Sound applicators produce an ultrasonic field in the vicinity of the applicator, which shows a characteristic interference pattern [13]. This interference results in nonuniform distribution of intensity along its direction of propagation in the form of maxima and minima as shown in Figure 2. The distinct pattern of maxima and minima spreads over a certain distance called the near field. Beyond this nonhomogeneous field, the distant field extends as a homogeneous sound field, the far field. Because of this pattern of interference, the nonuniform intensity distribution along the direction of ultrasound propagation is inevitable, especially within the near field. To further complicate this issue, the distribution of acoustic energy on a cross-sectional area of ultrasound beam is not homogeneous either. Great caution must therefore be exercised in the design of a phonophoresis device to ensure that the desired amount of acoustic energy is delivered to the stratum corneum, the skin barrier that is to be perturbed. The ultrasonic beam also diverges as it travels away from the surface of an ultrasonic therapy applicator. The beam divergence is related to the frequency of the ultrasound and the size of the applicator. The lower the ultrasound frequency and the smaller the applicator, the greater the beam divergence.

D. Acoustic Impedance

As an ultrasound beam passes through a medium or a tissue, its intensity is reduced because of absorption of ultrasonic energy. The loss of acoustic energy is due to reflection and attenuation. The acoustic energy absorbed is converted to thermal energy, causing an increase in temperature.

The acoustic impedance (Z) of a material is its characteristic resistance to the propagation of ultrasound. Acoustic impedance of a material is directly proportional to the propagation velocity of ultrasound (c) in the material and the density of the material (p), i.e., $Z = p \times c$. The acoustic impedances of some materials are listed in Table 1 [12].

E. Reflection

When an ultrasound beam passes across the interface of two media that differ in acoustic impedance, reflection occurs, which results in a loss of acoustic energy. The amount of ultrasound reflected from the interface can be calculated with the equations [14]

$$I_r/I_i = [(Z_2 - Z_1)/(Z_2 + Z_1)]^2 \tag{1}$$

and

$$I_t/I_i = 4Z_2Z_1/(Z_2 + Z_1)^2 \tag{2}$$

where I_r, I_i, and I_t are the reflected intensity, incident intensity, and transmitted intensity, respectively, and Z_1 and Z_2 are the acoustic impedances of media 1 and 2. Equations (1) and (2) apply only at normal incidence, i.e., when the incident ultrasound beam is perpendicular to the interface. It can be seen from equation (1) that the larger the difference in acoustic impedance between two materials making up the interface, the more significant is the reflection. For instance, because of a large difference in the acoustic impedance between bone and periosteum tissue, a significant amount of acoustic energy is reflected at the interface and absorbed by the periosteum tissue. The absorbed energy thus warms the tissue (up to 40–43°C) for the desired therapeutic effect [11].

Table 1 Impedance Values of Various Media

Medium	Impedance, Z ($\times 10^5$ g cm^{-2} sec^{-1})
Bone	6.0
Liver	1.68
Fat	1.43
Brain	1.56
Blood	1.65
Air	0.0004
Normal saline	1.55
Water	1.54
Muscle	1.64
Forearm	1.55
Calf	1.55
Face	1.65
Upper arm	1.65

Source: Wadsworth and Chanmugan [12].

F. Attenuation

The absorption or attenuation of acoustic energy occurs at the molecular level. The compressional waves of ultrasound force molecules to oscillate to and fro at extremely high frequency (e.g., 1 million times per second with 1 MHz ultrasound). A certain amount of energy has to be spent to cause these movements, leading to a progressive loss of ultrasonic intensity. In the therapeutic frequency range, the attenuation rate increases directly with frequency. When the frequency is doubled, the rate of attenuation is doubled. Consequently, an ultrasound of higher frequency penetrates tissues to a smaller depth than low-frequency ultrasound.

G. Cavitation

Acoustic cavitation is the formation and activity of gas- or vapor-filled cavities (bubbles) in a medium exposed to an ultrasound field. There are two types of cavitation: stable cavitation and collapse cavitation. Stable cavities vibrate in accordance with the ultrasound field and generate high shear force. Collapse cavities oscillate in an unstable manner about their equilibrium radius, grow to several times the equilibrium size, and collapse violently. The large amount of energy released during the collapse phase may be associated with the high temperature and chemical reactivity [15].

Cavitation tends to be unpredictable in its occurrence because it requires far more energy to cause a bubble or cavity to be formed than it takes to drive a preexisting bubble or cavity into oscillation [16]. The occurrence of cavitation also depends on the ultrasound frequency and the viscosity of the medium: the higher the frequency and medium viscosity, the less likely the occurrence of cavitation. Cavitation is believed to be one of the causes of the biological effects of ultrasound. Because the occurrence of cavitation can be prevented by application of a sufficiently high pressure to the system under investigation, the absence or presence of cavitation can be tested experimentally by examining whether the biological effect of ultrasound exists under increased pressure. Experimental evidence suggests that cavitation is more likely to occur when pulsed ultrasound is used, provided that the ultrasound intensity during the pulses exceeds the threshold of cavitation occurrence and the duration of the pulses is long enough for the cavitation to develop [13].

III. POSSIBLE MECHANISMS OF PHONOPHORESIS

Despite the fact that phonophoresis has been successfully used by clinicians for over three decades, its mechanism of action is still a subject of speculation. Although it is not difficult to postulate various mechanisms that may be responsible for the enhanced topical drug absorption, it is often difficult to confirm a hypothesis experimentally or to isolate one parameter from another, because they are not always mutually exclusive (e.g., collapse cavitation always involves the release of heat—the thermal effect). The possible mechanisms for phonophoretic drug delivery are discussed below.

A. Mechanical Effect

1. Acoustic Radiation Pressure

Some researchers believe that radiation pressure may be responsible for the successful administration of drugs percutaneously via ultrasound [1,17]. Radiation pressure is the static pressure exerted by an ultrasonic wave on any interface or medium across which there is a decrease in ultrasonic intensity in the direction of wave propagation. For complete absorption of a finite ultrasonic beam of a plane wave,

$$F = W/c \qquad (3)$$

where F is the force due to radiation pressure, c is the velocity of ultrasound, and W is the ultrasonic power [14]. The force F acts in the direction of wave propagation. The force acting on a perfect reflector at normal incidence is equal to twice the force that would act on a perfect absorber.

2. Oscillating Motion

The oscillating motion of particles of a medium about a fixed point in an ultrasonic field is sometimes referred as the "first-order effect" of ultrasonic energy, as compared to the "second-order effect" of ultrasound, the shear stress caused by the oscillating cavities. The amplitude of the oscillation of particles is proportional to the square root of the acoustic energy at that point [16]. The effect of the oscillating motion on tissues has been described as a "micromassage" because of the alternate compression and relaxation of tissues caused by the propagation of ultrasound [12].

The forces of sound pressure establish a stress pattern that produces reciprocating movement of the cells. The pressure maxima and minima are separated by one-half wavelength. For ultrasound of 1-MHz frequency, the distance in soft tissues is about 750 μm with 1 million oscillations per second; for 2 MHz, 375 μm and 2 million oscillations; and for 10 MHz, 75 μm and 10 million oscillations. The amplitude of the displacement of the particles is only about 0.018 μm for an ultrasound wave of 1 MHz and 1 W/cm^2. The amplitude of displacement is inversely proportional to the frequency, because particles vibrate faster at higher frequencies and thus require the input of more energy to be driven at the same amplitude. If the energy input remains the same and the frequency is increased, the amplitude of displacement will decrease accordingly. For an ultrasound of 10 MHz and 1 W/cm^2, the displacement is approximately 0.0018 μm for each of 10 million vibrations occurring within a second. Such vigorous perturbation conceivably has a profound effect on any mass transfer process.

Although the transfer of acoustic energy does not require the actual migration of medium particles along the direction of ultrasound propagation, but only the oscillation of these particles within a very small range, the kinetic energy provided to the tissues will undoubtedly accelerate certain processes favored by thermodynamic conditions, such as the diffusion process brought upon by a concentration gradient (or a chemical potential gradient to be precise) during phonophoresis. On the other hand, the kinetic energy level of diffusing drug molecules is also enhanced when subjected to an ultrasound field, which may lead to increased skin permeation of the drug.

3. Shear Stress from Oscillating Cavitation

As noted above, the "second-order effect" refers to a steady-state hydrodynamic shear field generated by stabilized oscillating cavities [16]. Because of the high-energy characteristics, many biological effects of ultrasound are thought to be linked to the oscillating cavities. The effect of ultrasound on the diffusion process across artificial membranes was recently reported by Levy et al. [18], who used cellulose and microporous polypropylene membranes and NaCl, KIO$_3$, urea, and bovine serum albumin as permeants. Using a pair of thermostated diffusion cells with an ultrasound probe placed upstream, they observed an enhancement of membrane permeability when ultrasonic energy was applied. This enhancement was reversible. Since the enhanced permeability in the presence of ultrasound was reduced more than one-half (from 55% to 23%) after the medium was degassed while other conditions were kept the same, acoustic cavitation appeared to play an important role in the enhancement of membrane permeation.

Experimental evidence indicates that cavitation occurs in vivo in mammalian tissue when the irradiating ultrasound intensity exceeds 0.08 W/cm^2 [19]. The effect of high shear stress on thixotropic structures can also be observed when ultrasonic energy is applied to such materials. Some commercial coupling gels used in ultrasound physiotherapy are thixotropic materials for better "holding" capability.

B. Thermal Effect

1. Temperature Elevation Within Tissues

The therapeutic effect of ultrasound in physiotherapy and sports medicine is believed to be attributable primarily to ultrasound's superb capability in selectively heating deep-seated tissues [5,11]. The acoustic energy that is removed from the compressional wave by attenuation is converted into heat, and so the temperature rises within that tissue. The low ultrasound attenuation in both subcutaneous fat tissue and skeletal muscle allows therapeutic ultrasound beams to penetrate these tissues with little loss of acoustic energy. Up to 30% of the acoustic energy may be reflected at the soft tissue–bone interface to raise the temperature in the adjacent area. Polymeric implants may exhibit a similar phenomenon when subjected to an ultrasound field, which is one of the possible mechanisms for polymeric implantable drug delivery systems regulated by ultrasound [20]. The temperature increase measured on the skin surface during phonophoresis was only about 1–2°C. Histological examination revealed that no difference was found between the ultrasound-exposed skin and control skin [18].

2. Nonlinear Effect

The nonlinear effect of acoustic energy is a phenomenon in which uneven heating occurs in a homogeneous medium or tissue due to nonlinear transmission properties of the medium. Normally, ultrasonic intensity decreases exponentially as a function of penetration distance. When a high-frequency, high-intensity pulsed ultrasound is used, however, a nonlinear effect may occur at a finite distance through the tissue where an abrupt increase in absorption of acoustic energy causes the formation of a "hot spot." The thermal effect in the deep tissues during phonophoresis should therefore always be taken into consideration when one attempts the development of phonophoretic delivery systems.

When focused ultrasound is used, it has been demonstrated that the ultrasonic energy may be delivered to a specific point within tissues to exert its heating effect. The trackless lesions produced by ultrasound within brain tissues are such an example [21]. This property of ultrasound may be useful for targeted drug delivery.

C. Ultrasound-Induced Biological Change

1. Effect on Blood Circulation

There is some discrepancy in the literature as to whether ultrasound treatment affects blood circulation. Bickford and Duff [22] reported that a consistent, sustained increase in blood flow occurred as a result of ultrasound treatment with only high intensity (>3 W/cm^2), whereas with more tolerable ultrasonic intensities (2 W/cm^2), vasodilation was detected in only about one-half of the cases. Abramson et al. [23] demonstrated that an increase in local blood flow may persist up to an average of 26 min after termination of 18–21 min ultrasound treatment. The effect of ultrasound on the blood flow of cutaneous, subcutaneous, and muscular tissues was investigated by Paaske et al. [24] on normal human subjects with a local ^{133}Xe washout technique. Ultrasonic irradiation was conducted for 3 min at 0.25, 0.5, and 0.75 W/cm^2 intensities, each intensity being employed as continuous as well as pulsed irradiation. No correlation between the ultrasound dose and blood flow or change in skin temperature could be demonstrated in their study. Murphy and Hadgraft [25] reported that the blood flow under the skin area exposed to 3-MHz, 1-W/cm^2 ultrasound did not cause any change in the local cutaneous blood flow, which was measured with laser-Doppler velocimetry.

2. Effect on Biological Membranes

Application of ultrasound may change the permeability of biological membranes, as demonstrated by the ultrasound-irradiated plasma membranes of mammalian erythrocytes [26,27]. Coble and Dunn [28] applied ultrasound to frog skin with a focused beam of 1 MHz and observed reversible intensity-dependent changes in both the membrane potential and short-circuit current (a property proportional to the flux of sodium ions through the membrane). Lehmann and Krusen [29] reported an irreversible increase in the permeability, a decrease in the active transport of sodium ions, and an increase in the isoelectric point of isolated frog skin after exposure to continuous-wave (1.8 and 3 W/cm^2) and pulsed (1.8 W/cm^2 time average) 1-MHz ultrasound. These effects could be duplicated by increasing the temperature of the membrane to 41°C in the absence of ultrasound.

Very limited quantitative information exists in the literature about the skin permeability change as a result of ultrasound exposure. Brucks et al. [30] reported an enhancement of ibuprofen permeation across human skin in vitro in the presence of ultrasound that could not be attributed to an increase in temperature. They concluded that no permanent damage of the barrier properties of the skin was found after the ultrasound exposure (1 W/cm^2, 1 MHz, continuous wave for 30 min).

IV. TRANSDERMAL DRUG DELIVERY BY PHONOPHORESIS

Phonophoresis has been successfully used to deliver anti-inflammatory medication to inflamed subcutaneous tissues [4,5,7,31]. This technique has also been used to administer various drugs including local anesthetics [32,33], antibiotics [34], and medication for the treatment of herpes simplex [35,36]. With the mounting interest in the development of novel transdermal drug delivery systems for systemic medication, several recent studies have attempted to understand some fundamental parameters related to phonophoretic drug delivery.

The effect of ultrasound on transdermal drug delivery was studied by Levy et al. [18] by administering three substances in vivo—D-mannitol, a highly polar sugar alcohol; physostigmine, a lipophilic anticholinesterase drug; and inulin, a macromolecular polysaccharide (MW 5000)—across the skin of two animal models, Sprague-Dawley rats and albino guinea pigs. Phonophoresis for 3 min (1 MHz, 1.5 W/cm^2, continuous wave) resulted in an approximately fourfold increase in D-mannitol absorption in comparison with the controls (without ultrasound treatment) in the 5-hr experiments. The application of ultrasound for 5 min (1 MHz, 3.0 W/cm^2, pulsed wave 4:1) increased inulin absorption approximately fourfold within 2 hr of ultrasound treatment. Topical absorption of D-mannitol and inulin into rat skin was measured by cumulative urinary excretion of ^{3}H-labeled drugs. Evaluation of the effects of phonophoresis for transdermal delivery of physostigmine was measured by the decrease of whole blood cholinesterase (ChE). Their results indicate that phonophoretic delivery of physostigmine (3 W/cm^2 pulsed wave, 5 min) increased the level of whole blood ChE inhibition from approximately 2% to 15% in guinea pigs and from 35% to 53% in rats within 1 hr in comparison with the controls. The application of ultrasound eliminated completely the lag time usually associated with transdermal delivery of drugs. The reversibility of the effect of ultrasound on skin was demonstrated by the observation that ultrasound treatment of guinea pig skin 1 hr before drug application did not change physostigmine absorption and also that 5 hr after ultrasound treatment no difference in physostigmine absorption was found between the treated and control subjects. A small increase in surface skin temperature immediately after ultrasound treatment was reported but was believed unlikely to cause dramatic changes in skin permeability.

Kost and coworkers [37] conducted in vitro phonophoresis of salicylic acid and hydrocortisone through hairless mouse skin. The apparatus used in their

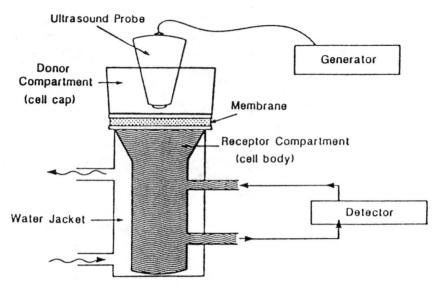

Figure 3 A schematic diagram of a typical experimental setup for in vitro phonophoresis study. (From Kost et al. [37].)

study is shown in Figure 3. An attempt was made to elucidate the mechanism of ultrasonically enhanced skin permeability in terms of the lipoidal and hydrophilic pathways of the stratum corneum. Salicylic acid (pK_a 2.97) in solutions of pH 2.65 and pH 9.9 was delivered by phonophoresis for 90 min (1 MHz, 3 W/cm^2, 20% duty cycle). The results showed that ultrasound enhanced the permeation of both un-ionized (pH 2.65) and ionized (pH 9.9) salicylic acid, indicating that ultrasound may have an effect on both lipophilic and hydrophilic routes. Analysis of ultrasound-exposed stratum corneum using differential scanning calorimetry and Fourier transform infrared spectroscopy detected no changes in comparison with unexposed stratum corneum.

Bommannan et al. [38] used ultrasound to increase the penetration of salicylic acid across hairless guinea pig skin in vitro. Phonophoresis of ^{3}H-labeled salicylic acid (pH 5.5) with ultrasound (0.2 W/cm^2, 16 MHz) for 5–20 min was found to enhance the drug permeation two- to threefold in comparison with the control. The reason for using 16-MHz ultrasound was based on the hypothesis that higher frequency ultrasound would better localize the acoustic energy within the stratum corneum and would therefore provide more perturbation in the skin barrier layer to facilitate drug permeation. The permeation results appear to support the authors' hypothesis; both the extent and the rate of absorption of salicylic acid were observed to be improved with higher ultrasound frequency (reflected by the higher amount and faster excretion of the radioisotope compared with the control). Their observation that increasing ultrasound frequency from lower values up to 10 MHz resulted in consistent enhancement of drug permeation but the permeation with 16-MHz ultrasound was unexpectedly lower than that with 10-MHz ultrasound indicates the need for further investigations to find an optimal frequency range for phonophoresis.

Murphy and Hadgraft [25] investigated the interaction of ultrasound with normal human skin in vivo by two techniques: (1) pretreating the skin with ultrasound of 3.0 MHz and 1.0 W/cm,^{2} for 5 min, followed by 15-sec passive diffusion of the model drug methyl nicotinate and (2) passive diffusion of methyl nicotinate and hexyl nicotinate for 3 min prior to 5-min application of ultrasound, with the drug being removed before the ultrasound treatment. The influence of ultrasound on the drug penetration across the skin was assessed by measuring the blood flow under the exposed area with laser-Doppler velocimetry (LDV). Ultrasound treatment alone was found not to affect local cutaneous blood flow under the experimental conditions. Three parameters evaluated from LDV response vs. time graphs were peak height, time to onset of erythema (t_0), and time to peak (t_p). The data from ultrasound skin pretreatment show an increase in peak height and a decrease in both t_0 and t_p, compared with the control (without ultrasound treatment). The extent of enhanced absorption was greater for the less lipophilic methyl nicotinate. The authors concluded that the stratum corneum is modified by ultrasound pretreatment in some way, as reflected by enhanced drug absorption, and that this modification is reversible and lasts for a short period of time. Since the application of ultrasound to drug-pretreated skin was shown to enhance the absorption of hexyl nicotinate, ultrasonic energy seems capable of enhancing the rate of partitioning of lipophilic drugs from the stratum corneum reservoir.

V. TECHNIQUES OF APPLICATION OF ULTRASOUND

What makes phonophoretic drug delivery different from the other novel drug delivery methods is the application of ultrasound as a driving force. Because of the characteristics of ultrasonic energy, there are several unique concerns about the technique of ultrasound application.

A. Coupling Agent and Drug Delivery Media

Because ultrasound is conducted through the propagation of compressional waves in a medium, a medium of high transmissivity to ultrasound (defined as the percentage of acoustic energy transmitted)—a coupling agent—must be used for an effective application of ultrasound. Degassed water is an excellent coupling agent for transfer of acoustic energy from the surface of a transducer into a patient because of the small difference in acoustic impedance between water and soft tissues, and also because the possibility of cavitation is minimized owing to the absence of dissolved gas. Many commercially available coupling agents are aqueously based thixotropic gels. It was reported by Warren et al. [39] that the transmissivities of some commercial coupling agents are 90–100% as efficient as water, with the transmissivity of glycerol being 75% that of water and mineral oil 90% that of water.

For phonophoresis, the drug to be delivered may be incorporated into a coupling agent. The elimination of any air bubbles, even microscopic ones, in the coupling agent is crucial because the presence of air bubbles causes cavitation and the loss of acoustic energy, which leads to a significant decrease in ultrasound transmission.

B. Moving Sound Head Technique

The sound head of the ultrasound applicator is frequently placed in direct contact with the skin in the presence of a coupling agent during physiotherapy and phonophoresis. With this technique, the sound head is kept in continuous slow and steady motion over the skin area to be treated, in either a circular or parallel pattern, in order to (1) achieve a more uniform application of ultrasonic energy, (2) cover a larger skin area, and (3) avoid building up "hot spots" or standing waves that could lead to tissue damage. A standing wave is the interference of a reflected sound wave with the incident sound wave which results in an increase in the energy level at certain points in an ultrasound beam [40]. The drug to be delivered is incorporated into the coupling agent, which may be either a thixotropic gel of an aqueous base or an oil-based emulsion or ointment. Tissue damage is unlikely to occur if the intensity used on the trunk or proximal extremity does not exceed 1.5 W/cm^2 or that on the distal extremity does not exceed 0.5 W/cm^2 with 150-cm^2 treated skin area in a 5-min treatment [5].

C. Stationary Technique

The stationary technique is used when the treated area is localized and small. The patient's tolerance to ultrasound intensity is quite different with the stationary technique from that observed with the moving sound head technique. Whereas intensities up to 2 W/cm^2 are common with the moving sound head technique, very few patients can safely tolerate even 0.2 $W/cm,^2$ for more than 2 or 3 min with the stationary technique. The potential risk of periosteal overheating (i.e., to 45°C or higher) is also increased [5].

D. Immersion Technique

For certain body areas that have a difficult contour for an ultrasound applicator to work on, such as the ankle or finger joints, the immersion technique may be used. Both the area to be treated and the ultrasound applicator are immersed in a coupling agent, and ultrasound is applied by moving the applicator at a distance of 1–2 cm over the area to be treated. The drawback of this technique is that a relatively large amount of a coupling agent is required.

E. Water Applicator Technique

The drawback of the immersion technique can be overcome by a modified method: immersing the ultrasound applicator in a durable plastic bag filled with degassed water, then applying the flexible bag surface to the treatment area covered with coupling agent. Both the moving sound head and stationary techniques can be used with this method.

F. Choice of Ultrasound Parameters

1. Frequency

The relationship between penetration depth and frequency of ultrasound in soft tissues is well established; for example, at 0.09 MHz, approximately 50% of acoustic energy penetrates to a depth of 10 cm; with 1 MHz, 5 cm; and with 4 MHz, 1 cm [5]. Griffin and Touchstone [6] studied the effect of ultrasound frequency on phonophoretic delivery of hydrocortisone into pig skin in vivo (1 W/cm^2, 17 min). Of five frequencies investigated (0.09, 0.25, 0.5, 1.0, and 3.6 MHz), 0.25-MHz ultrasound yielded the highest mean hydrocortisone concentration in tissues, and 3.6 MHz yielded the second highest value, whereas 1.0 MHz, the frequency used most commonly in physiotherapy, exhibited the least recovery of hydrocortisone. Due to the uncomfortable sensation associated with 0.25-MHz ultrasound revealed by human subject tests, 3.6-MHz frequency was recommended as a preferable frequency for phonophoresis because of minimal possibility of causing skin damage [6]. On the other hand, a study reported by Bommannan et al. [38] indicated that ultrasound frequencies higher than those used in physiotherapy (i.e., >3 MHz), such as 10–16 MHz, may achieve higher phonophoretic drug delivery.

2. Continuous and Pulsed Ultrasound

The ultrasonic energy output from an ultrasound applicator can be produced on a continuous basis or pulsed (i.e., discontinuous waveforms). When pulsed ultrasound is used, the ultrasonic energy output is the average output over one cycle of on-and-off mode. The total energy output of the pulsed ultrasound is reduced to a fraction of the continuous counterpart with the same instantaneous peak energy output (amplitude of compressional waves), depending on the duty factor (the percentage of "on" time in a cycle) or on/off ratio of the pulsed ultrasound. An "off" period of pulsed ultrasound allows the heat generated during the previous "on" period to dissipate, thus avoiding potential tissue damage due to overheating. Under certain circumstances, such as when the stationary technique is used, pulsed ultrasound appears to be appropriate.

3. Intensity and Duration

Although the bioeffects committee of the American Institute of Ultrasound in Medicine issued brief statements in both 1976 and 1978 regarding the safety levels for diagnostic ultrasound exposures [41], no regulation has been set in respect to the ultrasound "dose," e.g., the maximal safe intensity and treatment duration for physiotherapy and phonophoresis. Wadsworth and Chanmugam [12] provide general guidelines for the selection of intensity and duration under various circumstances in physiotherapy. It is believed that the selection of intensity and duration should also be based on the patient's sensation of and tolerance to the ultrasound applied in the particular instance [5]. This aspect of biomedical ultrasound application merits further investigation.

VI. COMPARISON BETWEEN PHONOPHORESIS AND IONTOPHORESIS FOR TRANSDERMAL DRUG DELIVERY

Phonophoresis differs from iontophoresis in several respects. Phonophoresis is more versatile than iontophoresis for several reasons.

1. Ultrasound enhances the skin penetration of both nonionic and ionic drug species, whereas iontophoresis can only be used to deliver ionic drugs (with the exception of electro-osmosis; however, the quantity of drug delivered by electro-osmosis is very low).
2. Phonophoresis can be used for both aqueous media (e.g., aqueous solutions and gels) and oily media (e.g., ointments and creams), whereas iontophoresis is restricted to aqueous media.
3. It is theoretically possible to develop an ultrasonic skin penetration enhancement device that could be used to increase the drug delivery rate of transdermal devices (passive diffusion) currently in existence and to shorten their onset time (lag time).

The penetration depth of phonophoretically delivered drugs is over 5 cm [42], in comparison with a few millimeters for iontophoresis. On the other hand, phonophoresis may not be as efficient as iontophoresis in delivering a significant quantity of a drug across the skin barrier. While one to two orders, or even higher, enhancement in transdermal drug delivery is common for iontophoresis, only a fewfold enhancement is usually accomplished by phonophoresis. From a practical viewpoint, miniaturization of phonophoretic drug delivery systems is much more difficult to achieve than that of iontophoretic drug delivery systems.

For iontophoretic drug delivery systems, it is quite feasible to develop a "wrist watch" type of device, because the electronic circuit involved is rather simple and the only bulky parts may be associated with the battery and drug reservoir. On the other hand, the need for the proper electronic parts to obtain an alternating voltage of high frequency and voltage for the conversion of electric energy into mechanical energy and the structure of a transducer would put a constraint on size reduction.

VII. CHALLENGES AND FUTURE PROSPECTS FOR THE DEVELOPMENT OF PHONOPHORETIC DRUG DELIVERY SYSTEMS

The techniques of phonophoresis currently used in physiotherapy as summarized in the preceding sections may not be readily adapted for phonophoretic transdermal drug delivery systems for systemic medication. As for the development of any novel drug delivery systems, there are several criteria that have to be met to ensure acceptable risk/benefit and cost/benefit ratios. One of the main purposes of controlled drug delivery is to improve safety and minimize side effects by providing a better and more controlled drug absorption process and by reducing the fluctuation in the drug concentration in the blood. To develop a successful phonophoretic drug delivery system, it is therefore essential to have both precision in the amount of drug delivered and reproducibility of the delivery process. The device should also be convenient for physicians and patients to use. None of the current phonophoresis procedures and techniques have yet met such requirements. Research into the development of phonophoretic transdermal delivery systems is only in its infancy. Much more research must be done to understand the mechanisms of phonophoresis for maximization of drug delivery, to set standards for the safe use of ultrasonic energy levels for drug delivery (e.g., for long-term daily use), and to investigate the impact of acoustic energy on formulation parameters such as drug stability and choice of pharmaceutical excipients.

Since ultrasound has been known to cause chemical reactions [43], drug degradation reactions and interactions with excipients may be triggered and/or accelerated in the presence of an ultrasonic field. To achieve accurate and reproducible drug delivery, the drug formulation (in solution form or, preferably, semisolid form for easy loading) in a phonophoretic drug delivery system will probably have to be placed in a drug reservoir to maintain a constant skin contact area and a consistent level of exposure to ultrasonic energy. If a more versatile phonophoresis device is to be designed to enhance the performance of other transdermal drug delivery systems (e.g., transdermal patches), research is needed to develop a device design that permits efficient transfer of ultrasonic energy across the transdermal drug delivery systems.

We thank Dr. M. Kara for his kind assistance in the preparation of this chapter.

REFERENCES

1. D. M. Skauen and G. M. Zentner, *Int. J. Pharm.* 20, 235 (1985).
2. K. Fellinger and J. Schmid, *Klinik und Therapie des Chronicshen Gelenkerumatismus*, Maudrich, Vienna, 1955, p. 549.
3. P. Tyle and P. Agrawala, *Pharm. Res.* 6(5), 355 (1989).
4. J. A. Kleinkort and F. Wood, *Phys. Ther.* 55, 1320 (1975).
5. J. E. Griffin and T. C. Karselis, *Physical Agents for Physical Therapists*, Charles C. Thomas, Springfield, IL, 1988, p. 263.
6. J. E. Griffin and J. C. Touchstone, *Am. J. Phys. Med.* 51(2), 62 (1972).
7. J. C. McElnay, T. A. Kennedy, and R. Harland, *Int. J. Pharm.* 40, 105 (1987).
8. G. Wanet and N. Dehon, *J. Belge Rhum. Med. Phys.* 31, 2 (1976).
9. J. E. Griffin, Phonophoresis: a review, *Proc. Int. Symp. Ther. Ultrasound*, 1982, pp. 180–192.
10. M. Moll, *USAF Med. Ser. Dig. 30* (May-June), 8 (1979).
11. J. F. Lehmann and B. J. De Lateur, in *Krusen's Handbook of Physical Medicine and Rehabilitation*, F. J. Kottke, G. K. Stillwell, and J. F. Lehmann, Eds., W. B. Saunders, Philadelphia, 1990, p. 313.
12. H. Wadsworth and A. P. P. Chanmugan, in *Electrophysical Agents in Physiotherapy*, Science Press, Marrickville, Australia, 1983, Chap. 5.
13. J. F. Lehmann and B. J. De Lateur, in *Therapeutic Heat and Cold*, J. F. Lehmann, Ed., Williams & Wilkins, Baltimore, 1990, Chap. 9.
14. P. N. T. Wells, *Biomedical Ultrasonics*, Academic Press, London, 1977, p. 17.
15. G. R. ter Har, in *Physical Principles of Medical Ultrasonics*, C. R. Hill, Ed., Ellis Horwood, West Sussex, 1986, p. 388.
16. A. R. Williams, *Ultrasound: Biological Effects and Potential Hazard*, Academic, New York, 1983, pp. 126–136.
17. W. Summer and M. Patrick, *Ultrasonic Therapy*, Elsevier, New York, 1964.
18. D. Levy, J. Kost, Y. Meshulam, and R. Langer, *J. Clin. Invest.* 83, 2074 (1989).
19. G. R. ter Haar and S. Daniels, *Phys. Med. Biol.* 26(6), 1145 (1981).
20. J. Kost, K. Leong, and R. Langer, Ultrasonically controlled drug delivery in vivo, *Proc. Int. Symp. Controlled Release Bioact. Mater.* 14, 186–187 (1987).
21. D. L. Carstensen, M. W. Miller, and C. A. Linke, *J. Biol. Phys.* 2, 173 (1974).
22. R. B. Bickford and R. S. Duff, *Circ. Res.* 1, 534 (1953).
23. D. I. Abramson, C. Burnett, Y. Bell, S. Tuck, H. Bejal, and C. J. Fleischer, *Am. J. Phys. Med.* 39, 51 (1960).
24. W. P. Paaske, H. Hovind, and P. Sejrsen, *Scand. J. Clin. Invest.* 31, 389 (1973).
25. T. M. Murphy and J. Hadgraft, in *Prediction of Percutaneous Penetration—Methods, Measurements, Modelling*, R. C. Scott, R. H. Guy, and J. Hadgraft, Eds., IBC Technical Services, London, 1990, p. 333.
26. M. J. Lota and R. C. Darling, *Arch. Phys. Med.* 36, 282 (1955).

27. M. L. Bundy J. Lerner, D. L. Messier, and J. A. Rooney, *Ultrasound Med. Biol. 4*, 259 (1978).

28. A. J. Coble and F. Dunn, *J. Acoust. Soc. Am. 60*, 225 (1976).

29. J. F. Lehmann and F. J. Krusen, *Arch. Phys. Med. Rehabil. 35*, 20 (1954).

30. R. Brucks M. Nanavaty, D. Jung, and F. Siegel, *Pharm. Res. 6*(8), 697 (1989).

31. J. E. Griffin, J.L. Echternach, R. E. Price, and J. C. Touchstone, *Phys. Ther. 47*, 594 (1967).

32. E. J. Novak, *Arch. Phys. Med. Rehabil.* May, 231 (1964).

33. H. A. E. Benson, J. C. McElnay, and R. Harland, *Int. J. Pharm. 44*, 65 (1988).

34. S. Ragelis, *Antibiotiki 26*(9), 699 (1981).

35. M. Fahim, T. Brawner, L. Millikan, M. Nickell, and D. Hall, *J. Med. 6*(3), 245 (1978).

36. M. S. Fahim, T. A. Brawner, and D. G. Hall, *J. Med. 11*(2/3), 143 (1980).

37. J. Kost, M. Machlf, and R. Langer, Experimental approaches to elucidate the mechanism of ultrasonically enhanced transdermal drug delivery, *Proc. Int. Symp. Controlled Release Bioact. Mater. 17*, 29–30 (1990).

38. D. Bommannan, H. Okuyama, P. Stauffer, and R. Guy, Sonophoresis: enhancement of transdermal drug delivery using ultrasound, *Proc. Int. Symp. Controlled Release Bioact. Mater. 17*, 31–32, (1990).

39. C. G. Warren, J. N. Koblanski, and R. A. Sigelmann, *Arch. Phys. Med. Rehabil. 57*, 218 (1976).

40. A. R. Williams, *Ultrasound: Biological Effects and Potential Hazard*, Academic, New York, 1983, p. 23.

41. A. R. Williams, *Ultrasound: Biological Effects and Potential Hazard*, Academic, New York, 1983, p. 291.

42. J. E. Griffin, J. C. Touchstone, and A. Liu, *Am. J. Phys. Med. 44*, 20 (1965).

43. E. C. Friedrich, J. M. Domek, and R. Y. Pong, *J. Org. Chem. 50*, 4640 (1985).

IV

DRUG PERMEATION ENHANCEMENT VIA THE NASAL ROUTE

16

Permeability and Metabolism as Barriers to Transmucosal Delivery of Peptides and Proteins

Bruce J. Aungst
The DuPont Merck Pharmaceutical Company,
Wilmington, Delaware

I. BIOAVAILABILITY OF TRANSMUCOSALLY ADMINISTERED PEPTIDES AND PROTEINS

Peptides and proteins are being increasingly considered as drug candidates. Many physiological processes are naturally regulated by peptide or protein factors. Growth, immune responses, blood pressure, blood clotting, and bone calcification are some examples. Improved methods of obtaining these peptides and proteins and the identification of more potent or more stable analogues have enhanced the feasibility of using peptides and proteins therapeutically. One problem that commonly limits the development of peptide and protein drugs, though, is that they are relatively ineffective when given orally. Almost all peptide and protein drugs currently on the market must be administered by injection.

Various ways to enhance the bioavailability of orally administered peptides and proteins have been studied, and administration via other noninjection, nonoral routes has been attempted. These alternative routes employ application of the formulation directly to the mucosal membrane of the nasal cavity, the rectum, or the buccal or sublingual areas of the mouth, through which the drug can be absorbed. We can refer to those routes of absorption as transmucosal, a term that also includes intestinal absorption. The difference between intestinal and other transmucosal routes of administration is that it is very difficult to control the site or area of delivery of an orally administered formulation. This is important to do when the membrane metabolizes the drug or when coadministration of adjuvants to enhance bioavailability is required. Other mucosal sites allow this to be accomplished much more easily.

Transmucosal delivery could offer the advantage of a being a noninjection route of administration. Presumably, patients usually prefer to avoid needles. Another common problem is that peptides and proteins usually have short durations of action. Any requirement of frequent dosing would probably be less of a limitation to patient acceptance if injections were not required. Under certain conditions it may also be possible to sustain the release of transmucosally administered drugs to prolong their duration of action.

Unfortunately, the bioavailabilities or relative potencies of transmucosally administered peptides and proteins are usually quite low, unless absorption-promoting adjuvants are coadministered. Some representative data illustrating this are given in Table 1. For the data included in this table, no absorption-promoting adjuvants were used. Under these conditions transmucosally administered peptides and proteins almost always have poor bioavailability, as depicted by these data. Therefore, for transmucosal delivery of peptide and protein drugs to become clinically acceptable, it is necessary to improve their bioavailability. To improve their bioavailability, it is necessary to understand why it is low.

As described in the sections that follow, both metabolism and lack of membrane permeation can contribute to the poor bioavailability of transmucosally administered peptides and proteins. Metabolism might occur within the lumen of the nasal, rectal, oral, or intestinal cavities, at the surfaces of these membranes, or within the cells. After rectal and intestinal absorption, the peptide or protein must pass the additional metabolic barrier presented by the liver before finally reaching the systemic circulation. The contribution of poor membrane permeation to low bioavailability is not unexpected considering that peptides and proteins are often relatively high molecular weight, hydrophilic compounds. Nasal and gastrointestinal bioavailabilities of oligomers of polyethylene glycol (PEG) decrease from approximately 60% to 30% as molecular weights increase from 400 to 700 [25]. PEGs with molecular weights greater than 1500 consistently have bioavailabilities less than 10%. Since PEG is excreted in the urine unchanged, metabolism does not contribute to the loss of bioavailability. A similar dependence of nasal bioavailability on molecular weight was shown in rats by Fisher et al. [26]. Sodium cromoglycate (MW 512) was 53% bioavailable, inulin (MW 5200) was 15% bioavailable, and dextran (MW 70,000) was 2.8% bioavailable. These are also nonmetabolized marker compounds.

The question that must be addressed for peptides and proteins is, What are the relative contributions of metabolism and poor membrane permeation to low transmucosal bioavailability? An understanding of the relative importance of these barriers is essential to formulating ways to overcome the barriers. If metabolism is primarily the problem, inhibitors of metabolism could be coadministered. If poor membrane permeation is the problem, membrane permeation enhancers could be used to temporarily increase permeability and increase the absorption rate. Both approaches might be required for certain peptide or protein drugs.

One way investigators have addressed the question of the relative contributions of metabolism and permeation barriers is by examining the effects of metabolism inhibition or membrane permeation enhancement. Therefore, it will be helpful to briefly review the areas of transmucosal permeation enhancers and metabolism inhibitors.

II. MEMBRANE PERMEATION ENHANCERS

A. Categories and Representative Data

Permeation enhancers are agents that are used to increase the permeability of some particular membrane. Many of these agents described in the literature can be included in one of the structural categories listed in Table 2. Examples and structures of some permeation enhancers in the surfactant, steroidal detergent, and enamine/*N*-acyl amino acid categories are given in Figures 1–3.

Usually, the utility of these agents has been demonstrated by measuring the increase in transmucosal bioavailability (*F*) or pharmacologic activity (potency) of the peptide or protein. A sampling of studies describing typical effects of permeation enhancers is given in Table 3. It is clear from these data that tremendous increases in bioavailability of transmucosally administered peptides and proteins are possible with these membrane permeation-enhancing adjuvants.

B. Mechanisms

The term ''permeation enhancer'' strictly implies that these compounds affect membrane permeability to peptides or proteins. This has often not been shown, however. The potential contributions of other mechanisms of absorption enhancement, as listed in Table 4, should be recognized even if permeability enhancement is suspected.

The agents in the categories of Table 2, and those listed as examples, clearly do affect membrane permeability. We know this because the transmucosal bioavailabilities of nonmetabolized drugs, including macromolecules, have been shown to be increased. Table 5 summarizes one such study in which the effects of several permeation enhancers were evaluated for the nonprotein compounds creatinine, inulin, and polyvinylpyrrolidone. In some cases these agents have been directly shown to increase the permeability of the mucosal membrane. For example, Wheatley et al. [32] showed that 0.1% sodium deoxycholate increased the in vivo fluxes of mannitol and inulin across a sheep nasal membrane 10–20-fold. Many of these compounds have also been shown to cause the rupture

Table 1 Bioavailability (F) or Relative Potency of Various Peptide and Protein Drugs Administered Transmucosally

Peptide/Protein	Approx. MW (#AA)	Route	Species	F	Relative potency	Ref.
Thyrotropin-releasing hormone	379	Oral	Rat	0.2–1.5%		1
		Oral	Dog	3.5–12.6%		1
		Oral	Human	2.0%		1
Metkephamide	661	Nasal	Rat	65–102%		2
D-Ala,D-Leu enkephalin	570	Nasal	Rat	59%		2
Somatostatin analogue (cyclic hexapeptide)	800	Oral	Dog	1–3%		3
		Duodenal	Rat	1%		4
His-D-Trp-Ala-Trp-D-Phe-Lys NH2	900	Oral	Rat		0.7% of IV	5
		Oral	Dog		0.8% of IV	5
Somatostatin analogue (Sandostatin)	1,000	Oral	Human	0.3%		6
Desmopressin (DDAVP)	1,100	Nasal	Human	9–20%		7
Arg vasopressin	1,100	Oral	Rat		0.3% of SC	8
		Rectal	Rat		5% of SC	8
Lys vasopressin	1,100	Oral	Rat		0.1% of IV	8
		Colonic	Rat		1.0% of IV	8
Luteinizing hormone releasing hormone (LHRH)	1,200	Nasal	Human		1% of IV	9
Nafarelin (LHRH analogue)	1,300	Nasal	Monkey	2%		10
		Nasal	Human	3.6%		11

	MW	Route	Species	F	F	Ref
Buserelin (LHRH analogue)	1,300	Nasal	Human	6%		12
Atrial natriuretic peptide fragment	(25)	Nasal	Human	0%	No effect	13
Growth hormone releasing hormone analogue	(29)	Nasal	Human		<1% of IV	14
Eel calcitonin analogue	(32)	Nasal	Dog	39%		15
Insulin	6,000	Nasal	Rat		0.4–2.0% of IM	16
		Rectal	Rat		3.2–17.0% of IM	16
		Buccal	Rat		0.7–3.6% of IM	16
		Sublingual	Rat		0.3% of IM	16
		Nasal	Rabbit	0.9%		17
		Nasal	Rat	0.3%		17
		Rectal	Rat	0.2%		18
Epidermal growth factor	6,200	Rectal	Rat	0%		19
Interferon β	17,000	Nasal	Rabbit	0%		20
				3%		21
Met growth hormone	22,000	Stomach	Rat	0.8%		22
		Duodenum	Rat	1.0%		22
		Ileum	Rat	0.7%		22
		Colon	Rat	0.2%		22
		Nasal	Rat	<1%		23
Growth hormone	22,000	Nasal	Rat	7.4%		24

Abbreviations: MW, molecular weight; AA, amino acid; F, bioavailability; IV, intravenous; SC, subcutaneous; IM, intramuscular.

Table 2 Structural Categories of
Transmucosal Permeation Enhancers

- Surfactants
- Steroidal detergents (bile salts)
- Salicylate and analogues
- EDTA and other chelators
- Enamines/*N*-acyl amino acids

of erythrocytes in vitro, and this has been used as an index of their relative potential to cause membrane irritation. But these studies also indicate that the agents affect the permeability of the erythrocyte membrane.

The mechanisms by which these agents increase mucosal membrane permeability have not been clearly established. However, mechanisms have been proposed for each of these categories. These are summarized in Table 6.

Polyoxyethylene ethers
    Example:
        Laureth-9 $CH_3(CH_2)_{10}CH_2(OCH_2CH_2)_9OH$
        [polyoxyethylene (9) lauryl ether]

Fatty acids (salts)
    Example:
        Na Caprate $CH_3(CH_2)_8COO^- \cdot Na^+$

Phosphoglycerides
    Example:
        Lysolecithin

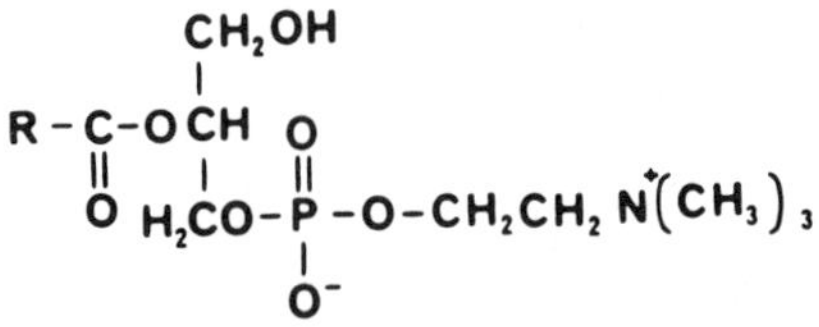

Figure 1 Major categories of surfactant membrane permeation enhancers and examples of their structures.

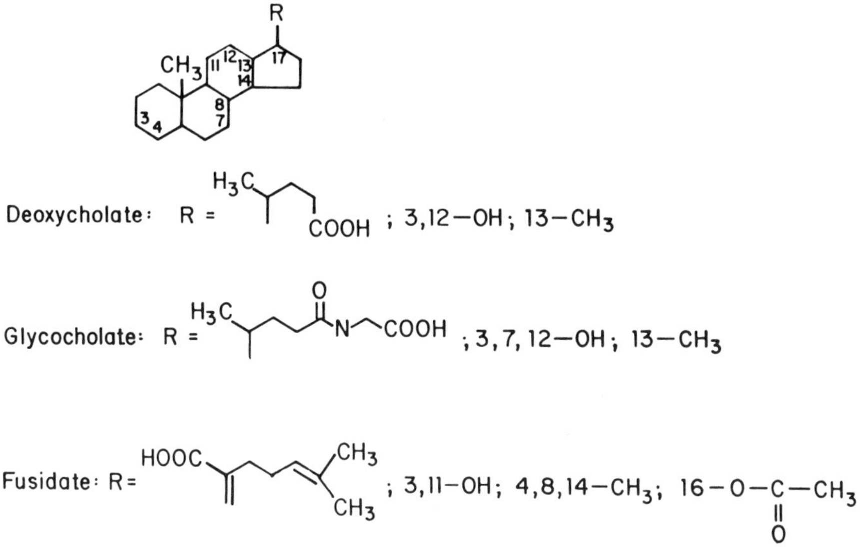
R
CH3
Deoxycholate: R =
H3C
COOH
; 3,12–OH; 13–CH3
Glycocholate: R =
H3C
O
N
COOH
; 3, 7, 12–OH; 13–CH3
Fusidate: R =
HOOC
CH3
CH3
; 3,11–OH; 4,8,14–CH3; 16–O–C–CH3
O

Figure 2 Structures of the most common steroidal detergent membrane permeation enhancers.

C. Differences Among Membranes

Whenever transmucosal drug delivery is proposed, it is important to understand the differences among the various potential sites available for transmucosal administration. Although orally administered tablets and capsules are generally the

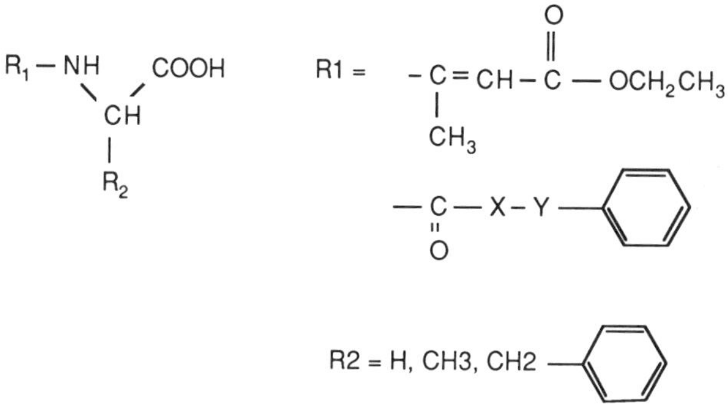
R1 – NH
COOH
CH
R2
R1 =
–C=CH–C — OCH2CH3
CH3
O
—C—X–Y
O
R2 = H, CH3, CH2

Figure 3 Structures of some enamine / *N*-acyl amino acids that are membrane permeation enhancers.

Table 3 Representative Preclinical Data Using Surfactants and Steroidal Detergents as Permeation Enhancers for Nasal Delivery of Protein Drugs

Adjuvant	Drug	Species	Result	Re
Various nonionic and ionic surfactants (1%)	Insulin	Rat	Potency increased up to 10× control	2
Na caprylate, Na caprate, Na laurate (1%)	Insulin	Rat	F increased from 10% (control) to 98% maximum	2
Laureth-9 (1%)	Human growth hormone	Rat	F increased from <1% (control) to 57–79%	2
Lysophosphatidylcholine (0.5%)	Insulin	Rat	Potency similar to that with laureth-9	2'
Various bile salts and saponin (1%)	Insulin	Rat	Potency increased almost 10× control	2
Na taurodihydrofusidate (1%)	Insulin	Rat	F increased from 0.3% (control) to 18%	1
		Rabbit	F increased from 0.9% to 5.2%	1
Glycyrrhetinic acid derivatives (0.1–2%)	Insulin	Rat	F increased from 2% (control) to 13% maximum	3
Na glycocholate (0.5%)	Human growth hormone	Rat	F increased from <1% (control) to 7–8%	2

most preferred dosage form, with this route of delivery it is probably most difficult to effectively coadminister a drug with permeation enhancers or metabolism inhibitors. This is because of the difficulty of concentrating the enhancer or inhibitor at the membrane surface. When the nasal, buccal, sublingual, and rectal transmucosal routes are compared, one may have certain advantages over

Table 4 Possible Mechanisms of Enhancing Transmucosal Peptide and Protein Absorption

A. Barrier disruption (permeability enhancement)
  1. Mucus layer
  2. Transcellular
  3. Paracellular (tight junctions)
  4. Epithelial cell loss
B. Altered physicochemical properties of drug in vehicle
C. Inhibition of metabolism

Table 5 Effects of Various Adjuvants on Rectal Absorption of Different Marker Compounds in Rats

Compound (MW)	Enhancement factor		
	5 mM sodium deoxycholate	5 mM sodium lauryl sulfate	25 mM EDTA
Creatinine (113)	43	51	27
Inulin (5500)	60	40	9
Insulin (6000)	35	31	9
Polyvinylpyrrolidone (35,000)	40	34	3

Source: Adapted from Nakanishi et al. [31].

the others. Among the considerations are patient preferences, the types of dosage forms required, capability of retaining the dose at the site of administration, and susceptibility to toxicity. These issues will not be discussed further here. These mucosal membranes can also be expected to differ with regard to the need for and the effects of permeation enhancers and metabolism inhibitors.

Consider the differences in permeability and the effects of permeation enhancers. Morphologically, mucosal membranes are not all alike. The rectal mucosa, like the intestinal membranes, is primarily a simple columnar epithelium: a single cell layer with tight junctions interconnecting neighboring cells and

Table 6 Proposed Mechanisms of Mucosal Membrane Permeability Enhancement for Various Categories of Compounds

Surfactants
    Extraction of membrane proteins or lipids
    Membrane fluidization
Steroidal detergents
    Extraction of membrane proteins or lipids
    Membrane fluidization
    Reverse micellization in membrane, creating aqueous channels
EDTA and other chelators
    Chelates calcium at tight junctions, increasing paracellular transport
Salicylate and analogues
    Decreases nonprotein sulfhydryls in membrane
    Interacts with membrane proteins
    Calcium chelation
Enamines/*N*-acyl amino acids
    Surface-active: membrane fluidization or extraction of membrane proteins or lipids
    Calcium chelation

Table 7 Mucosal Membranes Differ in Their Responses to Permeation Enhancers[a]

Permeation enhancer	Insulin potency relative to IM (%)		
	Rectal	Nasal	Buccal
None	9.5 ± 2.0	2.0 ± 0.5	1.9 ± 1.3
Glycocholate (Na salt, 5%)	40.1 ± 8.2	46.8 ± 4.7	25.5 ± 7.5
Laureth-9 (5%)	31.9 ± 11.0	28.7 ± 6.9	27.2 ± 10.3
Salicylate (Na salt, 5%)	41.7 ± 11.3	4.1 ± 2.4	2.0 ± 1.1
EDTA (Na$_2$ salt, 5%)	31.0 ± 6.7	3.5 ± 1.0	2.9 ± 1.4

[a]Insulin was administered transmucosally to rats by various routes, and the effects of permeation enhancers were evaluated.
Source: Adapted from Aungst et al. [16] and Aungst and Rogers [33].

functioning as the barrier to paracellular diffusion. The mucosal membrane of the nasal cavity is composed of several types of epithelia. A small portion extending into the nasal cavity from the nares is a stratified squamous epithelium. The remainder of the nasal membrane is made up of the respiratory epithelium, composed of ciliated cuboidal and columnar cells and goblet cells, and the olfactory epithelium, a pseudostratified neuroepithelium. In contrast, the buccal and sublingual membranes are stratified epithelia that are keratinized in some areas. Rather than tight junctions, the barrier to paracellular transport is an intercellular matrix derived from the membrane-coating granules.

Recognizing that mucosal membranes are morphologically different, my coworkers and I investigated the differences among these sites in their susceptibilities to the effects of permeation enhancers [16,33]. Results are summarized in Table 7. Insulin was administered to rats rectally, nasally, and buccally, and plasma glucose concentrations were measured over a 4-hr period. By comparing the magnitude of decrease in glucose concentrations to that after intramuscular insulin, using an IM insulin dose/response curve, we estimated the relative potency of transmucosally administered insulin. The effects of permeation enhancers representative of four of the categories listed in Table 2 were evaluated. Sodium glycocholate and laureth-9 enhanced insulin absorption from each of the sites examined. In contrast, sodium salicylate and EDTA affected only rectal insulin absorption. One reason for this may be that the nasal and buccal membranes are not affected by enhancers whose mechanisms involve calcium chelation or opening of the tight junctions. This is a reasonable explanation for the buccal membrane, because tight junctions contribute relatively little to the barrier to diffusion. Other factors could also be involved, though. These might include differences among the membranes in morphology unrelated to tight junctions, membrane uptake of the enhancers, membrane lipid composition, metabolic capacity, or mechanisms protecting against cellular injury.

III. METABOLISM INHIBITORS

A. Peptidases and Proteases of Mucosal Membranes

The permeability of mucosal membranes is somewhat predictable, theoretically, based on the partition coefficient and molecular weight (or volume) of the diffusant. Metabolism of peptides and proteins by mucosal membranes is less predictable. Any given peptide or protein has numerous possible sites of metabolism, depending on which enzymes it encounters. It is desirable, then, to learn what peptidases and proteases are associated with the mucosal membranes that could be sites of peptide and protein drug delivery. Although the peptidase and protease activities associated with the intestines have been characterized to some extent, only recently have studies been directed toward evaluating other mucosal membranes. A summary of these studies is compiled in Table 8 to illustrate what is known of how various peptide and protein substrates are metabolized by mucosal membranes.

Only the simplest of substrates and enzymes have been evaluated so far. Aminopeptidases are a group of enzymes that cleave the N-terminal amino acid from peptides. Clearly, aminopeptidases are present in mucosal membranes, and if a peptide is susceptible to aminopeptidases it will probably be rapidly metabolized when administered to these sites. Aminopeptidase activities of the different mucosal membranes have generally varied less than twofold. Inhibitors of aminopeptidases are available, and these can be used to retard metabolism. The metabolism of larger peptides and proteins by mucosal membranes (other than intestine) have not yet been studied to identify the enzymes involved. This generally requires identifying the metabolites and evaluating the effects of known inhibitors or activators of the proposed enzymes. Proteins such as proinsulin and insulin are known to be metabolized by mucosal membrane homogenates, and in these cases endopeptidases are probably involved [38].

B. Inhibitors

It is necessary to understand whether peptides and proteins are metabolized by mucosal membranes, and if so, what pathways and enzymes are involved. If these are known, then the effects of metabolism inhibitors on the bioavailability or metabolism rate of the drug can be evaluated. It will be useful then to also briefly examine how typical peptide or protein drugs are metabolized by other organs or tissues and to see examples of the inhibitors that are available for certain enzymes. In some cases routes of metabolism have been proposed based on the effects of certain enzyme inhibitors.

Leucine enkephalin and other enkephalins have been frequently used as model peptide drugs, as shown, for example, in Table 8. A scheme for leucine

Table 8 Peptidases and Proteases of Mucosal Membranes

Substrate	Membrane	Enzyme	Other findings	Inhibitor	Ref.
Various amino acid methoxynaphthylamides	Duodenal, ileal, rectal, nasal, buccal	Aminopeptidase N, aminopeptidase A, aminopeptidase B, leucine aminopeptidase	Differences among membranes not great, except for aminopeptidase A	Bestatin, puromycin	34
Met-enkephalin (TGGPM), Leu-enkephalin (TGGPL), D-Ala^2-Met-enkephalin (TAGPM)	Ileal, rectal, nasal, buccal	Aminopeptidases, dipeptidyl peptidase, dipeptidyl carboxypeptidase	Differences among membranes not great; aminopeptidases contribute most; TGGPM rate > TGGPL >> TAGPM		35
Leu-enkephalin	Nasal	Aminopeptidases		Bestatin, puromycin, aminoboronic acid derivatives	36
Thymopentin	Nasal	Aminopeptidases		Boroleucine	37

enkephalin metabolism is shown in Figure 4. The initial metabolic step can be mediated by aminopeptidases, dipeptidyl aminopeptidase, angiotensin-converting enzyme (ACE), or enkephalinase. Enkephalinase is also more properly known as endopeptidase 24.11 or as neutral endopeptidase. We have shown that in rat blood, plasma, and brain and skeletal muscle homogenates, aminopeptidases make the greatest contribution to leucine enkephalin metabolism [39]. Inhibitors of aminopeptidases are listed in Table 8. Captopril and other ACE inhibitors are well known. Thiorphan is the most commonly used inhibitor of endopeptidase 24.11.

Endopeptidase 24.11 also plays a major part in the metabolism of atrial natriuretic factor (ANF) and atrial natriuretic peptide (ANP). ANF is a 128-amino-acid peptide found in atrial homogenates. ANP usually refers to the fragment of ANF (amino acids 99–126) that is found in the circulation. Thiorphan, when administered with ANP to rats, increased plasma ANP concentrations and enhanced its diuretic and natriuretic activities, compared to ANP administration alone [40]. Another study [41] measured kidney trichloroacetic acid–precipitated radioactivity in mice administered ^{125}I-ANP, as an index of ANP levels in vivo. Thiorphan, as well as two other inhibitors of endopeptidase 24.11, acetorphan and kelatorphan, increased ANP levels. Less significant increases were seen with the aminopeptidase inhibitors bestatin and carbaphethiol, and boroleucine had no effect. Inhibitors of carboxypeptidases, serine peptidases, and aspartic peptidases also had no effect. Captopril reduced ANP levels. Several other publications have also shown the importance of endopeptidase 24.11 in ANP metabolism, and other inhibitors of endopeptidase 24.11 and of ANP metabolism have been identified. However, ANP metabolism by mucosal membranes and the effects of inhibitors have not been well studied.

For a third example, consider luteinizing hormone-releasing hormone, or LHRH (pGlu-His-Trp-Ser-Tyr-Gly-Leu-Arg-Pro-Gly-NH$_2$). In tissue homogenates, endopeptidase 24.15 cleaves the Tyr^5-Gly^6 peptide bond. Inhibition of this enzyme with N-[1-(RS)-carboxy-3-phenylpropyl]-Ala-Ala-Phe-p-aminobenzoate (compound I) increased LHRH recovery in the brain after ICV injection [42] and increased its pharmacologic activity after ICV or IV dosing [43]. Inhibitors of either endopeptidase 24.15 (compound I) or endopeptidase 24.11 (N-[1-(RS)-carboxy-3-phenylpropyl]-Phe-p-aminobenzoate) prolonged the half-life of plasma LHRH after IV injection, and the effects of these inhibitors were synergistic [42]. Endopeptidase 24.11 cleaves LHRH at Gly^6-Leu^7. Various rat tissue homogenates had greatly differing activities of endopeptidases 24.15 and 24.11 [42]. Table 1 lists nasal LHRH as having only 1% the activity of LHRH administered intravenously. Do endopeptidases 24.15 and 24.11 contribute to LHRH metabolism by mucosal membranes? We don't know yet.

LHRH also is an example of a compound whose metabolic stability was enhanced by analoging at the site of metabolism. Nafarelin and buserelin have substitutes for the Gly^6 amino acid. Interestingly, these have nasal bioavailabil-

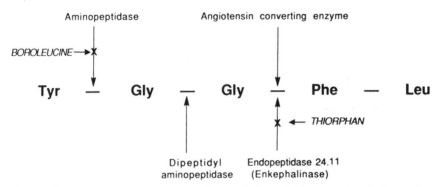

Figure 4 Scheme for leucine enkephalin metabolism, the enzymes involved, and inhibitors of those enzymes.

ities somewhat greater than that of LHRH, but bioavailability is still quite low (Table 1).

These three examples are given to make the point that if the route of metabolism and the enzymes involved are known, then metabolism can probably be inhibited. There are numerous peptidase inhibitors available in addition to those discussed here. The design of specific, very potent peptidase inhibitors, such as the aminoboronic acid derivative aminopeptidase inhibitors, is an emerging area of research. For example, novel compounds have been prepared as inhibitors of carboxypeptidases [44], aminopeptidases [45], and endopeptidase 24.11 [46]. To be able to take advantage of agents such as these for transmucosal delivery of peptides and proteins, we must have an understanding of the metabolism of the peptide or protein at the absorption site.

IV.   METABOLISM AND MEMBRANE IMPERMEABILITY AND INCOMPLETE BIOAVAILABILITY

A.   Evidence Based on the Effects of Enhancers or Inhibitors In Vivo

One of the ways we can examine the metabolism and permeability barriers to transmucosal absorption is by studying how absorption is affected by altering metabolism or membrane permeability. As discussed in the previous section, it is known that nasal, rectal, buccal, and other mucosal membranes have peptidase activity. But relatively little has been done so far to inhibit metabolism or to see how that affects transmucosal bioavailability. However, in one example [24], the nasal bioavailability of human growth hormone in rats was determined in the presence of metabolism inhibitors or permeation enhancers. The aminopeptidase inhibitor amastatin increased bioavailability from 7% to 29%, but bestatin, another aminopeptidase inhibitor, did not promote absorption. The permeation enhancers palmitoyl carnitine and lysophosphatidylcholine increased bioavailability to 22% and 26%, respectively. One could conclude from these data that membrane permeation and metabolism each contribute to the barrier to absorption (in this case of human growth hormone).

Another study [47] led to a similar conclusion for the dodecapeptide desenkephalin-gamma-endorphin (DEgE). DEgE bioavailability after rectal dosing without adjuvants in rats was 0–4%. EDTA prevented DEgE degradation but did not alone improve rectal bioavailability. A medium-chain glyceride permeation enhancer increased rectal bioavailability to 8–20%, and EDTA further increased it to 10–44%.

There are numerous studies showing the effects of permeation enhancers on transmucosal bioavailability or pharmacologic activity (Table 3 lists some). These certainly suggest that membrane permeability is consistently a factor limiting peptide and protein absorption. This conclusion is especially valid when the absorption of nonmetabolized marker compounds has also been enhanced (as shown in Table 5).

B. Many Permeation Enhancers Also Inhibit Metabolism

When permeation enhancers have been shown to improve the transmucosal absorption of a peptide or protein, the implied conclusion often has been that membrane permeability is the primary barrier to absorption. Although this could be true, the evidence is complicated by the fact that many permeation enhancers also have inhibitory effects on mucosal membrane peptidases. Sodium glycocholate and laureth-9 each inhibited insulin metabolism in rat nasal mucosal homogenates and also inhibited leucine aminopeptidase [48]. Sodium glycocholate also inhibited insulin metabolism in homogenates of rabbit nasal, buccal, rectal, and intestinal mucosal membranes [38]. The promoting effects of bile salts on human calcitonin absorption through the rat oral mucosa were related to the inhibition of degradation of calcitonin in mucosal homogenates [49]. Sodium glycocholate also inhibited the degradation of human β-interferon in homogenates of rabbit nasal mucosa [50]. These data raise doubts about conclusions with respect to the roles of the permeability and metabolism barriers when the effects of permeation enhancers on absorption are described. Clearly, models with which metabolism and permeability can be separately evaluated will be more useful for identifying how these contribute to the loss of transmucosal bioavailability.

C. Evidence from Separate Measurements of Permeation and Metabolism

The simultaneous measurement of metabolism and membrane permeation in one experiment allows one to compare the relative rates of these processes. This, then, may indicate why certain peptides or proteins are not well absorbed transmucosally. In vitro models with isolated or perfused membranes have been used almost exclusively for these experiments.

The model tetrapeptide Leu-Gly-Gly-Gly was metabolized in perfusates of rat jejunum, but nearly 50% was apparently absorbed, at least into the cells, intact [51]. It was speculated that cytoplasmic peptidase activity could complete the hydrolysis. D-Ala^2, D-Leu^5 enkephalin and Tyr-D-Ala-Gly-Phe were also metabolized by rat jejunum mucosal cells in vitro, and metabolism was inhibited by bestatin or phenylalanine [52]. However, in no case did the peptide accumulate in the mucosal tissue. In contrast, the renin inhibitor Pro-His-Pro-Phe-His-Leu-Phe-Val was transported across rabbit jejunum in vitro in the presence of phosphoramidon, which decreased its metabolism [53]. Similarly, the opioid peptide Tyr-Pro-Phe-Pro-NH$_2$ crossed the rabbit ileal epithelium when dipeptidylpeptidases were inhibited with diisopropylfluorophosphate [54]. Arg-vasopressin did not diffuse across isolated ileal mucosa, even under conditions wherein it was metabolically stable [55]. Buccal mucosa of the hamster was also shown to be metabolically active in vitro, as the hydrolysis rate of L-leucine-p-nitroanilide was greater than the diffusion rate across the membrane [56].

The rates of metabolism and permeation can, of course, each vary from membrane to membrane. Insulin absorption from the rat colon in the presence of sodium deoxycholate was little affected by a soybean trypsin inhibitor, but absorption from the ileum was enhanced by it [57].

V. OPTIMIZING TRANSMUCOSAL DELIVERY

It is certainly possible for peptide or protein drugs to be rapidly metabolized at nasal, rectal, buccal, and intestinal mucosal sites of administration and for these membranes to be relatively poorly permeable to the compounds. This makes achieving adequate bioavailability a challenge. The studies listed below could provide a pathway toward a solution for such problems.

1. Determine transmucosal bioavailability (without adjuvants) to see whether there is a problem. Because membranes differ, various sites should be compared.
2. If bioavailability is low, evaluate membrane permeation and metabolism in vitro to determine if one of these factors alone contributes to the problem.

3. Evaluate the effects of permeation enhancers and metabolism inhibitors in vitro. Choice of metabolism inhibitors depends on the enzymes involved. Identify which adjuvants might enable absorption.
4. Evaluate the adjuvants in vivo. Good luck in the toxicology tests!
5. Optimize the formulation. Not discussed in this review are the various formulation approaches (e.g., particles, microspheres, sprays, infusion devices), which also affect transmucosal bioavailability.

REFERENCES

1. S. Yokohama, K. Yamashita, H. Toguchi, J. Takeuchi, and N. Kitamori. Absorption of thyrotropin-releasing hormone after oral administration of TRH tartrate monohydrate in the rat, dog and human, *J. Pharm. Dyn.* 7, 101–111 (1984).
2. K. S. E. Su, K. M. Campanale, L. G. Mendelsohn, G. A. Kerchner, and C. L. Gries. Nasal delivery of polypeptides. I. Nasal absorption of enkephalins in rats, *J. Pharm. Sci.* 74, 394–398 (1985).
3. D. F. Veber, R. Saperstein, R. F. Nutt, R. M. Freidinger, S. F. Brady, P. Curley, D. S. Perlow, W. J. Paleveda, C. D. Colton, A. G. Zacchei, D. J. Tocco, D. R. Hoff, R. L. Vandlen, J. E. Gerich, L. Hall, L. Mandarino, E. H. Cordes, P. S. Anderson, and R. Hirschmann. A superactive cyclic hexapeptide analog of somatostatin, *Life Sci.* 34, 1371–1378 (1984).
4. J. A. Fix, K. Engle, P. A. Porter, P. S. Leppert, S. J. Selk, C. R. Gardner, and J. Alexander. Acylcarnitines: drug absorption-enhancing agents in the gastrointestinal tract, *Am. J. Physiol.* 251, G332–G340 (1986).
5. R. F. Walker, E. E. Codd, F. C. Barone, A. H. Nelson, T. Goodwin, and S. A. Campbell. Oral activity of the growth hormone releasing peptide His-D-Trp-Ala-Trp-D-Phe-Lys-NH_2 in rats, dogs and monkeys, *Life Sci.* 47, 29–36 (1990).
6. E. Kohler, M. Duberow-Drewe, J. Drewe, G. Ribes, M. M. Loubatieres-Mariani, N. Mazer, K. Gyr, and C. Beglinger. Absorption of an aqueous solution of a new synthetic somatostatin analogue administered to man by gavage, *Eur. J. Clin. Pharmacol.* 33, 167–171 (1987).
7. A. S. Harris, M. Ohlin, S. Lethagen, and I. M. Nilsson. Effects of concentration and volume on nasal bioavailability and biological response to desmopressin, *J. Pharm. Sci.* 77, 337–339 (1988).
8. M. Saffran, C. Bedra, G. S. Kumar, and D. C. Neckers. Vasopressin: a model for the study of effects of additives on the oral and rectal administration of peptide drugs, *J. Pharm. Sci.* 77, 33–38 (1988).
9. G. Fink, G. Gennser, P. Liedholm, J. Thorell, and J. Mulder. Comparison of plasma levels of leutinizing hormone releasing hormone in men after intravenous or intranasal administration, *J. Endocrinol.* 63, 351–360 (1974).
10. S. T. Anik, G. McRae, C. Nerenberg, A. Worden, J. Foreman, J.-Y. Hwang, S. Kushinsky, R. E. Jones, and B. Vickery. Nasal absorption of nafarelin acetate, the decapeptide [D-Nal(2)^6]LHRH, in Rhesus monkeys. I, *J. Pharm. Sci.* 73, 684–685 (1984).

11. R. L. Chan, M. R. Henzl, M. E. LePage, J. LaFargue, C. A. Nerenberg, S. Anik, and M. D. Chaplin. Absorption and metabolism of nafarelin, a potent agonist of gonadotropin-releasing hormone, *Clin. Pharmacol. Ther. 44*, 275–282 (1988).

12. F. J. Holland, L. Fishman, D. C. Costigan, L. Luna, and S. Leeder. Pharmacokinetic characteristics of the gonadotropin-releasing hormone analog D-Ser(TBU)-[6]EA-[10]luteinizing hormone releasing hormone (Buserelin) after subcutaneous and intranasal administration in children with central precocious puberty, *J. Clin. Endocrinol. Metab. 63*, 1065–1070 (1986).

13. A. Delabays, M. Porchet, B. Waeber, J. Nussberger, and H. R. Brunner. Effects of intranasal administration of synthetic (4-28)human atrial natriuretic peptide to normal volunteers, *J. Cardiovasc. Pharmacol. 13*, 173–176 (1989).

14. M. L. Vance, W. S. Evans, D. L. Kaiser, R. L. Burke, J. Rivier, W. Vale, and M. O. Thorner. The effect of intravenous, subcutaneous, and intranasal GH-RH analog, $[Nle^{27}]GHRH(1-29)-NH_2$, on growth hormone secretion in normal men: dose–response relationships, *Clin. Pharmacol. Ther. 40*, 627–633 (1986).

15. C. Manzoni, C. Monti, and M. Valente. Bioavailability of elcatonin ($ASU^{1.7}$-eel calcitonin) after intranasal administration to rats and dogs, *Pharmacol. Res. 21*, 105–106 (1989).

16. B. J. Aungst, N. J. Rogers, and E. Shefter. Comparison of nasal, rectal, buccal, sublingual and intramuscular insulin efficacy and the effects of a bile salt absorption promoter, *J. Pharmacol. Exp. Ther. 244*, 23–27 (1988).

17. M. J. M. Deurloo, W. A. J. J. Hermens, S. G. Romeyn, J. C. Verhoef, and F. W. H. M. Merkus, Absorption enhancement of intranasally administered insulin by sodium taurodihydrofusidate (STDHF) in rabbits and rats, *Pharm. Res. 6*, 853–856 (1989).

18. E. J. van Hoogdalem, C. D. Heijlegers-Feijen, J. C. Verhoef, A. G. de Boer, and D. D. Breimer. Absorption enhancement of rectally infused insulin by sodium tauro-24,25-dihydrofusidate (STDHF) in rats, *Pharm. Res. 7*, 180–183 (1990).

19. T. Murakami, H. Kawakita, M. Kishimoto, Y. Higashi, H. Amagase, T. Hayashi, N. Nojima, T. Fuwa, and N. Yata. Intravenous and subcutaneous pharmacokinetics and rectal bioavailability of human epidermal growth factor in the presence of absorption promoter in rats, *Int. J. Pharm. 46*, 9–17 (1988).

20. Y. Maitani, T. Igawa, Y. Machida, and T. Nagai. Intranasal administration of β-interferon in rabbits, *Drug Des. Del. 1*, 65–70 (1986).

21. T. Igawa, Y. Maitani, Y. Machida, and T. Nagai. Enzyme immunoassay of human fibroblast interferon after intranasal administration with several excipients in rabbits, *Chem. Pharm. Bull. 36*, 3055–3059 (1988).

22. J. A. Moore, S. A. Pletcher, and M. J. Ross. Absorption enhancement of growth hormone from the gastrointestinal tract of rats, *Int. J. Pharm. 34*, 35–43 (1986).

23. A. L. Daugherty, H. D. Liggitt, J. G. McCabe, J. A. Moore, and J. S. Patton. Absorption of recombinant methionyl-human growth hormone (Met-hGH) from rat nasal mucosa, *Int. J. Pharm. 45*, 197–206 (1988).

24. D. T. O'Hagan, H. Critchley, N. F. Farraj, A. N. Fisher, B. R. Johansen, S. S. Davis and L. Illum. Nasal absorption enhancers for biosynthetic human growth hormone in rats, *Pharm. Res. 7*, 772–776 (1990).

25. M. D. Donovan, G. L. Flynn, and G. L. Amidon. Absorption of polyethylene glycols 600 through 2000: the molecular weight dependence of gastrointestinal and nasal absorption, *Pharm. Res. 7*, 863–868 (1990).
26. A. N. Fisher, K. Brown, S. S. Davis, G. D. Parr, and D. A. Smith. The effect of molecular size on the nasal absorption of water-soluble compounds in the albino rat, *J. Pharm. Pharmacol. 39*, 357–362 (1987).
27. S. Hirai, T. Yashiki, and H. Mima. Effect of surfactants on the nasal absorption of insulin in rats, *Int. J. Pharm. 9*, 165–172 (1981).
28. M. Mishima, Y. Wakita, and M. Nakano. Studies on the promoting effects of medium chain fatty acid salts on the nasal absorption of insulin in rats, *J. Pharmacobio-Dyn. 10*, 624–631 (1987).
29. L. Illum, N. F. Farraj, H. Critchley, B. R. Johansen, and S. S. Davis. Enhanced nasal absorption of insulin in rats using lysophosphatidylcholine, *Int. J. Pharm. 57*, 49–54 (1989).
30. M. Mishima, S. Okada, Y. Wakita, and M. Nakano. Promotion of nasal absorption of insulin by glycyrrhetinic acid derivatives. I, *J. Pharmacobio-Dyn. 12*, 31–36 (1989).
31. K. Nakanishi, M. Masada, and T. Nadai. Effect of pharmaceutical adjuvants on the rectal permeability to drugs. IV. Effect of pharmaceutical adjuvants on the rectal permeability to macromolecular compounds in the rat, *Chem. Pharm. Bull. 32*, 1628–1634 (1984).
32. M. A. Wheatley, J. Dent, E. B. Wheeldon, and P. L. Smith. Nasal drug delivery: an in vitro characterization of transepithelial electrical properties and fluxes in the presence or absence of enhancers, *J. Controlled Release 8*, 167–177 (1988).
33. B. J. Aungst and N. J. Rogers. Site dependence of absorption-promoting actions of laureth-9, Na salicylate, Na$_2$EDTA, and aprotinin on rectal, nasal, and buccal insulin delivery, *Pharm. Res. 5*, 305–308 (1988).
34. R. E. Stratford and V. H. L. Lee. Aminopeptidase activity in homogenates of various absorptive mucosae in the albino rabbit: implications in peptide delivery, *Int. J. Pharm. 30*, 73–82 (1986).
35. S. D. Kashi and V. H. L. Lee. Enkephalin hydrolysis in homogenates of various absorptive mucosae of the albino rabbit: similarities in rates and involvement of aminopeptidases, *Life Sci. 38*, 2019–2028 (1986).
36. M. A. Hussain, A. B. Shenvi, S. M. Rowe, and E. Shefter. The use of alpha-aminoboronic acid derivatives to stabilize peptide drugs during their intranasal absorption, *Pharm. Res. 6*, 186–189 (1989).
37. M. A. Hussain, C. A. Koval, A. B. Shenvi, and B. J. Aungst. An aminoboronic acid derivative inhibits thymopentin metabolism by mucosal membrane aminopeptidases, *Life Sci. 47*, 227–231 (1990).
38. A. Yamamoto, E. Hayakawa, and V. H. L. Lee. Insulin and proinsulin proteolysis in mucosal homogentates of the albino rabbit: implications in peptide delivery from nonoral routes, *Life Sci., 47*, 2465–2474 (1990).
39. M. A. Hussain, S. M. Rowe, A. B. Shenvi, and B. J. Aungst. Inhibition of leucine enkephalin metabolism in rat blood, plasma and tissues in vitro by an aminoboronic acid derivative, *Drug Metab. Disp. 18*, 288–291 (1990).

40. A. J. Trapani, G. J. Smits, D. E. McGraw, K. L. Spear, J. P. Koepke, G. M. Olins, and E. H. Blaine. Thiorphan, an inhibitor of endopeptidase 24.11, potentiates the natriuretic activity of atrial natriuretic peptide, *J. Cardiovasc. Pharmacol. 14*, 419–424 (1989).

41. C. Gros, A. Souque, and J. C. Schwartz. Inactivation of atrial natriuretic factor in mice in vivo: crucial role of enkephalinase (EC 3.424.11), *Eur. J. Pharmacol. 179*, 45–56 (1990).

42. A. Lasdun, S. Reznik, C. J. Molineaux, and M. Orlowski. Inhibition of endopeptidase 24.15 slows the in vivo degradation of luteinizing hormone-releasing hormone, *J. Pharmacol. Exp. Ther. 251*, 439–447 (1989).

43. A. Lasdun and M. Orlowski. Inhibition of endopeptidase 24.15 greatly increases the release of luteinizing hormone and follicle stimulating hormone in response to luteinizing hormone/releasing hormone, *J. Cardiovasc. Pharmacol. 252*, 1265–1271 (1990).

44. J. E. Hanson, A. P. Kaplan, and P. A. Bartlett. Phosphonate analogues of carboxypeptidase A substrates are potent transition-state analogue inhibitors, *Biochemistry 28*, 6294–6305 (1989).

45. B. Lejczak, P. Kafarski, and J. Zygmunt. Inhibition of aminopeptidases by aminophosphonates, *Biochemistry 28*, 3459–3555 (1989).

46. B. P. Roques and A. Beaumont. Neutral endopeptidase-24.11 inhibitors: from analgesics to antihypertensives? *Trends Pharmacol. Sci. 11*, 245–249 (1990).

47. E. J. van Hoogdalem, C. D. Heijligers-Feijen, A. G. de Boer, J. C. Verhoef, and D. D. Breimer. Rectal absorption enhancement of des-enkephalin-g-endorphin (DEgE) by medium-chain glycerides and EDTA in conscious rats, *Pharm. Res. 6*, 91–95 (1989).

48. S. Hirai, T. Yashiki, and H. Mima. Mechanisms for the enhancement of the nasal absorption of insulin by surfactants, *Int. J. Pharm. 9*, 173–184 (1981).

49. Y. Nakada, N. Awata, Y. Ikuta, and S. Goto. The effect of bile salts on the oral mucosal absorption of human calcitonin in rats, *J. Pharmacobio-Dyn. 12*, 736–743 (1989).

50. T. Igawa, Y. Maitani, Y. Machida, and T. Nagai. Effect of absorption promoters in intranasal administration of human fibroblast interferon as a powder dosage form in rabbits, *Chem. Pharm. Bull. 37*, 418–421 (1989).

51. Y. C. Chung, D. B. A. Silk, and Y. S. Kim. Intestinal transport of a tetrapeptide, L-leucylglycylglycylglycine, in rat small intestine in vivo, *Clin. Sci. 57*, 1–11 (1979).

52. G. A. Kerchner and L. E. Geary. Studies on the transport of enkephalin-like oligopeptides in rat intestinal mucosa, *J. Pharmacol. Exp. Ther. 226*, 33–38 (1983).

53. K. Takaori, J. Burton, and M. Donowitz. The transport of an intact oligopeptide across adult mammalian jejunum, *Biochem. Biophys. Res. Commun. 137*, 682–687 (1986).

54. S. Mahe, D. Tome, A. M. Dumontier, and J. F. Desjeux. Absorption of intact morphiceptin by diisopropylfluorophosphate-treated rabbit ileum, *Peptides 10*, 45–52 (1989).

55. B. Matuszewska, G. G. Liversidge, F. Ryan, J. Dent, and P. L. Smith. In vitro study of intestinal absorption and metabolism of 8-L-arginine vasopressin and its analogues, *Int. J. Pharm. 46*, 111–120 (1988).
56. K. W. Garren, E. M. Topp, and A. J. Repta. Buccal absorption. III. Simultaneous diffusion and metabolism of an aminopeptidase substrate in the hamster cheek pouch, *Pharm. Res. 6*, 966–970 (1989).
57. M. Kidron, H. Bar-On, E. M. Berry, and E. Ziv. The absorption of insulin from various regions of the rat intestine, *Life Sci. 31*, 2837–2841 (1982).

17

Toxicological Evaluation of Intranasal Peptide and Protein Drugs

Michael A. Dorato
Lilly Research Laboratories, Division of Eli Lilly and Company, Greenfield, Indiana

I. INTRODUCTION

The historical development of intranasal drug administration and the developing recognition of the importance of the nasal passages have been reviewed by Chien and Chang [1] and Proctor [2,3]. Ancient cultures have employed the nasal route for therapy and for the administration of psychotropic and hallucinogenic substances. The importance of the nose in conditioning inspired air has been recognized since at least the time of Galen (the second century). In humans, the nose primarily serves to warm and humidify inspired air and to remove entrained particles. The nose (Fig. 1) also serves in olfaction, though not as importantly in humans as in most common laboratory animals. The attributes of the nasal cavity that allow for the efficient conditioning of inspired air, i.e., a large blood supply and surface area, also allow for the systemic absorption of pharmacologic agents.

Those agents particularly suited for intranasal administration are those that may be subject to significant first-pass metabolism, possess poor stability in the gastrointestinal tract, and/or show poor oral absorption [4,5]. Insulin, for example, was studied in intranasal delivery systems as early as 1922 [6]. Most commonly, drugs have been administered intranasally for their local effect on the nasal mucosa (e.g., antihistamines, decongestants).

The advent of recombinant DNA technology has facilitated the development of peptide and protein drugs as important therapeutic agents [7]. Because many

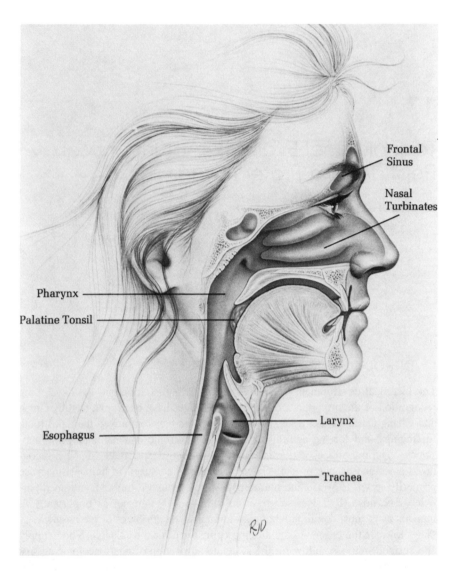

Figure 1   The human upper respiratory tract, showing position of nasal turbinates.

protein and peptide drugs are incompatible with the environment of the gastro-intestinal tract, they are usually administered parenterally. It has been recognized that the intranasal administration of peptide and protein drugs such as insulin [8], desmopressin [9], luteinizing hormone-releasing hormone (LHRH) [10], and others [4] provides a reasonable alternative to injection and protects the protein and/or peptide from the gastrointestinal tract. As experience is gained with intranasal formulations, it is expected that over the next ten years more drugs, peptides and proteins included, will be given by the intranasal route for systemic effects [7,11].

In evaluating laboratory studies of nasal irritation in animal models, one must understand the similarities and differences in anatomy between humans and animals. For example, most laboratory animals (which are macrosmatic, i.e., have a well-developed sense of smell) have a higher percentage of olfactory epithelium than do humans (microsmatic). This may account for the apparently greater sensitivity to the irritant potential of intranasal drug formulations in macrosmatic species. Though the macrosmatic species used in laboratory evaluations of intranasal irritation and toxicity may be more sensitive than humans, they still have relevance in evaluating effects of chronic use formulations. Differences in nasal anatomy between humans and laboratory animals may also affect dose and safety margins, particularly when dose is referenced to nasal surface area. The differences in sensitivity and safety margins must be kept in mind when extrapolating data from animals to humans.

A. Bioavailability of Peptides and Proteins

The bioavailability of peptide and protein drugs administered intranasally is often quite low. For example, LHRH, a low molecular weight polypeptide, had to be administered at significantly higher doses intranasally than parenterally [12]. The bioavailability of peptide and protein drugs administered intranasally generally decreases with increasing molecular weight [13–15]. Lee and Longenecker [13] reported that proteins composed of more than 27 amino acids have bioavailabilities of generally less than 1% (Fig. 2). The apparent multimodal nature of these data may be due to secondary and tertiary structure of the protein.

B. Penetration Enhancers

It has been found that the addition of surface-active agents appears to increase the permeability of the nasal mucosa to peptides and proteins [7,13,16–18]. Early in the development of intranasal insulin formulations, saponin was used to enhance the penetration of insulin into the nasal mucosa [8]. The addition of penetration enhancers to intranasal peptide and protein drug formulations affects toxicological evaluations. In most cases, the local and systemic effects of both the drug and the penetration enhancer should be evaluated, especially if the penetration enhancer is a new or little-known substance. Insulin alone applied

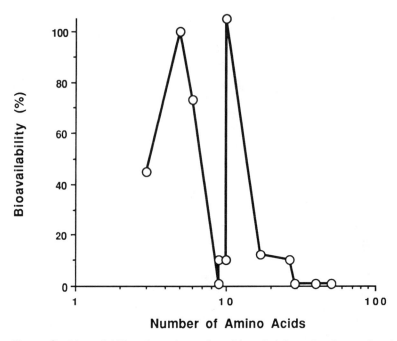

Figure 2 Bioavailability of proteins and peptides administered to the nasal cavity without penetration enhancers. (From [13].)

to the nasal mucosa is relatively nonirritating. Insulin in combination with common penetration enhancers has been reported to produce local toxicity, i.e., irritation, at the site of application (Table 1).

The mechanism of action of nasal penetration enhancers is largely unknown. Possible mechanisms include protein solubilization, protease inhibition, erosion of mucous membranes, membrane pore formation, and loosening of tight junctions. The chemical nature of penetration enhancers is diversified, and it is unlikely that any one mechanism will define the action of all agents. However, any of the mechanisms listed translate into concerns for the toxicologist, especially when the duration of use approaches that of an individual's lifetime.

II. METHOD OF INTRANASAL DRUG ADMINISTRATION

Drugs can be applied to the nasal mucosa in several ways: by dropper (direct nasal instillation); spray devices containing propellants, i.e., metered dose inhalers (MDIs); or spray devices without propellants, i.e., pump sprays and dry

Table 1 Local Toxicity of Intranasal Penetration Enhancers

Enhancer	Species	Local toxicity	Ref.
Bile salts	Human	Nasal irritation	18
		Ciliotoxicity	19
		Nasal burning and discomfort	20
Sodium glycocholate	Human	Nasal irritation and congestion	21
	Dog	Nasal irritation	22
	Rat	Nasal irritation	17
Laureth-9	Human	Nasal irritation	23
		No adverse effects	24
	Rat	Nasal irritation	25
Increased membrane temperature	Human	Rhinitis and nasal congestion	26
Glycyrrhetinic acid derivatives	Rat	No adverse effects	27
Sodium taurodihydrofusidate	Sheep	Minimal mucosal irritation	28

powder inhalers (DPIs). Significant differences in intranasal drug distribution have been reported depending on the method of intranasal administration [29–32]. Therefore the method of intranasal administration may affect the therapeutic efficacy and the toxicity of intranasal formulations. However, the literature does not present a unified view of advantages and disadvantages of common modes of intranasal drug administration. The mode of administration requires consideration prior to the design of toxicology studies. One must be aware of the potential differences in nasal deposition related to the method of delivery.

A. Drops vs. Sprays

Relative to distribution in the nasal cavity, both sprays and drops have had their supporters. Using the rabbit as a test model, Gundrum [29] found good distribution of instilled sulfanilamide nasal drops. In early studies of nasal deposition, drops were also found to be more effective than sprays in covering the nasal mucosa [30]. Others have found drops to be less efficient in delivering vasoconstrictor drugs to the normal nose [31]. Sprays were also reported to produce less nasal pathology than drops. Spray delivery systems were chosen in later studies because they distributed small volumes throughout the nasal cavity better than did drops [32]. In clinical studies of intranasal distribution of human serum albumin labeled with technetium-99m (^{99m}Tc), a significantly higher level of good nasal distribution was found after instillation as drops rather than as a spray [33]. Other workers using ^{99m}Tc labeled thiomersal [34] and beclomethasone [35] agreed that penetration of sprays was limited to the anterior portions

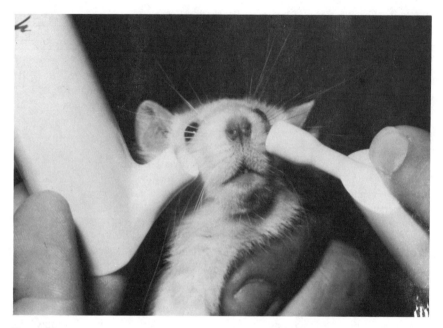

Figure 3 Size relationship of commercially available intranasal delivery system and a Fischer 344 rat.

of the nose, whereas drops spread more evenly. It was also reported that the better coverage of nasal mucosa seen with drops was independent of volume over the range of 0.1–0.75 mL [34]. Using ^{99m}Tc-labeled desmopressin [36], it was found that in humans, sprays deposited anteriorly in the nose and cleared back toward the nasopharynx. Drops were deposited posteriorly and cleared very rapidly, whereas sprays were absorbed better and had enhanced effects. The benefits of drops in comparison with sprays in terms of increased efficacy and decreased adverse effects are a major consideration in clinical and toxicological evaluations.

B. Special Considerations for Toxicology Studies

The administration of intranasal drug formulations to common laboratory animals (rats and dogs) presents a number of barriers to the use of commercially available spray devices. Commercial metered dose and pump spray aerosols are not compatible with the nasal anatomy of the rat (Fig. 3). Nasal instillation techniques utilizing microliter syringes with ground and polished 22 gauge needles have been used to administer intranasal compounds to the rat. The insertion depth of the syringes should be marked at about 7 mm. A dose volume of 20–50 μL/kg per nostril one to several times daily is common for conscious F-344 rats (approx. 200 g). Others have used total dose volumes of 50 μL [15] in anesthetized Wistar rats (260 g) and 30–40 μL [37] in anesthetized Sprague-Dawley rats (350–500 g).

Since the rat is an obligate nose-breathing animal, standard inhalation technology techniques could be used to study the effects of intranasal drugs on the rat nasal cavity. For example, nose-only inhalation chambers (Fig. 4) could be used effectively. Flow-past chambers (Fig. 5) providing fresh aerosol flow past each exposure port and immediate exhaust of exhaled air may provide an improved system for the study of intranasal drugs in rodents [38]. One must bear in mind that instillation and nose-only exposure techniques differ from clinical usage in that complete formulations are generally not used; that is, propellants are absent. The exposure pathlength is much greater in nose-only chambers than in the clinical application of an intranasal spray of any type. What is studied, however, is the effect of the drug and/or penetration enhancer on the nasal mucosa. For larger animals, the DeVilbiss atomizer administration system [39] was found to be quite appropriate (Fig. 6). This system is calibrated to deliver a known volume at a specified pressure and is marked for depth of insertion (1 cm for rabbits, 1.5 cm for dogs). Again, the test material may not exactly represent the final formulation (i.e., freons, etc.), but it will still give an evaluation of the effects of the drug and/or penetration enhancer on the nasal mucosa. In fact, the nasal anatomy of the rabbit may preclude the use of freon-propelled aerosols, and the alar fold in the dog nose makes for difficult and painful application using commercial metered dose inhalers.

III. PARTICLE SIZE

Particle size distribution is an important parameter relative to the action of inhaled aerosols in the respiratory tract. Particle size distribution determines the major sites of deposition in the respiratory tract. The emphasis on particle size distribution changes in consideration of the target site, nasal or pulmonary. Larger particles are preferable for nasal delivery because most will deposit in the target area of the nasal cavity and few will penetrate nontarget areas such as the lower respiratory tract.

A. Particle Deposition and Clearance

The nose is a well-designed filter for inhaled particulates. The principal mechanism of aerosol deposition in the nasal passages is impaction [40]. Aerosol deposition in the regions of the human respiratory tract (Fig. 7) has been ad-

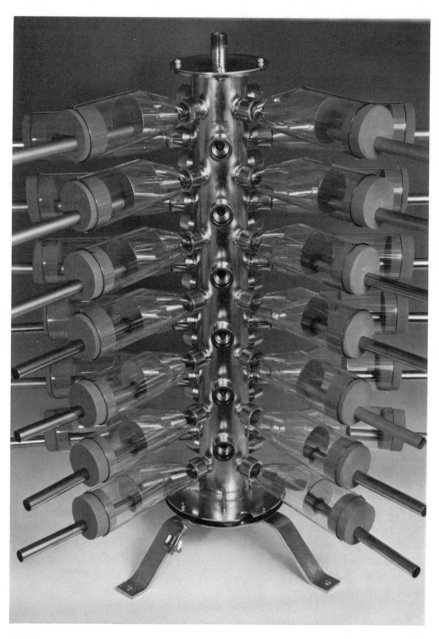

Figure 4   The flow-past nose-only inhalation exposure chamber and individual rat nose-only restraining tubes. (Lilly Research Laboratories.)

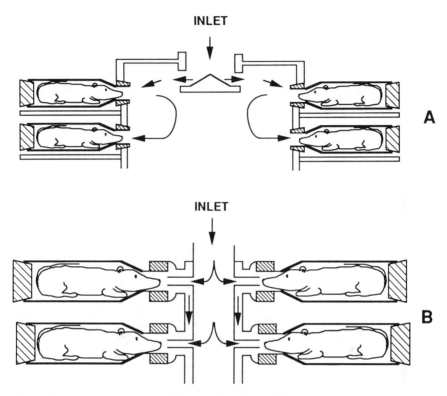

Figure 5 Schematic diagram of (A) traditional and (B) flow-past nose-only exposure chambers. (From [38].)

dressed by the Task Group on Lung Dynamics [41]. In general, deposition in the nasopharyngeal (N-P) region is limited to large particles [42,43]. Clearance of the anterior portion of the nose is generally slow and in a forward direction [42]. Material deposited on the ciliated portion of the nose clears to the nasopharynx and is either swallowed or expectorated [42]. Data reported by Mokler et al. [44] show a pattern of deposition in the respiratory tract regions of the F-344 rat similar to that shown in humans; however, the rat is shown to be more efficient in clearing inhaled particles in the nasal passages (Fig. 8). Most laboratory animals are more efficient in upper respiratory tract deposition, an important factor when choosing experimental models to study pulmonary toxicity. For intranasal aerosols, the disadvantage of differences in deposition characteristics between humans and animals is somewhat reduced. In fact, unlike adult humans, rodents and rabbits are obligate nose breathers and their exposure to aerosols is primarily via the nasal route [45]. This provides an advantage in

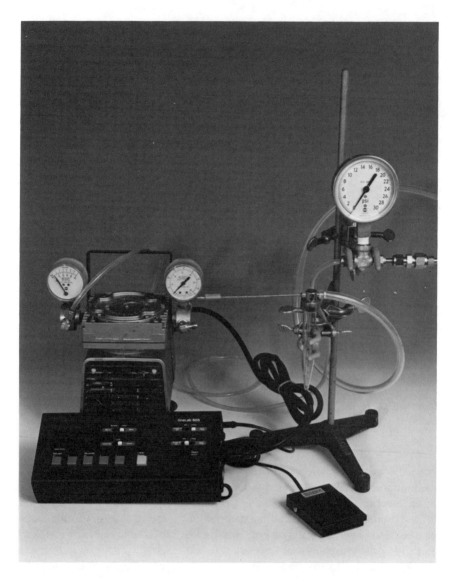

Figure 6   DeVilbiss 151 atomizer system used for intranasal administration in large animals. (Lilly Research Laboratories.)

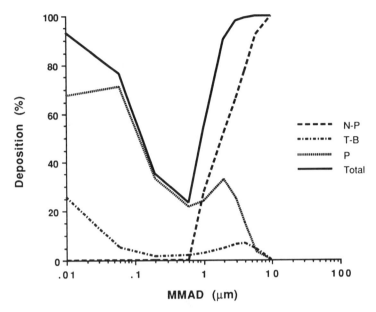

Figure 7   Size-related aerosol deposition in the nasopharyngeal (N-P), tracheobronchial (T-B), and pulmonary (P) regions of the human respiratory tract. Tidal volume = 1.45 liters. (From [41].)

that standard nose-only inhalation techniques could be used to evaluate the effect of intranasal drug formulations on the nasal mucosa.

B. Particle Size Distribution Measurements for Intranasal Aerosols

In studies of intranasal aerosols, particle size evaluations are conducted to demonstrate a high probability for nasal deposition in animals and humans and a low probability for penetration of the nasal chamber. Atomizers, by definition, produce relatively large aerosol particles, providing advantages relative to nasal deposition. MDIs generally produce smaller particles, which change in diameter with distance from the aerosol actuator due to the evaporation of the freon propellants. The cascade impactor provides a convenient source of particle size distribution data for all types of aerosols, including MDIs, DPIs, and pump sprays.

A primary concern in formulating intranasal aerosols is the relative proportions of small and large particles. Methods published on the use of cascade impactors in sizing metered dose aerosols generally use large-volume glass chambers to allow for droplet evaporation [46,47]. In actual use, the distance

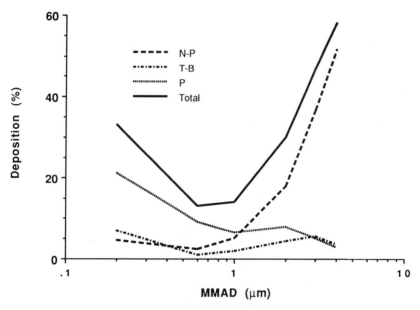

Figure 8 Size-related aerosol deposition in the nasopharyngeal (N-P), tracheobronchial (T-B), and pulmonary (P) regions of the F-344 rat respiratory tract. (From [44].)

traveled from actuator to impaction surface in the nose is probably insufficient to allow a significant decrease in particle size due to evaporation [48]. The use of large-volume chambers to estimate particle size, particularly when nasal penetration is of primary interest, may be unrealistic [35]. Although not identical to the nose, the cascade impactor cyclone provides a device with a vestibule, valve, and relatively short impaction pathlength. When an intranasal aerosol is evaluated with a system approximating nasal anatomy and airflow (i.e., a cascade impactor cyclone), a better estimation of nasal penetration and potential pulmonary exposure may be obtained (Table 2). The favorable comparison of the cascade impactor cyclone with the nose may be due to the sudden enlargement from the valve to the main chamber. Sudden enlargement in cross section, as from the nasal ostium (valve) to the main nasal chamber, is consistent with the conclusion that turbulent flow occurs in this region [43]. When operated at a flow rate of 10 liters/min, the impactor cyclone provides velocities at the vestibule and valve relatively similar to those estimated for the human nose (Table 2). The comparison is approximate, however, as velocity at the human nasal vestibule may be as high as 2–3 m/sec, and at the nasal valve may be as high as 12–18 m/sec [50].

Table 2 Comparison of Cascade Impactor Cyclone with the Human Nose

	Flow rate (cm³/sec)	Cross section		Velocity	
		Vestibule (cm²)	Valve (cm²)	Vestibule (cm/sec)	Valve (cm/sec)
Cascade impactor cyclone	166.67	4.15	0.64	40.16	260.42
Human nose	93.75[a]	1.4[b]	0.3[c]	66.96	312.5

[a]Task Group on Lung Dynamics [41]
[b]Schreider [49].
[c]Cole [50].

The particle size distribution of a freon-propelled MDI aerosol determined with a cascade impactor could vary with the sizing technique (Fig. 9). Particle size distribution was evaluated with either a cyclone preseparator or a glass chamber similar to that described by Yu et al. [47]. Using the cyclone preseparator, 11.7% of the particles were shown to be less than 3.7 μm in diameter. Using the glass chamber, 86.7% of the particles were shown to be smaller than

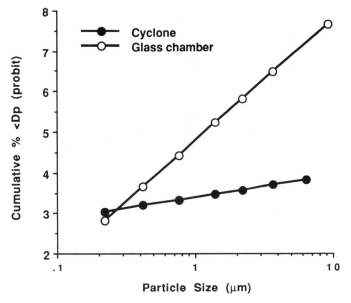

Figure 9 Particle size distribution of a metered-dose aerosol spray determined with a cascade impactor using a cyclone preseparator or a large-volume glass chamber.

3.7 μm. Since pulmonary exposure, as the result of nasal chamber penetration, is an undesirable factor with intranasal aerosols, this difference could be important when one is making decisions on nasal penetration and potential pulmonary exposure from an intranasal aerosol.

IV. NASAL ANATOMY AND DOSIMETRY

Preclinical toxicology evaluations are conducted in animals models. There is little doubt that the nasal cavities of common laboratory animals (e.g., rat, rabbit, dog, and monkey) differ from that of a human (Fig. 10). Excellent reviews of comparative nasal anatomy are available [49,51–53]. Humans and the higher apes have relatively simple noses, concerned primarily with conditioning inspired air through warming and humidification, and are therefore microsmatic [54]. Laboratory animals have more complex noses with highly developed olfactory epithelia and are therefore macrosmatic [51]. Gundrum [29] pointed out that the rabbit has a large olfactory area, probably more susceptible to injury than that of the human. The noses of humans and laboratory animals have major structural differences. For example, the nasal vestibule of rats contains atrioturbinates that act as effective particle impactors [51]. In addition, rats and other rodents have an opening in the nasal septum (septal window) that prevents either side of the nasal cavity from being treated separately [55]. Schreider [49] has presented a helpful comparison of the nasal anatomy of human, monkey, dog, and rat (Table 3). A comparison of nasal cavity surface area as a function of body weight shows the relationship rat > dog > monkey > human. Calculations of dose multiples in laboratory animals, relative to humans, are affected by these relationships. In a simplified example looking at a dose of 5 μL per nostril three times daily in human, monkey, rat, and dog, rats would be estimated to receive 300×, dogs 7.5×, and monkeys 10× the human dose on a body weight basis (Table 4). On a surface area basis, the multiples of human exposure for rats, dogs, and monkeys would be 15×, 0.5×, and 2.5×, respectively (Table 4). This represents a significant reduction in the safety margin of the local dose over the body dose. Although doses in toxicology studies are most often expressed on a mg/kg basis, expression of nasal dose on a surface area basis may be more appropriate when one is evaluating the nasal irritation potential of an intranasal formulation.

The relationship to clinical dose certainly changes dramatically based on weight or surface area. Nasal surface area, however, is difficult to derive. These relationships point out that the dose multiple difference between 1% and 10% formulations is not simply 10×. In actual use, however, the volumes administered in clinical studies can differ significantly from those used in toxicology studies, because the human nose more easily accommodates greater volumes.

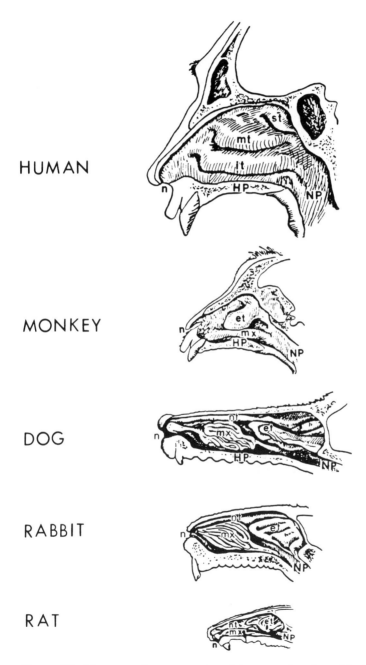

Figure 10 Diagrammatic representation of the mucosal surface of the lateral nasal wall and turbinates of the human, monkey, dog, rabbit, and rat. (Courtesy of Dr. J. Harkema.)

Table 3 Comparative Nasal Cavity Characteristics

	Rat	Dog	Monkey	Human
Weight (kg)	0.25	10.0	7.0	70.0
Nares cross section (mm^2)	0.7	16.7	22.9	140.0
Length (cm)	2.3	10.0	5.3	8.0
Surface area (cm^2)	10.4	220.7	61.6	181.0
Surface area/wt[a] (cm^2/kg)	41.6	22.1	8.8	2.6
Volume[b] (cm^3)	0.4	20.0	8.0	19.0
Turbinate complexity	Double scroll	Membranous scroll	Simple scroll	Simple scroll

[a]Both sides
Source: Schreider [49].

The mode of intranasal drug administration in preclinical toxicology studies is affected by test species. The nasal anatomy of rats, rabbits, dogs, and sometimes monkeys is not compatible with most commercially available metered dose units of either the pump spray or freon-propelled design. In rabbits, for example, studies conducted with a modified freon-propelled MDI produced significant turbinate and epithelial necrosis of similar severity and frequency in all treatment and control groups. Nasal drop instillation of the same formulation, absent freon, had no effect on the test animals. The damage in the MDI study occurred primarily in the area of the maxilloturbinate and was attributed to the anatomy of the rabbit nose (Fig. 10) and impaction of relatively large freon droplets. In the dog, the maxilloturbinate is located more posteriorly in the nasal cavity (Fig. 10), and the same freon-propelled MDI produced no adverse effects. The use

Table 4 Comparison of Dose on the Basis of Body Weight and Surface Area, Assuming Equivolume Administration, 5 μL/Nostril Three Times Daily, in Humans and Laboratory Animals

Species	Weight (kg)	Agent (% w/v)	mg/kg/day	mg/cm^2/nostril/day
Rat	0.25	1	1.2 (300×)	0.03 (15×)
Dog	10.0	1	0.03 (7.5×)	0.001 (0.5×)
Monkey	7.0	1	0.04 (10×)	0.005 (2.5×)
Human	70.0	1	0.004 (—)	0.002 (—)

of freon-propelled aerosols for direct intranasal spray in small laboratory animals, rather than nasal drop instillation, must be carefully considered.

Studies designed to qualitatively evaluate the distribution of dye instilled in the nasal cavity of small laboratory animals (i.e., rats) have emphasized the effect of technique on delivered dose. Intranasal instillations were conducted with a 22 gauge needle. In one case a blunt, smooth needle for instillation was used, whereas in the other an oral gavage tube was used. The blunt needle was placed 7 mm into the nostril, and the gavage tube was placed up against the external nares. The distribution of dye in the turbinal areas was greater using the 7-mm insertion depth. In intranasal toxicity studies performed in our laboratory, using the same protein/penetration enhancer formulation, groups of rats were dosed using the oral feeding tube technique or the 7-mm insertion depth technique. A significant difference in nasal irritation between the groups was attributed to the administration technique. The group dosed with the oral feeding tube did not show frank nasal pathology, but the other group did. In dogs, a modified Devilbiss 151 atomizer (Fig. 6) was found to pass the alar fold of the dog nose more easily than any available MDI actuator and provide good distribution in the turbinal region.

V. TOXICOLOGY STUDIES

The general objectives of toxicology studies with intranasal drugs are similar to those for drugs administered by any other route. In support of an Investigational New Drug Application (INDA), toxicology studies should (1) provide a preliminary working profile of the drug and/or other formulation components, (2) rule out possible cumulative or irreversible side effects, and (3) provide a database that will support early clinical trials and guide the design of subsequent toxicology studies. Post-INDA objectives are to confirm known adverse effects, expand the database to include long-term and developmental toxicity evaluations, and permit unimpeded expansion of ongoing clinical trials. The toxicology data should also provide information to make a reasonable product decision. The toxicology program for intranasal drugs (Table 5) differs from that used for any other type of therapy primarily in that the intranasal route of administration is used.

The use of penetration enhancers may complicate toxicity evaluations of intranasal drugs. Some penetration enhancers have been used in the food industry for long periods of time; some are essentially unknown. Even though a penetration enhancer may have GRAS (Generally Recognized As Safe) status in the food industry and thus be considered an excipient by formulation developers, this does not obviate the need for toxicology studies, including oncogenicity, when the substance is used in pharmaceutical formulations. The Commission of the European Communities [56] has stated that an excipient used for the first

Table 5   Proposed Toxicology Studies to
Support Development of an Intranasal
Formulation

Genetic toxicology
   Protein + penetration enhancer
Acute toxicology
   Parenteral and intranasal dosing
   Nasal irritation and mucociliary clearance
      Protein + penetration enhancer
Absorption, distribution, metabolism, and
   excretion
   Parenteral and intranasal dosing
      Protein + penetration enhancer
Medium-term toxicology
   Parenteral and intranasal dosing
      Protein + penetration enhancer
         clinical signs of irritation
         progression of toxic signs
         mucociliary clearance
Long-term/oncogenic toxicology
   Intranasal and other routes
      Protein and/or penetration enhancer
Developmental toxicology (fertility/teratology)
   Route to ensure systemic and fetal exposure
      Protein + penetration enhancer
Cardiovascular toxicology
   Intravenous route
      Protein + penetration enhancer

---

time in the pharmaceutical field should be treated like an active ingredient. Some
novel and known penetration enhancers have been combined with active ingredients that have a long clinical history, such as insulin. The missing information,
however, is often a database including years of clinical experience and/or long-
term toxicity data with a relevant route of administration, for the penetration
enhancer.

A.   Studies Supporting Clinical Trials

Toxicology studies supporting the clinical use of intranasal peptide and protein
drugs should address the systemic and local effects of both the drug and the
formulation components (Table 5). Local effects such as irritation, cell damage,
and altered clearance mechanisms can be exerted by either the drug or the penetration enhancer. If absorbed, either has the potential to produce systemic tox-

icity. Genetic toxicology screens are conducted with the drug, the penetration enhancer, and the complete formulation when possible. Acute studies are conducted using intranasal and intravenous routes, considering the formulation and its components. Absorption, distribution, metabolism, and excretion (ADME) studies are conducted intranasally, and the results are compared to what may already be known for oral and parenteral routes. The nose is known to be metabolically active, and ADME data will help to establish the utility of systemic exposure data from other routes [57–59]. Medium-term studies of various durations, from 2 weeks to 6 months, are conducted, with the duration dependent upon the proposed clinical study duration. These studies can be conducted with the drug and/or penetration enhancer and may involve intranasal plus other routes of administration. In the medium-term studies, it is important to evaluate the progression of clinical signs of toxicity and histopathologic findings. As an example, studies were conducted in our laboratory with an intranasal protein/penetration enhancer formulation administered to rats. Clinical signs of nasal irritation, including struggling, sneezing, salivation, head shaking, and nose rubbing, were seen in studies of less than 90 days. In studies of 90 days duration, histologic signs of nasal irritation were seen, including inflammation of septal and turbinate mucosal surfaces (Fig. 11), epithelial and submucosal infiltration of inflammatory cells, purulent exudate, and secondary mucosal hyperplasia. The progression of clinical signs of irritation to frank histopathology from 30 days to 90 days indicates a potential problem with increasing duration of use. Studies of the penetration enhancer alone indicated only goblet cell hypertrophy (Fig. 12). Goblet cell changes in the respiratory epithelium may result from irritation, as a direct or adaptive response (e.g., increased efficiency of mucociliary clearance) [60]. The difference in intensity of response between the protein/penetration enhancer formulation and the penetration enhancer alone was attributed to differences in intranasal instillation technique, as outlined above. Studies of the same intranasal formulation in dogs indicated severe clinical signs of nasal irritation at 30 days, related to the concentration of the penetration enhancer (Fig. 13).

It must be remembered that, owing to the greater percentage of olfactory epithelium, the nasal mucosa of laboratory animals may well be more sensitive to potential irritants than that of humans [29]. Laboratory animals may therefore present a more severe response in a shorter period of time. This becomes less important when the intranasal drug is to be administered for the lifetime of an individual. Long-term fertility/teratology and oncogenic studies should also be planned relative to concern over local and systemic effects. Depending on the clinical history of the protein involved, the focus may be on the penetration enhancer. The combination of a drug with growth-promoting properties (e.g., insulin, growth hormone) and a penetration enhancer believed to be a nasal

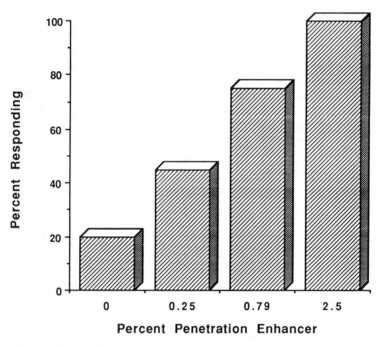

Figure 11 Nasal turbinate inflammation in Fischer-344 rats treated for 90 days with an intranasal protein/penetration enhancer formulation, via nasal instillation with a 22 gauge polished needle inserted to a depth of 7 mm.

irritant may require the evaluation of the complete formulation in oncogenic studies.

In most studies, with an intranasal formulation, intranasal administration would be the most appropriate route. However, in developmental and cardiovascular toxicity studies one may wish to administer the test material parenterally in order to maximize exposure of the test system. Regardless, specific protocols for intranasal toxicity studies are similar to those for any other route of administration. The major variation is in histopathology. It has been suggested that gross examination of the nasal cavity at necropsy severely limits useful histopathologic examination for nonneoplastic effects [61]. However, fixed, decalcified nasal tissue can be examined without destroying anatomic relationships.

B. Screening Procedures for Nasal Irritation

There are many approaches to identifying the toxic potential of intranasal formulations. Short-term tests, while having distinct disadvantages when compared

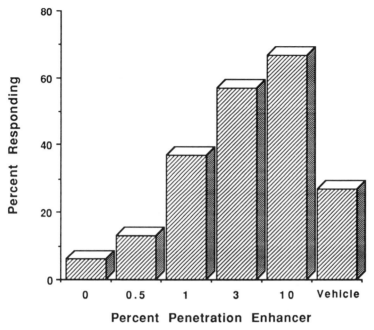

Figure 12 Goblet cell hypertrophy in Sprague-Dawley rats treated for 90 days with an intranasal penetration enhancer, via nasal instillation with a 22 gauge oral feeding tube positioned at the external nares.

to repeat dose studies, can provide a basis for early decisions about intranasal formulations.

1. Acute Effect on Nasal Mucosa

A convenient method for studying nasal absorption and irritation has been described by Hussain et al. [62] and Hirai et al. [16]. Briefly, anesthetized rats are surgically prepared to allow retrograde perfusion of the nasal cavity (Fig. 14). The nasopalatine is closed with a surgical adhesive to prevent drainage of the nasal cavity to the mouth. The animals breathe through a tracheal cannula during the course of the procedure. Histologic evaluation of nasal sections allow evaluation of dose-related epithelial cell necrosis and sluffing. This procedure has been used to show a dose/concentration response in damage to the nasal mucosa from intranasal clofilium tosylate (Fig. 15). Intranasal penetration enhancers have also been evaluated for short-term irritation to the nasal mucosa. One percent solutions of either polyoxyethylene 9-lauryl ether (Fig. 16) or sodium deoxycholate (Fig. 17) were used to flood the nasal cavity of rats. The solutions remained in the nasal cavity for 5 min before fixing. A comparison with rats

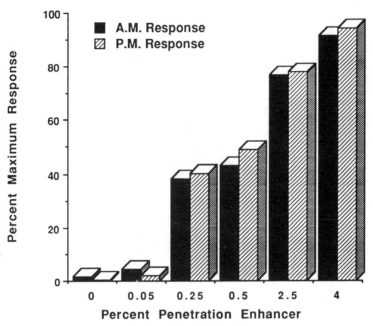

Figure 13 Clinical response in beagles treated for 30 days with an atomized intranasal protein/penetration enhancer formulation. The maximum response was determined as the total number of positive incidences of struggling, sneezing, salivation, head shaking, and nose rubbing, observed twice daily in four dogs for 30 days (max. response = 1200).

treated for 15 min with phosphate-buffered saline (Fig. 18) shows the dramatic effect of intranasal penetration enhancers on nasal mucosa.

2. Sensory Irritation of the Upper Airway

Reflex inhibition of respiratory rate, characterized by an expiratory pause, in response to nasal inhalation of irritating substances is a well-established response and has been reported in a number of species [64,65]. The observed decrease in respiratory rate was demonstrated to depend on irritant concentration [66]. Stimulation of trigeminal nerve endings in the nasal mucosa (Fig. 19) has been shown to exert a modulating effect on respiratory rate [68]. Responses in the mouse were shown to correlate very well with responses in humans in tests with a series of chemicals [69]. A standard procedure for estimating the sensory irritation of airborne chemicals, in mice, has been established [70]. Briefly, groups of four mice are placed in plethysmographs (Fig. 20) and conditioned to the exposure apparatus for about 10 min. The mice are then exposed nose-only

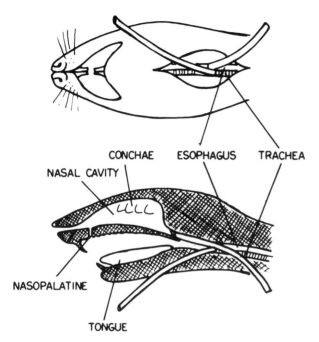

Figure 14 Diagram of the surgical procedure and cannulation arrangement for acute nasal irritation studies in the rat. (From [62]); reproduced with permission of the copyright owner, the American Pharmaceutical Association.)

for 10 min to increasing concentrations of the test substance. The exposure period is followed by a recovery period of approximately 5 min. Each aerosol exposure level is evaluated in triplicate ($n = 12$). The mouse, being an obligate nose-breathing animal, is a relevant model for aerosol effects on the nasal mucosa. A concentration-related decrease in respiratory rate was found for those substances that stimulate free nerve endings in the nasal mucosa (e.g., sodium lauryl sulfate). The concentration that produces a 50% decrease in respiratory rate (RD_{50}) is then calculated from the concentration response data [70,71].

The upper airway response of two potential intranasal penetration enhancers, sodium deoxycholate (Fig. 21) and a 1:1 combination of Tween-85 and oleic acid (Fig. 22), shows that sodium deoxycholate is about 4–5 times as irritating to the nasal mucosa as is the Tween-85/oleic acid system (Table 6). When faced with evaluating many chemicals within a structure–activity relationship or a number of potential intranasal penetration enhancers, this procedure provides comparative information quickly, at early stages of development, in a system that has been shown to be predictive for humans.

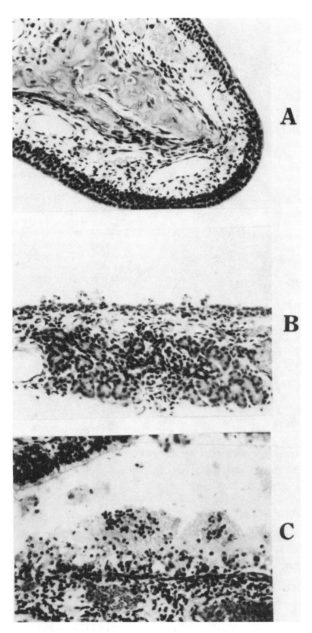

Figure 15 Nasal mucosa of Sprague-Dawley rats given intranasal clofilium tosylate. (A) Control, (B) 0.6 mg/kg, (C) 1.2 mg/kg. (From [63], reproduced with permission of the copyright owner, the American Pharmaceutical Association.)

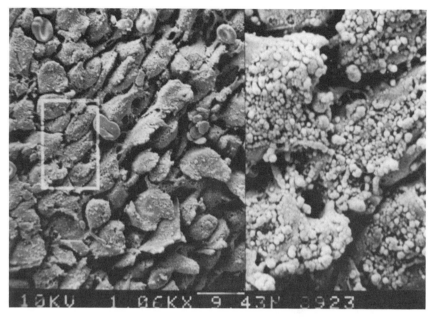

Figure 16 Scanning electron micrograph of rat nasal mucosa treated with a 1% solution of polyoxyethylene 9-lauryl ether for 5 min. (Courtesy of California Biotechnology, Inc., Mountain View, CA.)

3. Airway Lavage

Bronchoalveolar lavage from animals exposed for a short time to various chemical agents, either by inhalation or by intratracheal instillation, has proved useful as a rapid screen for lung injury [72,73]. This procedure has been useful in mice, gerbils, hamsters, rats, guinea pigs, and rabbits [72]. Lactate dehydrogenase (LDH) activity and isozyme patterns have been well established as indicators of tissue injury [74]. Many parameters can be evaluated in lavage procedures (Table 7). Although they were effective in determining relatively specific injury to the lower respiratory tract, it has been reported that lavage techniques were not effective in detecting injuries to the upper respiratory tract [76]. The upper respiratory tract epithelium is, however, the site of first contact of inhaled materials with the body. The nose is potentially a major target of toxic damage. If damage occurs, indicators of adverse effects (enzymes released from cells, inflammatory cells, etc.) should be present in the fluid covering the respiratory mucosa and thus be available for sampling by lavage [77]. A nasal lavage procedure has been developed for the upper and lower respiratory tract of the cat for the purpose of investigating cellular and humoral mechanisms of defense

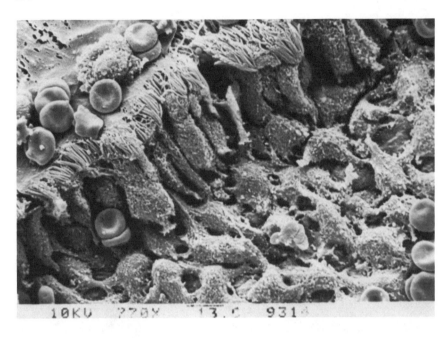

Figure 17 Scanning electron micrograph of rat nasal mucosa treated with a 1% solution of sodium deoxycholate for 5 min. (Courtesy of California Biotechnology, Inc., Mountain View, CA.)

and disease [78]. Nasal lavage may serve as a sensitive and reliable technique to detect inflammation in the upper airways in response to inhaled pollutants [79].

To evaluate the potential adverse effects of intranasal formulations on the upper respiratory tract, mice are placed in plethysmographs (as in sensory irritation studies, Fig. 20) and exposed nose-only to various concentrations of penetration enhancer. In order to compare nasal and bronchoalveolar lavage, LDH was evaluated in lavage fluid from both regions. Mice were anesthetized with ketamine (100 mg/kg) plus rompum (25 mg/kg) administered intraperitoneally. Nasal lavage was conducted according to the procedure described by Hussain et al. [62]. The nasal cavity was rinsed with warm saline solution (0.02 mL/g body weight) via a PE 90 cannula. Nasal lavage fluid from each of the four animals in each exposure group was pooled. The lower respiratory tract lavage was conducted as described by Mauderly [72]. The lungs were lavaged with warm saline solution (0.02 mL/g body weight). After 1 min, the lavage fluid was slowly aspirated. Lavage fluid recovery was generally greater than 80%. Pulmonary lavage fluid from each of the four animals in each exposure group was pooled. The lavage experiments were carried out in conjunction with upper

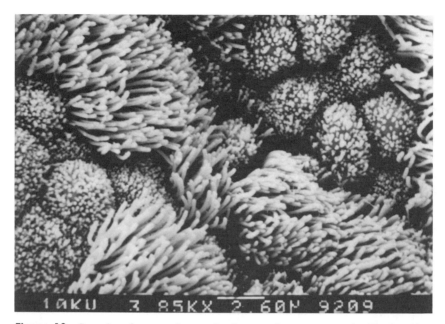

Figure 18 Scanning electron micrograph of rat nasal mucosa treated with phosphate-buffered saline for 15 min. (Courtesy of California Biotechnology, Inc., Mountain View, CA.)

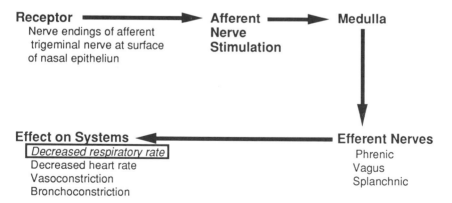

Figure 19 Pathway involved in producing the characteristic decrease in respiratory rate following exposure to a nasal irritant. (From [67].)

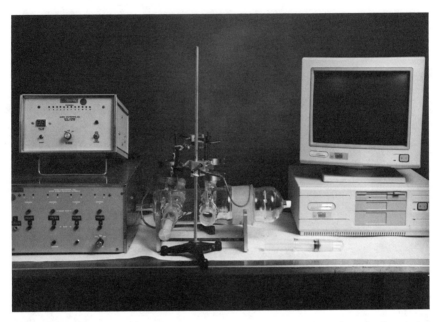

Figure 20 Glass exposure chamber (2.5 liters), plethysmograph, and monitoring equipment used to monitor sensory irritation of the upper airways in groups of four mice. (Lilly Research Laboratories.)

airway irritation studies and were conducted in triplicate ($n = 3$). LDH in the upper and lower airway lavage fluid, following exposure to sodium deoxycholate (Fig. 23) and Triton X-100 (Fig. 24) demonstrates the usefulness of upper airway lavage as an early indicator of adverse effects on the respiratory tract. An increase in lavage fluid LDH was seen for both surfactants. Sodium deoxycholate produced LDH elevations in both the upper and lower respiratory tract lavage fluid. Triton X-100 produced a much greater LDH effect in the upper respiratory tract lavage fluid. The data are expressed as percent LDH in lavage fluid from mice exposed to deionized water aerosol. The upper airway control was 17 IU LDH/liter, the lower airway control was 62 IU LDH/liter. The usefulness of lavage fluid analysis is greater as a comparative measurement of similar agents and somewhat less useful when comparing agents that act through different mechanisms [80].

4. Nasal Ciliary Function

Effect on ciliary function, in addition to frank damage, is a major concern relative to intranasal drug formulations. Little is known, however, about short- or long-term effects on nasal mucociliary activity as a result of intranasal drug

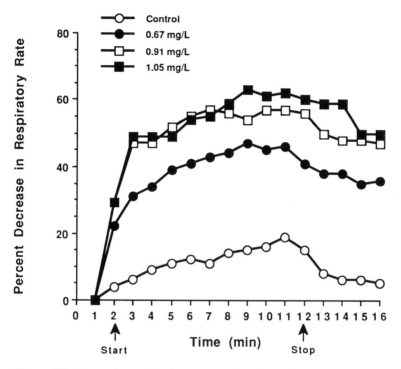

Figure 21 Upper airway irritation response in male Swiss mice exposed for 10 min to an aerosol of sodium deoxycholate, an intranasal penetration enhancer ($n = 12$).

administration. Ciliostatic effects have been reported for preservative components of intranasal formulations such as benzalkonium chloride [81]. In in vitro systems, ciliotoxicity of bile salts was shown to increase with increasing hydrophobicity [19]. Sodium deoxycholate, a bile salt used as an intranasal penetration enhancer, has been shown to be extremely ciliotoxic [19]. Mucociliary dysfunction is an important consideration for pathogenesis in the nasal cavity [82]. Therefore, both morphologic and functional effects of intranasal drug formulations on the nasal epithelium should be evaluated. In clinical studies, saccharin particles have been used to evaluate mucociliary clearance rates before and after intranasal drug administration [83]. This method, however, is not readily adaptable to studies in laboratory animals. In both clinical and laboratory studies, the movement of radioactive or radio-opaque tracers has been used to study the effect of intranasal drug administration on nasal ciliary function [84–86]. The need to study local side effects of intranasal drugs and other formulation components increases in importance for long-term use formulations such as insulin.

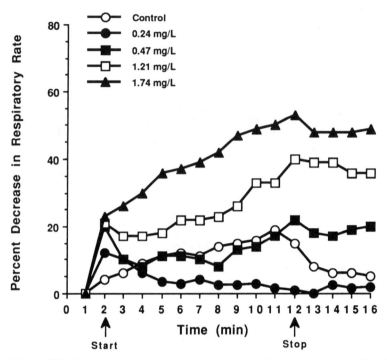

Figure 22 Upper airway irritation response in male Swiss mice exposed for 10 min to an aerosol of Tween-85/oleic acid (1:1), an intranasal penetration enhancer (n = 12).

VI. CONCLUSION

The nasal cavity serves primarily to condition and filter inhaled air in micros-matic species (humans and higher apes) and in addition plays an important olfactory role in macrosmatic species (most laboratory animals). It is the surface area and vascularity of the nasal cavity that make it an acceptable site for de-livery of peptide and protein drugs that might otherwise be poorly absorbed or

Table 6 Comparative Upper Airway Irritation of Selected Surfactants in the Mouse

Surfactant	RD_{50} (mg/liter)
Oleic acid/Tween-85	2.9
Sodium deoxycholate	0.71
Sodium lauryl sulfate	0.17

Table 7 Indicators of Acute Injury in Airway Lavage Fluid

Parameter	Location	Interpretation
LDH	Cytosol	Cell membrane permeability/lysis
Total protein	Extracellular	Transudation across capillary membranes
Sialic acid	Mucus and glycoproteins	Increased mucus secretion and transudation of serum glycoproteins

Source: Henderson et al. [74].

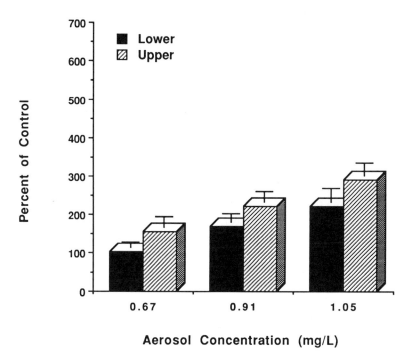

Figure 23 Lactate dehydrogenase in airway lavage fluid of male Swiss mice exposed for 10 min to an aerosol of sodium deoxycholate ($n = 3$).

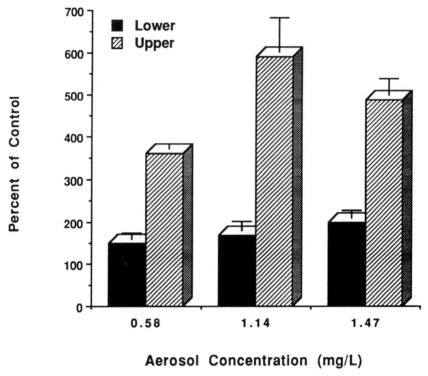

Figure 24 Lactate dehydrogenase in airway lavage fluid of male Swiss mice exposed for 10 min to an aerosol of Triton X-100, a surfactant ($n = 3$).

experience considerable metabolism and/or degradation in the gastrointestinal tract. Studies have shown that the nose is susceptible to injury when exposed to irritating environmental toxicants [87]. Adverse effects on structure and function of the nasal cavity are also a concern for intranasal drug formulations. The nasal mucociliary clearance mechanism is the respiratory tract's first line of defense against inhaled toxicants and infectious organisms.

The consequences of temporary effects on mucociliary activity related to the use of intranasal drug formulations are unknown. Therefore, effects on this system must be given attention in early toxicology evaluations and in subsequent clinical studies. The effects related to destruction and removal of cilia are relatively easily detected. Ciliary dysfunction, without major cell death, may only be evaluated using a functional assay, i.e., mucociliary clearance. The proposed mechanisms for surfactants used as penetration enhancers (e.g., erosion of mucous membrane, membrane pore formation, or loosening of tight junctions) may also aid in the transport of environmental toxicants and infectious agents as well as the intended peptide or protein drug. Therefore, susceptibility to infectious or toxic agents following short-term and long-term treatment with an intranasal formulation may become an issue [88].

In general, toxicology programs for the development of intranasal peptide and protein drug formulations are very similar to those used to support drug safety by other routes of administration. The unique aspects of intranasal administration focus on evaluation of local effects on nasal cavity epithelium, irritation, histopathology, and mucociliary function. Evaluation of effects of intranasal drug formulations on the nasal cavity begins with a battery of screening methods such as histologic evaluation of short-term effects on nasal mucosa [62,63], sensory irritation [65], airway lavage [73], and/or direct measurements of mucociliary function [86]. As a battery, these procedures are helpful in early detection of respiratory tract injury and in determination of the relative irritant and/or toxic potential of intranasal formulations and/or penetration enhancers.

Longer term studies (i.e., 30, 60, 90 days to one year) will provide a basis for evaluating the progression of toxic signs and symptoms with continued use of a particular formulation. As outlined above, 30-day studies with an intranasal protein/enhancer formulation provided information on dose-related clinical signs of nasal irritation but showed no histological effects. Ninety-day studies on the same formulation showed histologic changes in the nasal cavity. The progression of toxic effects is a significant finding for long-term use intranasal formulations and should be a major consideration in designing and evaluating toxicity studies.

A rational, reasonable approach to drug safety evaluation requires that proposed intranasal peptide and protein drug formulations be evaluated for potential local and systemic effects. Toxicology data may exist for other routes of administration and could be used to establish the potential for systemic toxicity. The nose, however, is known to be metabolically active [57–59]. Therefore, the use of existing toxicology data sets requires knowledge of metabolism via all relevant routes of administration.

Despite the long history that exists with some protein drugs (e.g., insulin), the addition of a penetration enhancer affects the complexity of the toxicologic evaluation of the formulation. Long-term toxicity studies with the entire formulation and with the penetration enhancer alone may be necessary. This is especially true if the local and systemic toxicity of the penetration enhancer is relatively unknown and if it is present in high concentration compared to the protein or peptide. Also, protein drugs with growth-promoting activity combined with potentially irritating penetration enhancers may be of particular concern, especially considering the relative lack of rotation sites for administration of intranasal formulations. There are no absolute answers about the most appropriate way to evaluate intranasal formulations, the strategy being dependent on the duration and frequency of use and the properties of the individual formulation components. Also, there are no specific regulatory guidelines relative to evaluating potential intranasal peptide and protein drug formulations. The goal of such evaluations is to evaluate potential local and systemic effects of the active ingredient and other components of the formulation.

REFERENCES

1. Y. W. Chien and S. F. Chang, in *Transnasal Systemic Medication*, Y. W. Chien, Ed., Elsevier, New York, 1985, pp. 1–100.
2. D. F. Proctor, in *The Nose: Upper Airway Physiology and the Atmospheric Environment*, D. F. Proctor and I. Andersen, Eds., Elsevier, New York, 1982, pp. 1–23.
3. D. F. Proctor, *Am. Rev. Resp. Dis. 115*, 97 (1977).
4. S. W. Bond, in *Drug Delivery to the Respiratory Tract*, D. Ganderton and T. Jones, Eds., Ellis Horwood, New York, 1987, pp. 133–139.
5. J. L. Colaizzi, in *Transnasal Systemic Medication*, Y. W. Chien, Ed., Elsevier, New York, 1985, pp. 107–119.
6. R. T. Woodyatt, *J. Metab. Res. 2*, 793 (1922).
7. K. S. E. Su, *Pharm. Int. 7*, 8 (1986).
8. W. S. Collens and M. A. Goldzieher, *Proc. Soc. Exp. Biol. Med. 29*, 756 (1932).
9. A. S. Harris, I. M. Nilsson, Z. G. Wagner, and V. Alkner, *J. Pharm. Sci. 75*, 1085 (1986).
10. G. Fink, G. Gennser, P. Liedholm, J. Thorell, and J. Mulder, *J. Endocrinol. 63*, 351 (1974).
11. M. Gibaldi, *Perspect. Clin. Pharm. 6*, 65 (1988).
12. S. Anik, G. McRae, C. Nerenberg, A. Worden, J. Foreman, H. Jiin-Hu, S. Kushinsky, R. Jones, and B. Vickery, *J. Pharm. Sci. 73*, 684 (1984).
13. W. A. Lee and J. P. Longenecker, *Biopharmacology 4*, 30 (1988).
14. C. McMartin, L. E. F. Hutchinson, R. Hyde, and G. E. Peters, *J. Pharm. Sci. 76*, 535 (1987).
15. A. N. Fisher, K. Brown, S. S. Davis, G. D. Parr, and D. A. Smith, *J. Pharm. Pharmacol. 39*, 357 (1986).
16. S. Hirai, J. Yashiki, and H. Mima, *Int. J. Pharm. 9*, 165 (1981).
17. Y. Hirata, T. Yokosuka, T. Kasahara, M. Kikuchi, and K. Oai, *Excerpta Med. Int. Congr. Ser. 468*, 319 (1979).
18. G. S. Gordon, A. C. Moses, R. D. Silver, J. S. Flier, and M. C. Carey, *Proc. Natl. Acad. Sci. U.S.A. 82*, 7419 (1985).
19. G. Duchateau, J. Zuidema, and F. Merkus, *Int. J. Pharm. 31*, 193 (1986).
20. R. D. Silver and J. S. Flier, *IDF Bull. 24*, 94 (1988).
21. A. C. Moses, G. S. Gordon, M. C. Carey, and J. S. Flier, *Diabetes 32*, 1040 (1983).
22. S. Hirai, T. Ikenaga, and T. Matsuzama, *Diabetes 27*, 296 (1978).
23. R. Salzman, J. E. Manson, G. T. Griffing, R. Kimmerle, N. Ruderman, A. McCall, E. I. Stultz, C. Mullin, D. Small, J. Armstrong, and J. C. Melby, *N. Engl. J. Med. 312*, 1078 (1985).
24. N. Paquot, A. J. Scheen, P. Franchmont, and P. J. Lefebvre, *Diabetes Metab. (Paris) 14*, 31 (1988).

25. B. J. Aungst, N. J. Rogers, and E. Shefter, *J. Pharmacol. Exper. Ther. 244*, 23 (1987).
26. W. S. Collens and M. A. Goldzieher, *Proc. Soc. Exp. Biol. Med. 29*, 756 (1932).
27. M. Mishima, S. Okada, Y. Wakita, and M. Nakano, *J. Pharmacobio-Dyn. 12*, 31 (1989).
28. J. P. Longenecker, A. C. Moses, J. S. Flier, R. D. Silver, M. C. Carey, and E. J. Dubevi, *J. Pharm. Sci. 76*, 351 (1987).
29. L. K. Gundrum, *Arch. Otolaryngol. 37*, 209 (1943).
30. V. E. Henderson, M. L. Beach, and J. F. A. Johnston, *Can. M.A.T. 24*, 684 (1931).
31. D. B. Butler and A. C. Ivy, *Arch. Otolaryngol. 39*, 109 (1944).
32. G. A. Elliott and E. N. DeYoung, *Ann. N.Y. Acad. Sci. 173*, 169 (1970).
33. F. Y. Aoki and J. C. W. Crawley, *Br. J. Clin. Pharmacol. 3*, 869 (1976).
34. J. G. Hardy, S. W. Lee, and C. G. Wilson, *J. Pharm. Pharmacol. 37*, 294 (1984).
35. G. W. Hallworth and J. M. Padfield, *J. Allergy Clin. Immunol. 77*, 348 (1986).
36. A. S. Harris, I. M. Nilsson, Z. G. Wagner, and U. Alkner, *J. Pharm. Sci. 11*, 1085 (1986).
37. G. C. Visor, E. Bajka, and E. Benjamin, *J. Pharm. Sci. 75*, 44 (1986).
38. W. C. Cannon, E. F. Blanton, and K. E. McDonald, *Am. Ind. Hyg. Assoc. J. 44*, 923 (1983).
39. G. A. Elliott, E. N. DeYoung, A. Purmalis, P. A. Triemstra, and B. A. Whited, in *Inhalation Toxicology and Technology*, B. K. J. Leong, Ed., Ann Arbor Science, Ann Arbor, MI, 1981, pp. 263–272.
40. R. F. Hoonan, A. Black, and M. Walsh, in *Inhaled Particles, III*, W. H. Walton, Ed., Unwin, London, 1971, pp. 71–80.
41. Task Group on Lung Dynamics, *Health Phys. 12*, 173 (1966).
42. O. G. Raabe, in *Mechanisms in Respiratory Toxicology*, Vol. 1, H. Witschi and P. Nettershein, Eds., CRC Press, Boca Raton, FL, 1982, p. 58.
43. D. L. Swift, *Ann. Biomed. Eng. 9*, 593 (1981).
44. B. V. Mokler, E. G. Damon, T. R. Henderson, R. L. Carpenter, S. A. Benjamin, A. H. Rebar, and R. K. Jones, in *Lovelace Inhalation Toxicology Research Institute Annual Report*, LF-66, NTIS, U.S. Dept. of Commerce, Springfield, VA, 1979.
45. O. G. Raabe, M. A. Al-Bayati, S. V. Teague, and A. Raselt, *Ann. Occup. Hyg. 32*, 53 (1988).
46. G. P. Polli, W. M. Grin, F. A. Backer, and M. H. Yunker, *J. Pharm. Sci. 58*, 484 (1969).
47. C. D. Yu, R. E. Jones, and M. Henesian, *J. Pharm. Sci. 73*, 344 (1984).
48. F. Moren and J. Andersson, *Int. J. Pharm. 6*, 295 (1980).
49. J. P. Schreider, in *Toxicology of the Nasal Passages*, C. S. Barrow, Ed., Hemisphere, Washington, DC, 1986, pp. 1–23.
50. P. Cole, in *The Nose: Upper Airway Physiology and the Atmosphere Environment*, D. Proctor and I. Andersen, Eds., Elsevier, New York, 1982, pp. 166–167.
51. D. F. Proctor and J. C. F. Chang, in *Nasal Tumors in Animals and Man*, Vol. 1, G. Reznik and S. Stinson, Eds., CRC Press, Boca Raton, FL, 1985, pp. 1–33.
52. E. A. Gross, J. A. Swenberg, S. Fields, and J. A. Popp, *J. Anat. 135*, 83 (1982).
53. A. Patra, *J. Toxicol. Environ. Health 17*, 163 (1986).

54. D. F. Proctor, *Am. Rev. Resp. Dis. 115*, 97 (1977).
55. G. Kelemen and F. Sargent, *Arch. Otolaryngeal. 44*, 24 (1946).
56. Directive 81/852/EEC, *Off. J. Eur. Commun. L317*, 16 (1981).
57. M. S. Bogdanffy, H. W. Randall, and K. T. Morgan, *Toxicol. Appl. Pharmacol. 88*, 183 (1987).
58. A. Dahl, in *Current Topics and Pulmonary Pharmacology and Toxicology*, M. A. Hollinger, Ed., Elsevier, New York, 1986, pp. 143–146.
59. R. E. Stratford and V. H. L. Lee, *J. Pharm. Sci. 74*, 731 (1985).
60. G. T. Burger, R. A. Renne, J. W. Sagartz, P. H. Ayres, D. R. E. Coggins, A. T. Mossberg, and A. W. Hayes, *Toxicol. Appl. Pharmacol. 101*, 521 (1989).
61. J. T. Young, *Fund. Appl. Toxicol. 1*, 309 (1981).
62. A. Hussain, S. Hirai, and R. Bawarshi, *J. Pharm. Sci. 69*, 1411 (1980).
63. K. S. E. Su, K. M. Campanale, and C. L. Gries, *J. Pharm. Sci.* 1251 (1984).
64. A. F. Kratschmer, *Akad. Wiss. Lit. Abh. Math. Naturwiss. Kl. 62*, 147 (1870).
65. Y. Alarie, *CRC Crit. Rev. Toxicol. 2*, 299 (1973).
66. Y. Alarie, *Arch. Environ. Health 13*, 433 (1966).
67. Y. Alarie, *Toxicol. Appl. Pharmacol. 24*, 279 (1973).
68. C. E. Ulrich and M. P. Haddock, *Arch. Environ. Health 24*, 37 (1972).
69. L. E. Kane, C. S. Barrow, and Y. Alarie, *Am. Ind. Hyg. J. 40*, 207 (1979).
70. *Annual Book of ASTM Standards*, ASTM, Philadelphia, 1985, pp. 569–584.
71. Y. Alarie, C. Kane, and C. Barrow, in *Toxicology: Principles and Practices*, A.L. Reeves, Ed., Wiley, New York, 1980, pp. 48–92.
72. J. L. Mauderly, *Lab. Animal Sci. 27*, 255 (1977).
73. R. F. Henderson, E. G. Damon, and T. R. Henderson, *Toxicol. Appl. Pharmacol. 44*, 291 (1978).
74. F. Wroblewski, *Am. J. Med. Sci. 234*, 301 (1957).
75. R. F. Henderson, *Environ. Health Perspec. 56*, 115 (1984).
76. R. F. Henderson, R. K. Wolff, A. H. Rebar, D. B. DeNicola, and R. L. Beethe, in *Lovelace Inhalation Toxicology Research Institute Annual Report*, LF-60, NTIS, U.S. Dept. of Commerce, Springfield, VA, 1978, pp. 352–355.
77. R. F. Henderson, J. M. Bensen, F. F. Hahn, C. H. Hobbs, R. K. Jones, J. L. Mauderly, R. O. McClellan, and J. A. Pickrell, *Fund. Appl. Toxicol. 5*, 451 (1985).
78. G. McCarthy and P. J. Quinn, *Irish Vet. J. 40*, 6 (1986).
79. H. S. Koren, G. E. Hatch, and D. E. Graham, *Toxicology 60*, 15 (1990).
80. B. A. Beck, B. Gerson, H. A. Feldman, and J. D. Brain, *Toxicol. Appl. Pharmacol. 71*, 59 (1983).
81. N. G. Toremalm, *Eur. J. Respir. Dis. 66*, 54 (1985).
82. Subcommittee on Pulmonary Toxicology, *Biologic Markers in Pulmonary Toxicology*, National Academy Press, Washington, DC, 1989, pp. 63–64.
83. D. F. Proctor, I. Andersen, and G. Lundquist, in *Respiratory Defense Mechanisms*, Part 1, *Lung Biology in Health and Disease*, J. Brain, D. Proctor, and S. Reid, Eds., Marcel Dekker, New York, 1977, pp. 427–452.
84. M. F. Quinlan, S. D. Salman, D. L. Swift, and H. W. Wagner, *Am. Rev. Resp. Dis. 99*, 13 (1969).
85. I. Andersen and D. F. Proctor, *Eur. J. Respir. Dis. 64*, 37 (1983).

86. S. L. Whaley, R. K. Wolff, B. A. Muggenberg, and M. B. Snipes, *J. Toxicol. Environ. Health 19*, 569 (1986).

87. J. R. Harkema, C. G. Plopper, D. M. Hyde, J. A. St. George, and D. L. Dungworth, *Am. J. Pathol. 127*, 90 (1987).

88. S. Yoshida, M. I. Golub, and M. E. Gershwin, *Reg. Toxicol. Pharmacol. 9*, 56 (1989).

V

DRUG PERMEATION ENHANCEMENT VIA THE OCULAR ROUTE

18

Permeation Enhancement for Ocular Route of Polypeptide Administration

George C. Y. Chiou and Yu-Qun Zheng

Institute of Ocular Pharmacology, Department of Medical Pharmacology and Toxicology, Texas A&M University College of Medicine, College Station, Texas

I. INTRODUCTION

Rapid developments in biotechnology have made it possible to produce a large number of peptide drugs at affordable prices. There is an intrinsic problem associated with the clinical uses of these peptide drugs, however; they are degraded in the gastrointestinal tract if they are administered orally. Most of these drugs are now given parenterally and are not appreciated by most patients. Numerous alternative routes of drug administration other than injections have been considered, yet none of them have been received with enthusiasm for various reasons [1–9]. Recently, the ocular route has been tested with favorable responses [10–15].

It has been reported that plain insulin eyedrops alone are unable to reach therapeutic concentrations in the systemic circulation to lower the blood sugar [10,14,15]. Neither changing the pH of the eyedrops nor adding aminopeptidase inhibitors to them can raise the insulin concentrations in the systemic circulation significantly [14]. A marked improvement in the systemic absorption of insulin through the eyes has been achieved, however, with the addition of permeation enhancers into insulin eyedrops [10,14,15]. Unfortunately, most of these enhancers are irritating to the eyes and are not suitable for use in ophthalmic solutions.

BL-9 and Brij-78 are the only two out of approximately 50 absorption enhancers studied to show no irritation to the eyes at concentrations up to 0.5%.

Therefore, it would be most useful to find out how potent these two agents are with respect to increasing insulin absorption into the systemic circulation through the eyes and lowering the blood glucose concentration.

Permeation enhancers can also be used to enhance the systemic absorption of other peptide drugs such as glucagon, ACTH, calcitonin, β-endorphin, met-enkephalin, and the like.

II. PHARMACOKINETICS

A three-compartment model has been developed in this laboratory for describing the pharmacokinetics of systemic absorption of various peptide drugs such as insulin, glucagon, luteinizing hormone-releasing hormone (LHRH), and leu-enkephalin through ocular routes. The three major compartments are (1) the precorneal area, (2) the peripheral regions, and (3) the systemic circulation. When radioactive peptides were used in these studies, the radioactivities determined included the intact peptide as well as its metabolites in the bloodstream. Therefore, the term "peptide equivalent" was used. Radioimmunoassay was used to determine the level of intact peptide molecules in the blood circulation.

When the radioactive peptide is instilled into the cul de sac of the rabbit eye (precorneal compartment), it is considered a bolus input of the drug onto the eyes. It is known that only a minute amount of the peptide drug can pass across the cornea to enter the eyeball; most of the drug is absorbed into the systemic circulation compartment via the conjunctival membrane and the nasolacrimal drainage system [11–14]. After the peptide is absorbed into the blood circulation, it is redistributed to other parts of the body, as represented by the peripheral compartment, or metabolized and excreted.

By using the ADAPT nonlinear parameter estimation computer program [16], a large discrepancy was found between the model simulation outputs and the experimental data. These results exclude the possibility that simple diffusion alone can be used to adequately describe the systemic absorption of peptide drugs through the eyes. On the other hand, insufficient evidence was available to indicate the involvement of active transport. Different approaches were therefore had to be taken by fitting only one out of five pharmacokinetic parameters, i.e., the transport constant between the precorneal compartment and the bloodstream compartment (K_{12}), with various concentrations of peptide solution instilled onto the precorneal compartment while keeping the other four parameters (K_{pc}, K_{23}, K_{32}, K_{el}) constant (Fig. 1). In this way, excellent agreement between model outputs and experimental data was obtained, indicating that a more elaborate transport mechanism such as facilitated diffusion might be involved.

Facilitated diffusion is a transport process in which the driving force for the movement of peptide molecules across the mucous membrane is the concentration gradient of the peptide molecules. The rate of diffusion is dependent on the

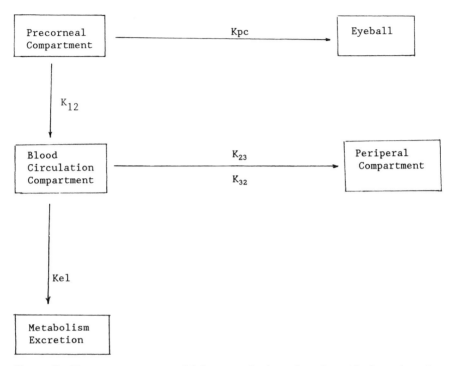

Figure 1 Three-compartment model for systemic absorption of peptide drugs through the eyes.

binding capacity of the peptide molecules and the hypothetical carriers and is limited by the availability of these carriers [17]. This hypothesis, with the limited number of carriers and the small area of mucous membrane partitioning the eye, nasolacrimal system, and bloodstream compartment, seemed to describe the penetration behavior of the peptide molecules and the inverse dependency of the parameter K_{12} on the peptide eyedrop concentration quite adequately.

Addition of permeation enhancers can increase the peptide absorption markedly [15]. However, the quality of the pharmacokinetics of the peptide absorption remained unchanged, indicating that the permeation enhancers could improve the availability of carriers to be bound by peptide molecules for facilitated transport across the mucous membrane.

III. EFFICACY OF PERMEATION ENHANCERS

New Zealand albino rabbits weighing 2–3 kg were anesthetized with 30 mg/kg of pentobarbital sodium administered intravenously. Additional pentobarbital so-

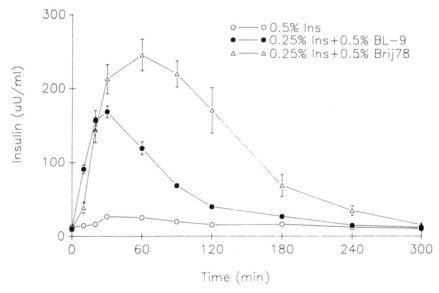

Figure 2 Effects of BL-9 and Brij-78 on insulin (0.25%) absorption through rabbit eyes. Each point is the mean ± SE of eight values.

dium was given throughout the experiment at the rate of 1 mg kg^{-1} hr^{-1} to maintain anesthesia. Fifty microliters of peptide solution was instilled into the left eye of the rabbit. Blood sample aliquots (1 mL) were collected from the femoral artery. The blood was centrifuged, and plasma aliquots were frozen for radioimmunoassay.

Blood concentrations of insulin, glucagon, ACTH, calcitonin, met-enkephalin, and β-endorphin were determined with radioimmunoassay using commercially available kits. Blood glucose concentration was determined with Glucoscan Test Strip read 1 min after fresh blood application by a Glucoscan 2000 meter (Lifescan, Mountain View, CA) at the time points indicated in the figures. All data were analyzed with a *t* test for two values. Each value was expressed as mean ± standard error of the mean. A *p* value of 0.05 or less was considered to be significant.

When plain insulin eyedrops at 0.25%, 0.5%, and 1.0% were administered, the insulin detected in the systemic circulation was very low, not exceeding 30 μU/mL. When the 0.5% BL-9 permeation enhancer was added, the peak concentration of insulin in the bloodstream reached 170, 240, and 270 μU/mL, respectively (Figs. 2–4). Another permeation enhancer, Brij-78, at the same concentration promoted the absorption of insulin eyedrops at 0.25%, 0.5%, and 1% even further, to 240, 250, and 320 μU/mL, respectively (Figs. 2–4). With

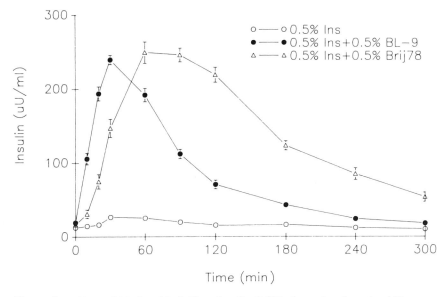

Figure 3 Effects of BL-9 and Brij-78 on insulin (0.5%) absorption through rabbit eyes. Each point is the mean ± SE of eight values.

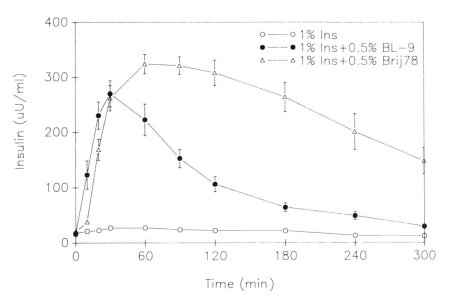

Figure 4 Effects of BL-9 and Brij-78 on insulin (1.0%) absorption through rabbit eyes. Each point is the mean ± SE of eight values.

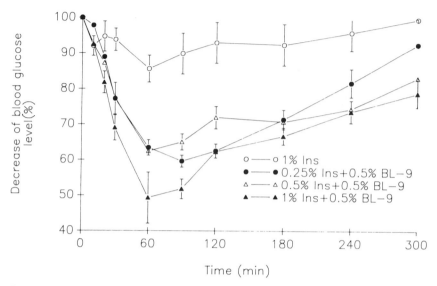

Figure 5 Effects of insulin with BL-9 (0.5%) on decrease of blood glucose level through rabbit eyes. Each point is the mean ± SE of eight values.

BL-9, the insulin concentration in the blood reached the peak at 30 min after instillation, whereas with Brij-78 the blood insulin levels reached the peak at 60 min after eyedrop instillation. The duration of insulin level in the bloodstream was much longer when Brij-78 was used than when BL-9 was used (Figs. 2–4).

Blood glucose concentration was not affected significantly by plain insulin eyedrops up to 1.0% concentration. When BL-9 and Brij-78 were added, marked reduction in blood sugar was noted. When 0.5% BL-9 was added to 0.25%, 0.5%, and 1.0% of insulin solutions, the blood sugar dropped 40%, 38%, and 51%, respectively, with a maximum effect seen at 60 min after eyedrop instillation and with a duration of approximately 5 hr (Fig. 5). These results indicate that the blood sugar responses observed were slower (30 min delay) than those induced by plain insulin absorption alone. Results obtained with insulin plus Brij-78 were similar to those obtained with BL-9 except that the blood glucose levels were suppressed for a longer period of time (Fig. 6).

Glucagon is used clinically in hypoglycemic crisis to raise the blood glucose concentrations. As the molecular weight of glucagon (3500) is only half that of insulin (6000), its absorption is more effective than insulin's. Thus plain glucagon eyedrops at a concentration of 0.2% could raise the blood glucose levels significantly [13]. With lower concentrations of 0.05% and 0.1%, plain glucagon

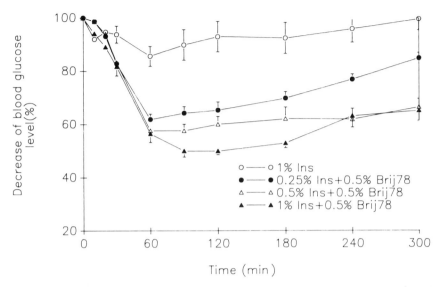

Figure 6 Effects of insulin with Brij-78 (0.5%) on decrease of blood glucose level through rabbit eyes. Each point is the mean ± SE of eight values.

without permeation enhancer could not raise the blood glucose levels significantly. When 0.5% of BL-9 or Brij-78 was added, however, the glucagon absorption was markedly enhanced and the blood glucose was raised. With 0.5% BL-9, 0.05% of glucagon absorption could be raised from 600 pg/mL to 2700 pg/mL (Fig. 7), and the blood glucose from 102 mg % to 160 mg % (Fig. 8). When 0.5% BL-9 was added to 0.1% glucagon, the glucagon in the bloodstream rose from 700 pg/mL to 4000 pg/mL (Fig. 7) and the blood glucose level rose from 114 mg % to 211 mg % (Fig. 8). Similar results were obtained with 0.5% Brij-78 except that it was more potent than BL-9 (Fig. 9).

The molecular weight of ACTH (4500) is slightly higher than that of glucagon (3500). Thus its systemic absorption should be enhanced by the addition of BL-9 and Brij-78 in the solution as well. When 0.5% of BL-9 was added to the 0.05% ACTH eyedrops, the blood level of ACTH rose from 168 pg/mL to 1030 pg/mL. With 0.05% ACTH and 0.5% Brij-78, the blood level of ACTH increased from 168 pg/mL to 1300 pg/mL. The absorption of ACTH with permeation enhancers was extremely effective and could reach almost the same level as with intravenous injection at a certain time point.

A study of the systemic absorption of calcitonin, met-enkephalin, and β-endorphin with permeation enhancers is under way and should be completed soon. These results clearly indicate that a sufficient amount of peptide drugs can

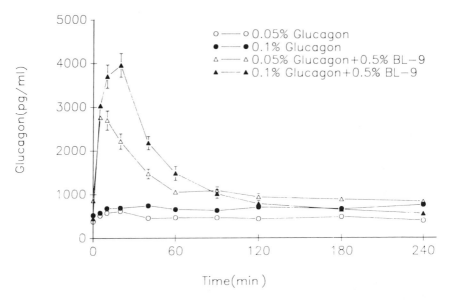

Figure 7   Effects of BL-9 (0.5%) on glucagon absorption through rabbit eyes. Each point is the mean ± SE of eight values.

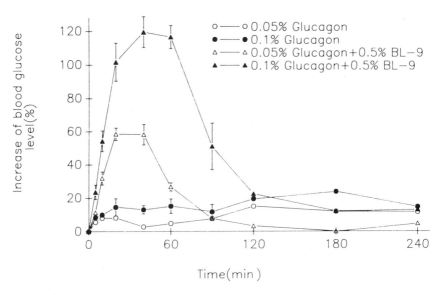

Figure 8   Effects of glucagon with or without BL-9 (0.5%) on blood glucose level. Each point is the mean ± SE of eight values.

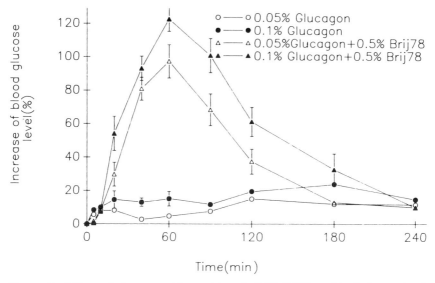

Figure 9 Effects of glucagon with or without Brij-78 (0.5%) on blood glucose level. Each point is the mean ± SE of eight values.

be absorbed systemically to achieve clinical usefulness with the use of permeation enhancers.

IV. ADVANTAGES OF THE USE OF PERMEATION ENHANCERS

Although systemic delivery of peptide drugs through the eyes is a good feasible method for drug delivery, it inherits a major problem of dosing limitations not to exceed 2.5 mg per eye per instillation (or 25 μL of 10% solutions). Actually, 5.0 mg per 2 eyes per instillation is sufficient for most potent peptide drugs if they are 100% absorbed through the eyes into the systemic circulation. However, for larger peptides with a molecular weight of 3000 or more, the percent absorption of peptide molecule into the systemic circulation is much less than complete. As a result, a permeation enhancer must be added to increase the peptide drug absorption.

Further, most peptide drugs are rather expensive. Therefore, permeation enhancers can cut down the absolute quantity of peptide drugs to be instilled into the eyes to save a considerable amount of money.

It is well known that high drug concentrations are closely related to local side effects, drug solubilities, peptide stabilities, and drug osmolarities. Therefore, the lower the concentrations used the better, and permeation enhancers can reduce the concentration required.

Of the approximately 50 permeation enhancers tested, only BL-9 and Brij-78 were found to be effective at the 0.5% concentration level, which did not produce ocular irritation [15]. When they were given along with peptide drugs, they were able to markedly enhance the systemic delivery of insulin (8–12-fold), glucagon (4–6-fold), and ACTH (6–8-fold). These results indicate that permeation enhancers can reduce the absolute amount of peptide drugs to be instilled into the eyes so that (1) lower doses of peptide drugs can be used to produce the desired effects, (2) the side effects of peptide drugs can be minimized, and (3) the price of the product can be reduced.

V. CONCLUSIONS

Systemic delivery of peptide drugs through the ocular route is a feasible alternative to parenteral injection. As the method is simple, economical, and painless, its clinical use in the future could become rather popular. One of the limiting factors of the ocular route is the absolute quantity of drug that can be instilled into the eyes and the poor penetrability of larger polypeptides across the mucous membrane. These problems can be solved by the addition of permeation enhancers such as BL-9 and Brij-78, which produce essentially no local irritation at concentration up to 0.5%.

The use of permeation enhancers can also reduce the amount of peptide drugs even of small molecular size. As a result, the side effects, instability, and high osmolarity of peptide eyedrops can be avoided.

It is hypothesized that peptide drugs are transported across the mucous membrane via facilitated diffusion. The use of permeation enhancers could make carriers more readily available to be bound by peptide molecules to enhance their transport across the mucous membrane.

Acknowledgment This work was supported in part by research grant EY 07511 from National Eye Institute/NIH and available university funds from Texas A&M University.

REFERENCES

1. H. P. Merkles, R. Anders, and J. Sandow, Buccal absorption of peptides in rats, *Proc. 32nd Annu. Congr. Int. Assoc. Pharm. Technol.* (APV), NL-Leiden, 1986, p. 57.
2. R. Anders, H. P. Merkle, W. Schurr, and R. Ziegler, Buccal absorption of protirelin: an effective way to stimulate thyrotropin and prolactin, *J. Pharm. Sci. 72,* 1481–1483 (1983).
3. N. F. Fisher, The absorption of insulin from the intestine, vagina, and scrota sac, *Am. J. Physiol. 67,* 65–71 (1923).

4. Y. Yamasaki, M. Shichiri, R. Kawamori, M. Kikuchi, T. Yagi, S. Arai, R. Tohdo, N. Hakui, N. Oji, and H. Abe, The effectiveness of rectal administration of insulin suppository on normal and diabetic subjects, *Diabetes Care 4*, 454–458 (1981).

5. R. R. Burnette and D. Marrero, Comparison between the iontophoretic and passive transport of thyrotropin releasing hormone across excised nude mouse skin, *J. Pharm. Sci. 75*, 738–743 (1986).

6. F. M. Wigley, J. H. Londono, S. H. Wood, J. C. Shipp, and R. H. Waldman, Insulin across respiratory mucosae by aerosol delivery, *Diabetes 20*, 552–556 (1971).

7. A. C. Moses, G. S. Gordon, M. C. Carey, and J. S. Flier, Insulin administered intravasally as an insulin–bile salt aerosol: effectiveness and reproducibility in normal and diabetic subjects, *Diabetes 32*, 1040–1047 (1983).

8. S. Hirai, T. Ikenaga, and T. Matsuzawa, Nasal absorption of insulin in dogs, *Diabetes 27*, 296–299 (1978).

9. R. Salzman, J. E. Manson, G. T. Griffing, R. Kimmerle, N. Ruderman, D. Phil, A. McCall, E. I. Stoltz, C. Mullin, D. Small, J. Armstrong, and J. C. Melby, Intranasal aerosolized insulin; mixed-meal studies and long-term use in type I diabetes, *N. Engl. J. Med. 312*, 1078–1084 (1985).

10. G. C. Y. Chiou, C. Y. Chuang, and M. S. Chang, Reduction of blood glucose concentrations with insulin eyedrops, *Diabetes Care 11*, 750–751 (1988).

11. G. C. Y. Chiou and C. Y. Chuang, Systematic delivery of polypeptides with molecular weights of between 300 and 350 through eyes, *J. Ocul. Pharmacol. 4*, 165–177 (1988).

12. G. C. Y. Chiou, C. Y. Chuang, and M. S. Chang, Systematic delivery of enkephalin peptide through eyes, *Life Sci. 43*, 509–514 (1988).

13. G. C. Y. Chiou and C. Y. Chuang, Treatment of hypoglycemia with glucagon eyedrops, *J. Ocul. Pharmacol. 4*, 179–186 (1988).

14. G. C. Y. Chiou, C. Y. Chuang, and M. S. Chang, Systematic delivery of insulin through eyes to lower the blood glucose concentration, *J. Ocul. Pharmacol. 5*, 81–91 (1988).

15. G. C. Y. Chiou and C. Y. Chuang, Improvement of systematic absorption of insulin through eyes with absorption enhancers, *J. Pharm. Sci. 78*, 815–818 (1989).

16. D.Z. D'Argenio and A. Schumitzsky, *Comput. Program. Biomed. 9*, 115–134 (1979).

17. R. R. Levine, *Pharmacology: Drug Actions and Reaction*, 3rd ed., Little, Brown, Boston, 1983, pp. 64–69.

19

Mechanisms of Ocular Peptide Absorption and Its Enhancement

Yongyut Rojanasakul
School of Pharmacy, West Virginia University, Morgantown, West Virginia

I. INTRODUCTION

During the past decade, significant progress has been made in the management of ocular diseases through the use of controlled delivery of medications using a number of improved methods of drug delivery. While this continues to be an important area of ocular drug research, increasing attention is now being focused on the development of specific novel delivery systems for the new generation of biotechnology-based peptide and protein drugs. Although these developments create new hope for improved treatment of certain ocular diseases, they also present a formidable challenge for scientists attempting to design appropriate delivery systems for these macromolecules. This chapter reviews recent findings and discusses problems and limitations associated with ocular peptide and protein delivery. Physiological and physicochemical factors that affect drug bioavailability and approaches to overcoming these obstacles are also discussed.

II. CONSTRAINTS AND APPROACHES TO IMPROVE OCULAR DRUG BIOAVAILABILITY

The eye is well protected from noxious substances in the environment by a variety of mechanisms, most notably a secretion of tears continuously flushing its surface, an impermeable surface epithelium, and a local immune defense system. Unfortunately, from a therapeutic standpoint, these mechanisms make it difficult to ensure an effective concentration of drug at the intended site. Thus, an understanding of these protective mechanisms is a prerequisite for the development of effective delivery systems.

The superficial corneal epithelium is covered by a mucopolysaccharide coating that is hydrophilic and maintains tear film continuity. Tears are secreted by lacrimal glands, from which they are conducted to the globe by numerous ducts in the upper tarsal plate in humans, but by a single duct closed to the lateral canthus in the rabbit [1]. The kinetics of tear formation and removal have been studied by many investigators [2–4]. In humans, the tear fluid is half replaced each 2–20 min, which corresponds to an average tear secretion rate of approximately 1 µL/min [5].

Tear drainage greatly influences the residence time for a drug and its availability for ocular absorption. Several drug delivery techniques ranging from simply increasing the vehicle viscosity to highly engineered devices to increase contact time and thus improve ocular bioavailability have been used. These include the use of high-viscosity gels [6,7], nanoparticles [8,9], liposomes [10,11], solid inserts [12], erodible inserts [13], soft contact lenses [14,15], latex systems [16], and bioadhesive systems [17]. At present, these techniques have met with only limited success because they have provided only a modest improvement in ocular drug bioavailability or have not gained patient acceptance [18]. The advantages and disadvantages of these methods were reviewed in detail by Lee and Robinson [19].

To achieve high ocular bioavailability, the instilled drug must move through the cornea, the major pathway for drug entry into the internal eye. Although a significant portion of the instilled drug can be absorbed across the conjunctiva and sclera, that portion is essentially lost owing to extensive vascularization of the underlying tissues, which removes drug via the circulatory system, causing unwanted systemic effects. The cornea, an avascularized tissue, is composed of three major layers: two boundary cellular layers, the epithelium and the endothelium, between which lies a thick connective tissue, the stroma. The epithelium of the cornea is highly lipophilic and is tightly closed by tight junctions, thus preventing direct penetration of most hydrophilic drugs to the deeper layers of the cornea. Attempts to improve corneal drug permeability generally fall into two categories—those that aim at modifying the structural integrity of the epithelium and those that aim at altering the chemical nature of the drug molecule, the so-called prodrug approach.

Ethylenediamine tetraacetic acid (EDTA), a calcium chelator, has been shown to increase corneal penetration of hydrophilic compounds, presumably by opening intercellular junctions [20]. Disruption of the epithelial barrier by benzalkonium chloride increases the ocular absorption of several compounds that vary in hydrophilicity and molecular weight [21–24]. Cetylpyridinium chloride enhances absorption of penicillin G with an efficacy equivalent to that of the deepithelialized cornea [25]. Chemical modifications of the drugs through the prodrug approach that result in more lipophilic derivatives have been shown to be effective at enhancing drug absorption. The prodrug approach has been used for a number of drugs, including timolol [26,27], pilocarpine [28], imidazolines [29], prostaglandins [30], and, probably the most successful case, epinephrine, with its prodrug ester, dipivalyl epinephrine [31–34]. The epinephrine prodrug is reported to be about 100 times as effective as its parent compound in the management of glaucoma and about 100–400 times less toxic to the cardiovascular system [31]. The prodrug approach has not been used for peptide and protein drugs. The complexity of these compounds' molecular structures may limit the use of this technique, especially for those with numerous charged groups. Chemical properties required for prodrug derivatization and the detailed methodology of this technique were reviewed by Lee and Li [18].

III. OCULAR PEPTIDE AND PROTEIN DELIVERY

Several biologically active peptides, including substance P [35], enkephalin [36], neurotensin [37], somatostatin [37], thyrotropin-releasing hormone (TRH) [38], leuteinizing hormone-releasing hormone (LHRH) [39], vasoactive intestinal polypeptide (VIP) [40], glucagon [41], and cholecystokinin [42], have been found in the ocular tissues. Although their exact pharmacologic effects are not well understood, these peptides have been shown to exhibit neurotransmitter or modulator functions. Antidiuretic hormone (ADH) influences aqueous humor dynamics and intraocular pressure (IOP) [43]. Oxytocin exerts a mitotic effect when large doses are employed [44]. The melanocyte-stimulating hormones have not been detected in the eye but are known to exert a positive IOP effect on the eye [45]. In addition, several polypeptide antibiotics such as gramicidin, bacitracin, polymyxins, cyclosporin, tryothricin, and tryocidine have been shown to be effective in the treatment of various ocular diseases. On the basis of these findings, it is conceivable that peptides will eventually become an important class of therapeutic agents in the management of certain ocular pathologic conditions such as glaucoma, circulation-related retinopathies, ocular inflammation, corneal wound healing, and ocular infection.

Despite their therapeutic potential, the use of peptides and proteins in the management of ocular diseases has not been fully realized. In fact, studies on ocular delivery of peptides and other macromolecules have been scarce, and, with few exceptions, the mechanisms by which these compounds permeate the ocular tissues are poorly understood. It is generally believed that the corneal epithelium is impermeable to the transport of macromolecules. Nonetheless, recent evidence indicates that inulin, a hydrophilic macromolecule with a molecular weight of 5000, can penetrate the cornea into the aqueous humor and anterior segment of the eye to the extent of 0.1–0.4% of the applied dose [46]. The transport of inulin appears to occur paracellularly instead of transcellulary, with no evidence of a carrier or active transport process. Results obtained from this laboratory indicate that thyrotropin-releasing hormone (TRH), a tripeptide with a molecular weight of 362, penetrates the cornea to the extent of slightly less than 0.1% of the total applied dose after 1 hr of in vitro perfusion. In vivo absorption is expected to be even lower owing to rapid precorneal loss of the compound. Theoretically, unless the corneal surface is structurally modified to allow more drug absorption, the majority of a dose would be lost from the ocular area and absorbed into the body's systemic circulation. Lee [47] reported systemic absorption of approximately 82% of the total applied dose after topical application for timolol, 36% for epinephrine, 21% for tyrosine, 22% for met-enkephalinamide, and 3% for inulin.

In addition to the transport barrier, the enzymatic barrier produced by peptidases is another important factor limiting ocular absorption of peptides and proteins. These enzymes are widely distributed throughout the eye and can be found in the tears, corneal epithelium, and iris-ciliary body [48]. While the ocular presence of these enzymes is known to be less extensive than that found in the GI tract, their degradative activity is still rather high. For example, as much as 90%, and in some cases almost 100%, of corneal leucine and methionine enkephalins are degraded within 5 min after topical application [49]. Among the peptidases, aminopeptidases, enzymes that cleave peptides and proteins at the N-terminus amide bond, are the most active enzymes found in the eye [47]. It was found that these enzymes can be inhibited by bestatin, a potent aminopeptidase inhibitor [49]. Successful delivery of peptides and proteins, therefore, depends on modifying not only the transport barrier but also the enzymatic barrier.

Perhaps the least known, least recognized barrier for ocular and most other types of epithelial drug delivery is the immunologic barrier. This is understandable, as most presently available drugs are relatively small molecules and possess low immunogenicity. However, this barrier may become important for peptides and proteins with a higher immunogenic potential. Immunologic defense mechanisms are known to be important in protecting the eye from infectious agents. Various immunologic components have been identified in ocular tissues, including secretory IgA [50], conjunctival associated lymphoid tissue (CALT) [51], and ocular surface Langerhans cells [52]. Immunologic defense systems incorporate a complex sequence of events in which the host recognizes that foreign molecules are present and then mobilizes a specific reaction against them. The initial processing of antigens involves antigenic presentation that is accomplished by two systems, CALT and Langerhans cells, both located locally in the epithelial surface [53]. The antigenic signals result eventually in T- and B-cell stimulation in regional lymph nodes. These stimulated lymphocytes then migrate via the bloodstream and eventually home in on particular mucosal sites. The T cells target submucosal sites in the conjunctiva, whereas B cells migrate to sites adjacent to lacrimal and accessory gland epithelia. The B cells then produce immunoglobulins, especially IgA, at these sites [54]. The IgA that appears in tears is unique in that it is dimerized with a polypeptide known as a secretory component acquired from the adjacent epithelia [55]. sIgA antibodies and T cells interact specifically with antigens and prevent them from adhering to and penetrating into the tissues [56,57].

Besides infectious agents, not much is known about how the eye processes macromolecules. However, it is expected that these immunologic defense mechanisms would have a significant effect on absorption of these macromolecules. In other epithelia such as the intestine, it has been shown that drastic reduction in absorption of the macromolecule horseradish peroxidase occurs upon long-term administration. This effect was found to be due to immunologic response of the gut epithelia, which was effective either by oral [58] or parenteral [59] immunization. Pang et al. [60] later found that oral immunization altered the distribution of another protein, bovine serum albumin, administered into the gut and enhanced intraluminal degradation of this compound. Abuchowski and Davis [61] showed that, by conjugating proteins to inert soluble polymers such as polyethylene glycol, polyvinylpyrrolidone, or dextran, the immune response can be abrogated. These conjugated proteins not only retain their biological activity but also are more resistant to proteolytic degradation, which results in prolonged retention of the compounds in the systemic circulation.

IV. PATHWAYS AND BARRIERS OF CORNEAL PEPTIDE ABSORPTION

There are two major pathways for drugs to be transported across the cornea: the transcellular and paracellular pathways. Transcellular drug transport can occur by a partitioning-controlled process, by diffusion through cellular pores, or by a carrier-mediated process. The paracellular pathway is anatomically composed of the intercellular spaces and tight junctions. Drug transport through this pathway can occur by passive diffusion or convective flow. Diffusive transport is a dissipative process that depends upon the difference in solute concentration and the permeability–surface area properties of the membrane. Convective transport is dominated by the balance of hydrostatic and osmotic gradients, the solute concentration, and the hydraulic and reflection coefficients of the restrictive barrier.

Partitioning is important for lipophilic drugs, which allow rapid movement into the "lipid-like" epithelial layers of the cornea. However, once entered into these layers, the drugs encounter an additional barrier corresponding to the diffusional resistance of the stroma. For very lipophilic drugs, this barrier can become the rate-limiting barrier owing to poor drug solubility, which lowers the effective drug concentration gradient and thus diffusion across this layer. Additionally, drug–tissue binding, which has been found to occur quite extensively in the stroma and particularly with very lipophilic drugs, can further impede the actual drug transport in this layer. Rojanasakul and Robinson [62] demonstrated that as much as 80% of the total drug progesterone entering the cornea was bound in the stroma. The extent of binding was also found to increase with increasing lipophilicity of the compounds.

The rate-limiting role of the stroma for lipophilic drugs has also been observed by several other groups. These studies established a parabolic relationship between drug lipophilicity and permeability, with the optimal drug lipophilicity (partition coefficient) for maximum corneal penetration in the range of 10–1000 [63–65]. In contrast to lipophilic drugs, the stroma offers relatively little resistance to hydrophilic drugs, and the epithelium, in this case, is rate-limiting. Transport of such drugs occurs predominantly via the paracellular pathway.

Other transport mechanisms such as cellular pore transport and carrier-mediated transport have not been considered for ophthalmic drugs. However, cellular pore transport has been shown to be important for ions and water and carrier-mediated transport for some metabolically important substances such as glucose and amino acids [66].

Unlike most conventional drugs, the transport mechanism of peptide and protein drugs in the cornea and other epithelia is relatively unknown. Depending on the amino acid composition, the molecules of these compounds can vary greatly in their lipophilicity. However, most peptides and proteins are generally hydrophilic with multiple charged groups and are thus expected to penetrate the cornea paracellularly. Because of the restrictive nature of this path, however, peptides may or may not be able to penetrate this region, depending on their molecular size and charge characteristics as well as on the degree of opening of the dynamic tight junction structures.

Tonjum [67] demonstrates that at normal physiological conditions horseradish peroxidase (HRP), a protein with a mass of 40,000 daltons, is unable to penetrate the corneal epithelium, suggesting that this barrier has dimensions of less than 3 nm. However, if the compound is given from the endothelial side, it can penetrate the endothelium, enter the stroma, and readily fill up the intercellular spaces of the epithelium, except in the top few layers. These results clearly demonstrate the rate-limiting role of the apical cell junctions and paracellular transport of the compound. Similar results were observed in the case of a highly charged polypeptide, poly-L-lysine (MW 15,000) [68]. In this study, it was also found that most of the compound was selectively taken up by the cornea through the epithelial surface defects caused by nonuniform shedding of the degenerating "old" cells.

Not all peptides are absorbed through the paracellular pathway. It has been suggested that peptides that are relatively lipophilic such as enkephalins permeate the cornea transcellularly and presumably by a partitioning process [49]. In this study, leucine enkephalin, a lipophilic enkephalin, was shown to penetrate the cornea to a greater extent than the less lipophilic analogue methionine enkephalin. Moderately lipophilic peptides, such as thyrotropin-releasing hormone (TRH) and phalloidin, have been shown to enter the cornea via both pathways, although the paracellular appears to be the predominant route [69]. Although their work is still in the preliminary stages, Rojanasakul et al. [68] interestingly have demonstrated transcellular uptake of a highly charged peptide, insulin, by the cornea. This process is followed by heavy nuclear accumulation of the compound, which can be found in both the epithelial and endothelial cell layers. The basis for this uptake is not yet clear, but it is believed to be due to the process of endocytosis since passive uptake via a partitioning process of large (MW$\approx$5700), hydrophilic, and charged molecules is unlikely. Interestingly, the transport of insulin in the intercellular spaces and stroma was found to be very limited, which is in contrast to that observed with other charged peptides such as polylysine, HRP, TRH, and phalloidin. Because both polylysine and HRP have a much larger molecular size than insulin, the size limitation effect cannot account for this discrepancy. Instead, it has been suggested to occur as a result of a charge discrimination effect of the cornea. The cornea, because of the charged groups lining its transport pathway, exhibits a permselective property that allows preferential passage of positively but not negatively charged compounds [70]. Since insulin is negatively charged at physiological pH, it is anticipated that this charge barrier may result in a decrease in its penetration. In contrast, polylysine, because of its excess free ϵ-amino groups, and phalloidin and TRH, because their basic guanidinium groups are protonated (positive) at this pH, would not be repelled by this barrier and would be expected to readily penetrate into any accessible spaces in the membrane.

V. PERMSELECTIVE PROPERTIES OF THE CORNEA

The transport barrier of the paracellular pathway has two properties that influence the absorption of charged compounds: (1) the general *permeability* (magnitude) of the barrier, which is mainly controlled by tight junctions, and (2) the *permselectivity* of the barrier, which is a quantitative measure of the ability of the membranes to discriminate or show preference for the transport of molecules of different charges.

Membrane permselectivity is a fairly general phenomenon that has been observed in a wide variety of epithelia in the body. It combines contributions from both passive electrostatic shunt activity, probably due to membrane fixed charges, and active cell membrane activity. The latter is generally a reflection of carriers and pumps residing in the membrane. In rabbit cornea, the active potential arises from an inward sodium transport from tears to aqueous humor [71,72] and an outward chloride transport in the reverse direction [73]. This results in a negative transcorneal potential (epithelial with respect to the endothelial side) with a magnitude of approximately 25 mV [74,75]. With regard to the passive permselectivity, our recent studies based on membrane diffusion and streaming potential measurements [70] indicate that the cornea contains both positively and negatively charged groups, with the magnitude and polarity depending on the degree of protonation. The cornea presents an isoelectric point (pI) of 3.2. At physiological pH and pH above pI, the cornea carries a net negative charge and allows preferential passage of positively charged molecules. Below pI, the reverse is valid. The basis for this phenomenon has been described as a result of electrostatic potential barrier generated by these charged groups, the so-called Donnan exclusion effect [76,77]. The nature of the membrane charges has not yet been identified, but it has been suggested that it results from ionizable protein amino acid residues, i.e., carboxylic acid and amine groups, that line the transport pathway.

In addition to being affected by the pH, membrane permselectivity is also influenced by the ionic strength of bathing solutions. Lowering the ionic strength of the solutions has been shown to increase the membrane charge discrimination [70]. This effect has been attributed to the increase in effective membrane charge density resulting from a lesser degree of electrostatic shielding.

VI. ACTIONS OF PENETRATION ENHANCERS

Because of the intrinsically poor penetrability of peptides and proteins across the epithelial membranes, methods to enhance their absorption are usually required. Several techniques, including modification of membrane integrity through the use of permeation enhancers, chemical manipulation of peptide structure, and iontophoresis, have been used. Among these, the use of penetration enhancers has probably received the most attention, mainly because of its simplicity and convenience—they can be directly incorporated into the formulation without the need of special delivery devices, and their use is not limited to accessible tissues as in the case of iontophoresis. They are also expected to work with a wide range of peptides and proteins and, perhaps, in various types of tissues.

Thus far, a wide variety of enhancers have been tested. However, most of these studies have been focused on promoting efficacy rather than on the mechanisms of action and their potential toxicity. To be of practical use, the enhancers must cause no harmful side effects in addition to being effective. Their actions also should be immediate, specific, and reversible. Many of the enhancers and their actions in various tissues are discussed in some detail in this book. This chapter concentrates on those currently in use or under investigation for ocular drug delivery.

Penetration enhancers can generally be classified as surfactants, bile salts, chelators, or salicylates. Of these, surfactants and chelators have been by far the most frequently studied enhancers for ocular delivery owing to their common use in ophthalmic formulations. Ionic surfactants such as benzalkonium chloride have been shown to increase ocular absorption of several compounds by disrupting the epithelial surface [21–24]. Corneas treated with this compound have been shown to allow the intercellular penetration of peroxidase, suggesting that the disruption effect is on the tight junctional complexes, which normally exclude the protein [24]. Scanning electron microscopic evaluation of the cornea indicates cellular uplifting and complete removal of the surface superficial layer if the concentration of benzalkonium chloride is raised above 0.05% [78]. Similarly, sodium lauryl sulfate has been shown to effectively promote drug absorption. However, this compound also causes severe irritation and damage to the eye even at low concentration [79].

Hazelton [80] and Draize and Kelley [81] noted that nonionic surfactants, unlike their ionic counterparts, are generally harmless to the eye except in some cases at very high concentrations. Marsh and Maurice [79] studied the effect of nonionic surfactants of various HLB values on corneal permeability and toxicity in humans. The surfactants with HLB values between 16 and 17, which correspond to Tween 20 and Brij 35, were found to be most effective in increasing corneal permeability. At 1% solution, these compounds were reported to increase fluorescein penetration fivefold without observed ocular irritation.

The mechanisms by which nonionic surfactants promote ocular absorption are not yet clear but probably involve several mechanisms such as removal of surface mucins, disruption of tight junction complexes, and structural damage to cell membranes. In recent studies, Rojanasakul et al. [82] demonstrated microscopically that digitonin, a natural nonionic surfactant, causes surface cell separation and cell membrane damage to the cornea. Electrophysiological studies conducted by the same group also indicate an increase in both paracellular and transcellular ion transport as demonstrated by a reduction in membrane electrical resistance and capacitance, respectively. These similar techniques were also used to study the promoting and toxic effects of several other enhancers, including the bile salt deoxycholate, calcium chelator EDTA, and various cytoskeleton-active agents, in the cornea [82,83]. Results obtained from these studies indicate that all enhancers significantly increase membrane permeability to an extent depending on concentration and exposure time. At an equimolar concentration of 1 mM, the rank order for efficacy is digitonin > EDTA > deoxycholate > cytochalasin B, with cytochalasin B being more effective than the bile salt and equally as potent as EDTA in the first 30 min after administration. Microscopic results, however, indicate that, with the exception of the cytoskeleton-active agent, all enhancers also cause severe surface cell separation and damage. Capacitance results, which show a substantial drop in membrane capacitance for the three compounds, but not cytochalasin, also support these findings.

In earlier studies, EDTA was shown to promote absorption of a number of compounds in epithelia including the cornea [20,84,85]. Its mechanism is to interfere with the ability of calcium to maintain intercellular integrity [84,86]. The fact that EDTA disrupts plasma membrane structures is somewhat unexpected. Although the mechanism of this effect is not clear, there is evidence suggesting that EDTA, by chelating calcium, can cause structural breakdown of the cell cytoskeleton, which in turn results in cell collapse and subsequent disintegration [83,87,88].

Nishihata et al. [89] demonstrated that EDTA can cause leakage of cell proteins from rectal epithelia. Like other surfactants, bile salts possess certain detergent characteristics and the ability to increase the permeability of membranes. These compounds have been shown to promote peptide absorption not only by a direct solubilizing effect but also by inhibiting cellular enzymatic activity [90].

Cytochalasins are a group of small, naturally occurring heterocyclic compounds that bind specifically to actin microfilaments, the major component of the cell cytoskeleton, and alter their polymerization [91,92]. In addition to its normal role in regulating cell contractility, mobility, and cell surface receptors, the cytoskeleton has been shown to participate in the regulation of epithelial tight junction permeability [93,94]. Using electron and confocal fluorescence microscopy, Rojanasakul and Robinson [83] demonstrated actin filament formation at the lateral borders of the superficial cells near the junctional complex of the cornea. Treatment with EDTA and cytochalasin B resulted in a disruption of these filaments and subsequent reduction in electrical resistance. This effect was fully reversible upon removal of the compounds, except for long-term exposure. Compounds that stabilize these filaments, for example, phalloidin and kinetin, exhibit the opposite effect on the corneal resistance. The high specificity to tight junctions and the relatively low toxicity of the cytoskeleton-active agents make these compounds attractive for enhanced peptide delivery, especially for those that permeate the membrane paracellularly.

VII. CONCLUSIONS

Several strategies have been used in an endeavor to optimize ocular drug bioavailability, most notably the prolongation of precorneal contact time through vehicle manipulation and the modification of corneal permeability through the prodrug approach or the use of penetration enhancers. The use of the enhancers has received increasing attention as a means of promoting peptide and protein absorption because of its simplicity and the difficulties in synthesizing prodrug analogues for peptides and proteins.

Many enhancers have been shown to be effective in promoting peptide absorption. However, their actions are rather nonspecific, and often they create some undesirable effects associated with tissue irritation and damage. Selection of an enhancer requires an understanding of basic transport mechanisms of peptides as well as the mechanisms of action of the enhancers. Understanding these mechanisms may enable the design of more useful agents that maximize the absorption-enhancing effects and minimize the irritating and toxic effects.

REFERENCES

1. A. M. Goldstein, A. de Palau, and S. Y. Botetho, *Invest. Ophthalmol. 6*, 498 (1967).
2. J. M. Conrad, W. A. Reay, R. E. Poleyn, and J. R. Robinson, *J. Parenter. Drug Assoc. 32*, 149 (1978).
3. F. J. Holly, *Int. Ophthalmol. Clin. 13*, 73 (1973).
4. N. Ehlers, *Acta Ophthalmol. 81*, 1 (1965).
5. S. Mishima, A. Gasset, S. D. Klyce, and J. L. Baum, *Invest. Ophthalmol. 5*, 264 (1966).
6. M. F. Saettone, B. Savigni, and A. Wirth, *J. Pharm. Pharmacol. 32*, 519 (1980).
7. A. Kupferman, W. J. Ryan, and H. M. Leibowitz, *Arch. Ophthalmol. 92*, 2028 (1981).
8. R. W. Wood, V. H. K. Li, J. Kreuter, and J. R. Robinson, *Int. J. Pharm. 23*, 175 (1985).
9. T. Harmia, J. Kreuter, P. Speiser, T. Boye, R. Gurny, and A. Kubis, *Int. J. Pharm. 33*, 187 (1986).
10. V. H. L. Lee, P. T. Urrea, R. E. Smith, and D. J. Schanzlin, *Surv. Ophthalmol. 29*, 335 (1985).
11. K. Singh and M. Mezei, *Int. J. Pharm. 16*, 339 (1983).
12. H. A. Quigley, I. P. Pollack, and T. S. Harbin, Jr., *Arch. Ophthalmol. 93*, 771 (1975).
13. S. E. Broomfield, T. Miyata, M. W. Dunn, N. Bueser, K. H. Stenzel, and A. L. Rubin, *Arch. Ophthalmol. 96*, 885 (1978).
14. S. R. Wattman and H. E. Kaufman, *Invest. Ophthalmol. 9*, 250 (1970).
15. F. T. Fraunfelder and S. M. Meyer, *Am. J. Ophthalmol. 99*, 362 (1985).
16. R. Gurny, *Pharm. Acta Helv. 56*, 130 (1981).
17. H. W. Hui and J. R. Robinson, *Int. J. Pharm. 26*, 203 (1985).
18. V. H. L. Lee and V. H. K. Li, *Adv. Drug Deliv. Rev. 3*, 1 (1989).
19. V. H. L. Lee and J. R. Robinson, *J. Ocul. Pharmacol. 2*, 67 (1986).
20. G. M. Grass, R. W. Wood, and J. R. Robinson, *Invest. Ophthalmol. Vis. Sci. 26*, 110 (1985).
21. R. R. Pfister and N. Burstein, *Invest. Ophthalmol. 15*, 246 (1976).
22. N. Keller, D. Moore, D. Carper, and A. Longwell, *Exp. Eye Res. 30*, 203 (1980).
23. N. L. Burstein, *Ophthalmol. Vis. Sci. 25*, 1453 (1984).
24. A. M. Tonjum, *Acta Ophthalmol. 53*, 335 (1975).

25. R. E. W. Godbey, K. Green, and D. S. Kull, *J. Pharm. Sci. 68*, 1176 (1979).
26. H. Bundgaard, A. Buur, S. C. Chang, and V. H. L. Lee, *Int. J. Pharm. 33*, 15 (1986).
27. S. C. Chang, H. Bundgaard, A. Buur, and V. H. L. Lee, *Ophthalmol. Vis. Sci. 28*, 487 (1987).
28. H. Bundgaard, E. Falch, C. Larsen, G. L. Mosher, and T. J. Mikkelson, *J. Pharm. Sci. 75*, 775 (1986).
29. E. Duzman, J. Anderson, J. B. Vita, J. C. Lue, C. C. Chen, and I. H. Leopold, *Arch. Ophthalmol. 101*, 1122 (1983).
30. L. Z. Bito, H. E. Kirby, R. A. Baroody, and O.C. Miranda, *Ophthalmol. Suppl. 27*, 178 (1986).
31. D. A. McClure, in *Prodrugs as Novel Drug Delivery Systems* (ACS Symp. Ser. 14), T. Higuchi and V. Stella, Eds., American Chemical Society, Washington, DC, 1979, p. 224.
32. M. A. Kass, A. I. Mandell, I. Goldberg, J. M. Paine, and B. Becker, *Arch. Ophthalmol. 97*, 1865 (1979).
33. M. B. Kaback, S. M. Podos, T. S. Harbin, Jr., A. Mandell, and B. Becker, *Am. J. Ophthalmol. 81*, 768 (1976).
34. C. P. Wei, J. A. Anderson, and I. Leopold, *Invest. Ophthalmol. Vis. Sci. 17*, 315 (1978).
35. J. Sternschantz, M. Sears, and H. Mishima, *Naunyn-Schmiedeberg's Arch. Pharmacol. 321*, 329 (1982).
36. H. Bjorklund, L. Olson, and A. Seiger, *Med. Biol. 61*, 280 (1983).
37. N. C. Brecha, H. J. Karten, and C. Schenker, *Neuroscience 6*, 1329 (1981).
38. E. Martino, M. Nardi, G. Vaudagna, S. Simonetti, A. Colotti, and A. Pinchera, *Experientia 36*, 622 (1980).
39. H. Munz, W. E. Stumpf, and L. Jennes, *Brain Res. 221*, 1 (1981).
40. H. Uusitalo, J. Lehtosalo, R. Palkama, and M. Toivanen, *Exp. Eye Res. 38*, 435 (1984).
41. K. Tornquist, I. Loren, I. Hakanson, and F. Sundler, *Exp. Eye Res. 33*, 55 (1981).
42. N. N. Osborne, D. A. Nicholas, A. C. Cuello, and G. J. Dockray, *Neurosci. Lett. 26*, 31 (1981).
43. S. Nagasubramznians, *Trans. Ophthalmol. Soc. U.K. 97*, 686 (1977).
44. J. D. Horowitz, Dissertation, Yale Univ. School of Medicine, New Haven, CT, 1981.
45. A. H. Neufeld, L. M. Jampol, and M. L. Sears, *Nature 238*, 158 (1972).
46. V. H. L. Lee, L. W. Carson, and K. A. Takemoto, *Int. J. Pharm. 29*, 43 (1986).
47. V. H. L. Lee, *Pharm. Technol. 11*, 26 (1987).
48. R. E. Stratford and V. H. L. Lee, *Curr. Eye Res. 4*, 995 (1985).
49. V. H. L. Lee, L. W. Carson, S. Dodda Kashi, and R. E. Stratford, *J. Ocul. Pharm. 2*, 345 (1986).
50. J. Mestecky, J. R. McGhee, and R. R. Arnold, *J. Clin. Invest. 61*, 731 (1978).
51. A. J. Axelrod and J. M. Chandler, in *Immunology and Immunopathology of the Eye*, A. M. Silverstein and G. R. O'Connors, Eds. Masson, New York, 1979, p. 292.

52. T. E. Gillette, J. W. Chandler, and J. V. Greiner, *Ophthalmology 1989*, 700 (1982).

53. J. W. Chandler and T. E. Gillette, *Ophthalmology 90*, 585 (1983).

54. W. B. Chodirker and T. B. Tomasi, Jr., *Science 142*, 1080 (1963).

55. M. R. Allansmith and T. E. Gillette, *Am. J. Ophthalmol. 89*, 353 (1980).

56. R. J. Gibbons, *Adv. Exp. Med. Biol. 45*, 315 (1974).

57. M. R. Allansmith, J. V. Greiner, and R. S. Baird, *Am. J. Ophthalmol. 86*, 250 (1978).

58. W. A. Walker, K. J. Isselbacher, and K. J. Bloch, *Science 177*, 608 (1972).

59. W. A. Walker, K. J. Isselbacher, and H. J. Bloch, *J. Immunol. 111*, 221 (1973).

60. K. Y. Pang, W. A. Walker, and K. J. Bloch, *Gut 22*, 1018 (1981).

61. A. Abuchowski and F. F. Davis, in *Enzymes as Drugs*, J. C. Holcenberg, Ed., Wiley, New York, 1981, p. 367.

62. Y. Rojanasakul and J. R. Robinson, *J. Ocul. Pharmacol. 4*(1), 51 (1988).

63. K. Kishida and T. Otori, *Jpn. J. Ophthalmol. 24*, 251 (1980).

64. R. D. Schoenwald and R. L. Ward, *J. Pharm. Sci. 67*, 786 (1980).

65. R. D. Schoenwald and H. S. Huang, *J. Pharm. Sci. 72*, 1266 (1983).

66. R. A. Thoft and J. Friend, *Invest. Ophthalmol. 11*, 723 (1972).

67. A. M. Tonjum, *Acta Ophthalmol. 52*, 650 (1974).

68. Y. Rojanasakul, S. W. Paddock, and J. R. Robinson, *Int. J. Pharm. 61*, 163 (1990).

69. Y. Rojanasakul, Ph.D. Thesis, Univ. Wisconsin-Madison, 1989.

70. Y. Rojanasakul and J. R. Robinson, *Int. J. Pharm. 55*, 237 (1989).

71. A. Donn, D. M. Maurice, and N. L. Mills, *Arch. Ophthalmol. 62*, 748 (1959).

72. K. Green, *Am. J. Physiol. 209*, 1311 (1965).

73. S. D. Klyce, A. H. Neufeld, and J. A. Zadunaisky, *Invest. Ophthalmol. 12*, 127 (1973).

74. A. M. Potts and R. W. Modrell, *Am. J. Ophthalmol. 44*, 284 (1957).

75. D. M. Maurice, *Exp. Eye Res. 6*, 138 (1967).

76. N. Lakshminarayanaiah, *Transport Phenomena in Membranes*, Academic, New York, 1969, p. 91.

77. F. Helfferich, *Ion Exchange*, McGraw-Hill, New York, 1962, p. 133.

78. N. L. Burstein, *Invest. Ophthalmol. Vis. Sci. 19*, 308 (1980).

79. R. J. Marsh and D. M. Maurice, *Exp. Eye Res. 11*, 43 (1971).

80. L. W. Hazleton, *Proc. Sci. Sect. Toilet Goods Assoc. 17*, 5 (1952).

81. J. H. Draize and E. A. Kelley, *Proc. Sci. Sect. Toilet Goods Assoc. 17*, 1 (1952).

82. Y. Rojanasakul, J. Liaw, and J. R. Robinson, *Int. J. Pharm. 66*, 131 (1989).

83. Y. Rojanasakul and J. R. Robinson, *Int. J. Pharm. 68*, 135 (1991).

84. M. E. Stern, H. F. Edelhauser, H. J. Pederson, and W. D. Staaz, *Invest. Ophthalmol. Vis. Sci. 20*, 497 (1981).

85. G. I. Kaye, S. Mishima, S. D. Cole, and N. W. Kaye, *Invest. Ophthalmol. Vis. Sci. 7*, 53 (1968).

86. R. B. Simpson and W. R. Loenstein, *Nature 267*, 625 (1977).

87. G. I. Kaye, C. M. Fenoglio, F. B. Hoefle, and J. Fischbarg, *J. Cell Biol. 61*, 537 (1974).

88. G. I. Kaye, F. B. Hoefle, and A. Donn, *Invest. Ophthalmol. 12*, 98 (1971).

89. T. Nishihata, H. Tomida, G. Frederick, J. H. Rytting, and T. Higuchi, *J. Pharm. Sci. 37*, 159 (1985).

90. S. Hirai, T. Yashiki, and H. Mima, *Int. J. Pharm. 9*, 173 (1981).

91. S. S. Brown and J. A. Spudich, *J. Cell Biol. 88*, 487 (1981).

92. M. D. Flanagan and S. Lin, *J. Biol. Chem. 255*, 835 (1980).

93. C. J. Bentzel and B. Hainau, *Mechanisms of Intestinal Secretion*, Alan R. Liss, New York, 1980, (H. J. Binder, ed.) p. 275.

94. W. S. Craig and J. V. Pardo, *J. Cell Biol. 80*, 203 (1979).

Index

Absorption
  cutaneous, 174
  dispersion protein aggregation, 30
  dissolution rate, 30
  drug solubility, 30
  formation of micelles, 30
  insulin, 338
  intestinal, 34, 323
  percutaneous, 12, 21
    intercellular, 174
  route of transmucosal, 323
Acanthosis, 53
Accumulation, charge, 262
Acid
  citric, 36
  fatty, 29
  oleic, 30
  phosphatase, 45
Acne, 12
Acoustic impedance, 316
Acoustic vibration, longitudinal
    compression waves, 304
ACTH, molecular weight, 391

Action
  duration of, 324
  intracellular lipid composition, 44
  mechanisms of alteration of the cell
    content, 44
Activation energy, iontophoresis, 219
Activity
  cellular enzymatic, 406
  chelating, 27
  endocytic, 45
  phagocytic, 45
  protease, 35
  proteolytic, 5
  regenerative, 48
  surface, 27
  thermodynamic, 52
Adhesion, intercellular, 51, 52
Adhesives, 12
  acrylics, 93
  aging properties of, 99, 102
  chemical compatibility with, 99
  design of, 99
  diffuse through, 99